Methods for Investigation

OF

AMINO ACID

AND

PROTEIN
METABOLISM

Methods in Nutrition Research

Edited by Ronald Ross Watson and Ira Wolinsky

Published Titles

Trace Elements in Laboratory Rodents, Ronald R. Watson
Methods for Investigation of Amino Acid and Protein Metabolism,
   Antoine E. El-Khoury

Methods for Investigation

OF

AMINO ACID

AND

PROTEIN
METABOLISM

EDITED BY

Antoine E. El-Khoury

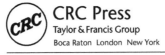

CRC Press
Taylor & Francis Group
Boca Raton London New York

CRC Press is an imprint of the
Taylor & Francis Group, an **informa** business

Contact Editor:	Lourdes Franco
Project Editor:	Steve Menke
Marketing Managers:	Barbara Glunn, Jane Lewis, Arline Massey, Jane Stark
Cover design:	Dawn Boyd

CRC Press
Taylor & Francis Group
6000 Broken Sound Parkway NW, Suite 300
Boca Raton, FL 33487-2742

First issued in paperback 2019

© 1999 by Taylor & Francis Group, LLC
CRC Press is an imprint of Taylor & Francis Group, an Informa business

No claim to original U.S. Government works

ISBN-13: 978-0-8493-9612-0 (hbk)
ISBN-13: 978-0-367-39983-2 (pbk)
Library of Congress Card Number 98-52452

Library of Congress Cataloging-in-Publication Data

Methods for investigation of amino acid and protein metabolism /
    edited by Antoine E. El-Khoury.
        p. cm. — (Methods in nutrition research)
        Includes bibliographical references and index.
        ISBN 0-8493-9612-3
        1. Proteins—Metabolism—Research—Methodology. 2. Amino acids—
        Metabolism—Research—Methodology. I. El-Khoury, Antoine E.
    II. Series.
    QP551.M387 1999
    612.3' 98—dc21   98-52452
                                                                       CIP

Visit the Taylor & Francis Web site at
http://www.taylorandfrancis.com

and the CRC Press Web site at
http://www.crcpress.com

Series Preface

Methods are critical to both good data and their correct interpretation. While there are methods series for biochemistry and other disciplines, nutritional sciences have suffered from the absence of such a resource. Many small but important techniques, procedures, and carefully tested methods make experiments easier and more accurate. This series, *Methods in Nutrition Research*, is designed to gradually fill this gap in research resources. It will provide published and unpublished details of technical procedures used by experts in different areas of nutrition research. It will also describe potential pitfalls to be avoided. The series is designed for the researcher with a focus on laboratory and field nutritional research methods and how to apply them precisely. It will contain books ranging from descriptions of studies of micronutrients in animal models to macronutrients in human studies. The overall aim of the series is to carry out nutritional research as efficiently as possible, without technical errors, from known procedural methods, ones which may not be easily found in the literature. Nutritional researchers will bring together their own as well as others' experiences to provide a single source of detailed, tested methods with complete descriptions on how to apply them.

We welcome *Methods for Investigation of Amino Acid and Protein Metabolism*. This well-conceived and crafted volume will surely contribute to the study of amino acid and protein metabolism.

Ronald Ross Watson
Ira Wolinsky
Series Editors

Preface

Because of the importance of research methods in the field of amino acid and protein nutrition and metabolism, it became clear to me that a book was very much needed to assemble and discuss the relevant aspects of those methods. My thoughts are directed toward an attempt to facilitate the reader's integration of the concepts involved in these investigative research methods and their corollaries. In addition to helping any nutrition investigator design and conduct appropriate research protocols in this area of nutrition, another objective is to assist doctoral students in nutrition who are planning to investigate amino acid and protein metabolism in humans or laboratory animals.

The pivotal role of amino acid transfer across tissue membranes in the compartmentation control of amino acid metabolism makes it essential that Chapter 1 discusses the available methods related to this aspect. The major expansion of the use of stable isotope-based techniques in the investigation of protein nutrition and metabolism highlights Chapters 6 and 7, on the discussion of mass spectrometry methods. Also, it is necessary to consider some specific conditions, in addition to healthy young adult subjects, where these methods can be applied, e.g., the elderly (Chapter 10), the fetus (Chapter 11), burn and trauma patients (Chapter 13), and diabetes mellitus (Chapter 14).

I hope that this book, a product of an excellent collaboration with national and international expert scientists, will permanently remove the shades of uncertainty related to these fundamental methods and inspire further investigation of amino acid and protein nutrition.

Antoine E. El-Khoury, M.D., Editor
Massachusetts Institute of Technology
Cambridge, Massachusetts

Editor

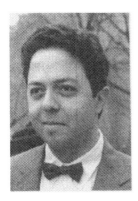

After earning a Doctor of Medicine's degree from St. Joseph University in Lebanon, Dr. Antoine E. El-Khoury moved to Paris, where he completed four years of clinical training in pediatrics. His interest in nutrition led him to undergo a year's training in Children Parenteral Nutrition at Hopital des Enfants Malades. Later, Dr. El-Khoury trained in Human Nutrition and Metabolism (Research Methods) at the University of Aberdeen and the Rowett Research Institute, Scotland. Since late 1991, Dr. El-Khoury has been a research scientist at the Massachusetts Institute of Technology Clinical Research Center and Laboratory of Human Nutrition, Cambridge, Massachusetts. His research activity with Prof. Vernon R. Young focused on amino acid and protein metabolism and nutrition in healthy young adult humans, with particular reference to the minimum dietary requirements for indispensable amino acids. Dr. El-Khoury has extensively used stable isotopes as tracers for *in vivo* nutritional and metabolic research investigations. He is a member of the American Society for Nutritional Sciences (ASNS), the American Society for Clinical Nutrition (ASCN), and the New York Academy of Sciences. He is an external reviewer for the *American Journal of Physiology (Endocrinology and Metabolism)*.

Contributors

Robert C. Albright Jr., D.O.
Department of Internal Medicine
Division of Nephrology
Mayo Clinic
Rochester, Minnesota

**Christine Bobin-Dubigeon,
Pharm.D., Ph.D.**
Centre de Recherche en Nutrition
  Humaine
Centre Hospitalier Universitaire
  Hotel-Dieu
Nantes, France

Douglas G. Burrin, Ph.D.
USDA/ARS Children's Nutrition
  Research Center
Department of Pediatrics
Baylor College of Medicine
Houston, Texas

Wei Cai, M.D.
Department of Surgery
Massachusetts General Hospital
and Harvard Medical School
and Shriners Hospital for Children
Boston, Massachusetts

Dominique Darmaun, M.D., Ph.D.
Centre de Recherche en Nutrition
  Humaine
Centre Hospitalier Universitaire
  Hotel-Dieu
Nantes, France

Teresa A. Davis, Ph.D.
USDA/ARS Children's Nutrition
  Research Center
Department of Pediatrics
Baylor College of Medicine
Houston, Texas

Marta L. Fiorotto, Ph.D.
USDA/ARS Children's Nutrition
  Research Center
Department of Pediatrics
Baylor College of Medicine
Houston, Texas

Dorothy Y. Fisher, B.S.
Department of Medicine
University of Vermont College of
  Medicine
Burlington, Vermont

Naomi K. Fukagawa, M.D., Ph.D.
Department of Medicine
University of Vermont College of
  Medicine
Burlington, Vermont

Peter Fürst, M.D., Ph.D.
Institute for Biological Chemistry and
  Nutrition
University of Hohenheim
Stuttgart, Germany

William W. Hay, Jr., M.D.
Department of Pediatrics
Division of Perinatal Medicine
University of Colorado School of
  Medicine
Denver, Colorado

L. John Hoffer, M.D., Ph.D.
McGill University
and Divisions of Internal Medicine and
  Endocrinology
Sir Mortimer B. Davis-Jewish General
  Hospital
Montreal, Quebec, Canada

Farook Jahoor, Ph.D.
USDA/ARS Children's Nutrition
  Research Center
Department of Pediatrics
Baylor College of Medicine
Houston, Texas

Katharina S. Kuhn, Ph.D.
Institute for Biological Chemistry and
  Nutrition
University of Hohenheim
Stuttgart, Germany

Clemens Kunz, Ph.D.
Research Institute of Child Nutrition
Dortmund, Germany

Sylvia Y. Low, Ph.D.
Department of Anatomy and
  Physiology
University of Dundee
Dundee, Scotland

Cornelia C. Metges, Dr. Agr.
Department of Biochemistry and
  Physiology of Nutrition
The German Institute of Human
  Nutrition
Bergholz-Rehbrücke, Germany

K. Sreekumaran Nair, M.D., Ph.D.
Department of Internal Medicine
Division of Endocrinology
Endocrine Research Unit
Mayo Clinic
Rochester, Minnesota

Bruce W. Patterson, Ph.D.
Washington University School of
  Medicine
St. Louis, Missouri

Klaus J. Petzke, Dr. Rer. Nat.
Department of Biochemistry and
  Physiology of Nutrition
The German Institute of Human
  Nutrition
Bergholz-Rehbrücke, Germany

Peter J. Reeds, Ph.D.
USDA/ARS Children's Nutrition
  Research Center
Department of Pediatrics
Baylor College of Medicine
Houston, Texas

Colleen M. Ryan, M.D.
Department of Surgery
Massachusetts General Hospital
and Harvard Medical School
and Shriners Hospital for Children
Boston, Massachusetts

Peter M. Taylor, Ph.D.
Department of Anatomy and
  Physiology
University of Dundee
Dundee, Scotland

Patti J. Thureen, M.D.
Department of Pediatrics
Division of Perinatal Medicine
University of Colorado School of
  Medicine
Denver, Colorado

Rhonda C. Vann, Ph.D.
USDA/ARS Children's Nutrition
  Research Center
Department of Pediatrics
Baylor College of Medicine
Houston, Texas

Yong-Ming Yu, M.D., Ph.D.
Department of Surgery Massachusetts
  General Hospital
and Harvard Medical School
and Shriners Hospital for Children
Boston, Massachusetts

Dedication

To my wife Maggie and my parents Elie and Vicky

Table of Contents

1 Investigation of Amino Acid Transfer Across Tissue Membranes

Peter M. Taylor and Sylvia Y. Low

CONTENTS

1.1 INTRODUCTION: FUNCTIONS OF AMINO ACID TRANSFERS

Plasma membrane of cells is the principal physical barrier limiting protein and amino acid (AA) movement between different metabolic compartments in an organism. Control of these movements is now recognised to be important for overall control of whole-body protein metabolism.[1-5] AA transport processes fulfill a number of specialised but essential body functions alongside their basic role in supplying cellular AAs for protein synthesis and cell metabolism. These include absorption/reabsorption

0-8493-9612-3/99/$0.00+$.50

of AAs (from intestinal/renal lumen, respectively),[6-8] control of neurotransmission (re-uptake of AA transmitters from synaptic cleft),[8-10] and inter-organ exchange of carbon and nitrogen.[1,2] The most quantitatively important sites of AA transfer in the human body are likely to be skeletal muscle, the kidneys, and tissues bathed by the splanchnic circulation (notably the liver and small intestine).[1,2,11] Dietary protein is hydrolysed to small peptides and AAs within the intestinal lumen; although peptide transport represents a considerable proportion of the total amino-N uptake across the brush-border membrane, intracellular peptide hydrolysis means that the overall trans-epithelial movement of amino-N is almost entirely in the form of AAs.[1,2,12] In this article, we provide a brief overview of the mechanisms involved in AA movements across cell membranes before describing methods available for their study, focusing on techniques applicable to *in vivo* or intact tissue/organ investigations.

1.2 MECHANISMS OF AMINO ACID TRANSFER

1.2.1 PASSIVE DIFFUSION

The simplest mechanism by which AAs cross cell membranes is by passive diffusion. Diffusional fluxes of solutes are proportional to the concentration difference across a permeable barrier (e.g., lipid bilayer of the cell membrane) and the concentration gradient lies within the barrier itself.[13] This relationship can be described quantitatively by a form of **Fick's First Law of Diffusion**:

$$J_{1 \to 2} = D.A.(c_1 - c_2)/x \tag{1}$$

where J = net diffusional flux (mol/sec), D = diffusion coefficient of substance across the barrier (cm^2/sec), A = barrier area (cm^2), c = concentration of substance (mol/cm^3), and x = barrier thickness (cm). The value of D is specific for both barrier *and* diffusing molecules. The flux J is directly proportional to this value and also to exchange area and solute concentration difference (Δc), whilst it is inversely proportional to membrane thickness. Both D and x are difficult to measure experimentally, so in practice the term permeability (P; cm/sec; where $P = D/x$) is generally used.[13] Thus:

$$J_{1 \to 2} = P.A.(\Delta c_{1 \to 2}) \tag{2}$$

Passive diffusion across the lipid bilayer is favoured for small lipophilic molecules. The selective permeability of the membrane depends on the relative tendency of a given solute to dissolve in lipid/water, given by the solvent-water partition coefficient (K_p), with molecular size playing a secondary role.[13] AAs are hydrophilic molecules with K_p values much lower than 1, and passive diffusion is usually much too slow for the required metabolic fluxes of AAs across membranes of living cells.[1,2] Cells have evolved "pores" (channels and transporters) which enable the membrane barrier to be bypassed for effective transmembrane exchange of polar solutes.[2,13] Important characteristics of these pores are:

(a) markedly greater solute flux than predicted by passive diffusion; (b) specificity for single or small structurally related group of substrates; (c) saturability (at least in theory); and (d) susceptiblility to specific inhibitors/inactivators.

1.2.2 Carrier-Mediated Transport

Metabolically important AA movements across cell membranes involve transporters (or "carriers") rather than channels (aqueous pores).[5,8,13,14] Transporters offer the required degree of substrate selectivity related to molecular interactions between solute "substrate" and binding site on the transporter protein, whereas channel selectivity is largely limited to discrimination between size and charge of potential substrates.[2,13,14] Transport mechanisms involve adsorption of solute from bulk fluid phase onto the binding site and a conformational change of the transport protein to move solute across the membrane. The binding site is alternately exposed to the two sides of the membrane during a transport cycle, in tandem with association or disassociation of the carrier-substrate complex.[13,14] The simplest carriers (facilitative transporters) act to "accelerate" (or facilitate) the process of diffusion down an (electro-) chemical gradient of solute. More complex carriers include co-transporters and counter-transporters, in which there is rigid coupling of the movement of two solutes either in the same or opposite directions.[13,14] Important factors influencing unidirectional flux through a transporter will include[13,14] the stoichiometry of a co-transport or counter-transport process, affinity of the binding site for each substrate, dependence on the membrane potential (particularly important if a net charge movement is involved), and the availability of substrates both at the *cis* and *trans* sides of the membrane (see Section 1.3). The physiological significance of coupling is that it allows the gradient of one solute to drive another solute uphill against an electrochemical gradient. Frequently, the gradient of Na^+ is used to drive accumulation of metabolically active substrates (including AAs) into cells. Transport stoichiometry is physiologically important.[1,2,13,14] For Na^+-coupled transport of solutes (e.g., AA), the equilibrium distribution ratio ($[S]_i/[S]_o$, where $[S]_i/[S]_o$ denote intra-/extracellular concentrations) or "concentrating power" of the transporter is related to both the Na^+- gradient (chemical + electrical) and coupling ratio (n); any increase in n markedly increases the achievable $[S]_i/[S]_o$.[13,14] Equilibrium $[S]_i/[S]_o$ values are not achieved *in vivo* because of energy losses, transporter "slippage" and dissipation of [S] gradient by other mechanisms.[13,14] The Na^+ gradient is generated largely by the Na^+ pump (Na^++K^+ATPase, a primary active transport process), and Na^+-coupled transporters utilising this gradient represent secondary active transport processes.[2,13,14] Solute gradients generated by the latter process can in turn be used to generate uphill transport of a different substrate by heteroexchanging carriers, although with low concentrating power (this is termed tertiary active transport).[1,2,12] Detailed descriptions of models of a variety of transport processes can be found elsewhere.[13,14] Although we focus exclusively on the plasma membrane in this article, it should be recognised that transport across intracellular membranes such as those of the mitochondria, lysosome and the endoplasmic reticulum also represent potentially important steps for control of AA metabolism.[2,12]

1.2.3 AMINO ACID TRANSPORT SYSTEMS

The pioneering work of Christensen and colleagues in the early 1960s led to the identification of a wide variety of amino acid transport mechanisms (or "systems") based on criteria of function[1,2,12] and, latterly, of structure after molecular cloning.[5,8] These transporter mechanisms differ in their substrate range, dependence on co-substrates such as ions (particularly Na$^+$), and their regulatory properties such as sensitivity to hormones, e.g., insulin.[2,5,12] AA transporters for the 20 common AAs are generally selective for a particular type of substrate. This selectivity is related to side-chain features, such as **charge** (anionic, cationic, zwitterionic or "neutral"), **size** (small or large neutral) and **structure** (e.g., extra N in glutamine, asparagine and histidine).[2,5,12] AA transporters may be functionally subdivided as follows:[2,8,9,12]

- Na$^+$-dependent: Systems A, ASC (ubiquitous), Systems B^0, B$^{0,+}$ (epithelial brush borders, embryonic tissue), System N (liver, muscle)
- Na$^+$ and K$^+$-dependent: System X$^-_{ag}$ (widespread, especially neural and epithelial tissues)
- Na$^+$ and Cl$^-$-dependent: GABA, taurine and glycine transporters (concentrated in neural tissue)
- Na$^+$-independent: Systems L, T, y$^+$, b$^{0,+}$

Suffixes + or - denote carriage of appropriately charged amino acid substrates. The "system"-based nomenclature is largely derived from **model** or **paradigm** substrates, and kinetic discrimination between systems has been aided by design and synthesis of "system-specific" non-metabolisable amino acid analogues, e.g., N-methylaminoisobutyric acid (MeAIB) for System A and 2-aminobicyclo [2,2,1] heptane-2-carboxylic acid (BCH) for System L.[1,2,12] A number of amino acid transporter proteins have now been cloned.[5,8,9]

1.3 KINETIC PROPERTIES OF AMINO ACID TRANSPORTERS

Kinetic properties of transport processes can be conveniently subdivided into those occurring at *cis*- or *trans*-faces of the membrane (i.e., at the same or opposite sides of the membrane, respectively, relative to the substrate under study).

The major *cis*-effects are (a) saturability and (b) stereospecificity.

Saturability results from competition between substrate molecules for a finite number of binding sites on transporter proteins. Saturable transport may be described by the **Michaelis-Menten** equation:

$$v = \frac{V_{max}\,[S]}{K_m + [S]}$$

(3)

where: v = velocity of reaction (rate of transport or *flux*; mol/min); [S] = substrate concentration on *cis* face of membrane (mol/l); V_{max} = maximum velocity (mol/min), all binding sites occupied; K_m = *Michaelis* constant (mol/l),[S] where 50% of sites are occupied. This relationship gives a single rectangular hyperbola for a uni-substrate transport process (see Figure 1.1A).[13,14] Physiologically important characteristics of this relationship are those at low substrate concentrations, when [S] << Km, v is directly proportional to [S], and at high substrate concentrations, when [S] >> K_m, v approaches V_{max}. For multi-substrate reaction mechanisms (where each co-substrate has a distinct binding site), K_m and V_{max} values for individual substrates will be dependent upon prevailing concentrations of co-substrate(s).[13,14]

A

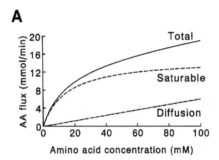

B

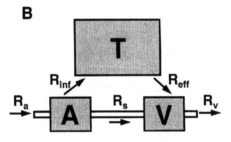

FIGURE 1.1A   Relationship between *cis*-[AA] and saturable or diffusional components of AA flux (for the example shown, K_m = 15 mM, V_{max} = 15 mmol/min). Total (saturable + diffusional) flux is also indicated. **FIGURE 1.1B**   Three-compartment model of tissue amino acid kinetics[3,4] representing fluxes between free amino acid pools in arterial inflow (A), venous outflow (V) and tissue (T). R_a, rate of AA delivery to tissue; R_s, rate of AA shunt from artery to vein; R_v, rate of AA exit from tissue; R_{inf} R_{eff}, rate of amino acid transport from artery to tissue (influx) and tissue to vein (efflux), respectively. (Modified from Biolo, G. Maggi, S.P, Williams, B.D, Tipton, K.D., and Wolfe, R.R., *Am. J. Physiol.*, 268, E514-520, 1995. With permission.)

Stereospecificity means structural features of the binding site favour association with certain stereoisomers of the substrate (usually biologically active forms); e.g., L-AAs are usually favoured over D-isomers, reflected in a lower K_m value ("higher affinity") without change in V_{max} (the translocation step is not impaired by substrates of same size and shape).[13,14]

The major *trans*-effects are:[13,14]

a) Exchange diffusion: where presence of *trans*-substrate accelerates exchange.
b) Counter transport: *trans*-acceleration mediated by a different substrate (hetero-exchange).

The overall magnitude of AA fluxes across tissue membranes will therefore depend both on the substrate concentration at *cis*- and *trans*- faces of the membrane, and the kinetic characteristics of the different carriers. Total flux will represent the sum of fluxes through individual transporters, plus a contribution from simple diffusion (see Figure 1.1A). A flux through a particular transport system will depend on the capacity of that system in the membrane (dictated largely by the amount of transport protein in the membrane), and by the affinity (K_m) of the transporter for the substrate. Values for transport affinity (K_m) and capacity (V_{max}) can be obtained experimentally, enabling flux at a given substrate concentration to be calculated.

1.4 TECHNIQUES FOR STUDYING AMINO ACID TRANSFERS: AN OVERVIEW

1.4.1 EXPERIMENTAL DESIGN AND RATIONALE

AA transporters and the substrate fluxes generated by them can be investigated by a variety of techniques using a range of preparations from molecular to the whole-body level, according to the type of information sought. An investigator may only require to measure the rate of AA transfer at physiological substrate concentrations, and with only minor perturbations of the experimental system (e.g., addition of a hormone such as insulin) in order to obtain the necessary information for studies of AA/protein turnover and metabolism, in which case *in vivo* preparations are appropriate.[3,15] For more detailed study of transport processes, it should be remembered that AAs are transported into cells in mammalian tissues by several distinct transport systems, with a variety of overlapping specificities.[1,2,12] The complement of AA transporters in a particular tissue membrane is an extremely important determinant of the rate of AA transfer across this membrane, and thus of the particular tissue's profile of AA metabolism.[2,12] Functional properties of different transport systems (e.g., K_m, concentrating power, exchange properties) are specialised for particular roles, and different cell types within a tissue may well express markedly different transporters with contrasting properties of major importance for channelling and regulating AA metabolism within the tissue[2,5,8,12] (e.g., along the liver sinusoid[11,16]). The apical and basolateral membranes of epithelial cells also possess different AA transporters, with overall properties promoting transepithelial transfers of substrates surplus to requirements of cellular metabolism.[2,5,8,12]

The complement of transporters in a given tissue can now be at least partly assessed by identifying transporter mRNA or protein (by Northern or Western blotting, respectively) when suitable nucleotide antibody probes and tissue samples are available. *In situ* hybridisation studies may be used to localise distribution of transporters within specific cell types of heterogeneous tissues.[5] Steady-state distribution ratios of solutes across membranes (usually expressed as [cell]/[plasma]) offer useful insights into whether passive or active processes are involved, but do not provide information on rates of movement.[1,2,12] AA movements are best measured by monitoring the unidirectional flux of tracers or the net movement of substrate across a membrane or tissue interface:[2,13,14] the tracers used may be either radioactively labelled AAs or, increasingly, stable-isotope labelled AAs. A small net AA flux may mask large unidirectional fluxes (net flux = influx - efflux) of considerable metabolic and physiological importance (reflecting the complement/reversibility/exchange properties of transporters in a membrane).[3,12,17] Techniques for studying AA transport mechanisms in tissue membranes include: (a) measuring net movement of bulk substrate across cell membranes; (b) measuring and analysing of tracer dilution profiles, or tissue extraction of tracer molecules from fluid perfusing tissues; (c) measuring tracer fluxes into or out of isolated cells/membrane vesicles or across cell layers; and (d) electrophysiological measuring of net ionic fluxes across membranes — these are only applicable to rheogenic transporters producing measurable current. All *ex vivo* preparations in which cellular integrity is maintained require to be bathed or perfused with an appropriate (preferably iso-osmotic) medium which is well buffered at the required pH, usually a physiological salt solution containing an energy substrate (e.g., glucose) if the experiment is to be prolonged. Oxygenation (using either air or 95% O_2/5% CO_2) and stirring of the medium may also be required. Major non-physiological changes in composition of the bathing medium (e.g., total replacement of Na^+ by a nominally non-permeant substitute cation such as choline, tetramethylammonium, or N-methyl-D-glucamine) may have indirect effects on transport by affecting factors such as membrane potential and viability of cells.

1.4.2　General Principles of Tracer Flux Methodologies

Tracers for study of AA transport and metabolism include both radioactive and stable-isotope labelled AAs. Radioactive tracers (usually with [^{3}H]- or [^{14}C]-labels) can be quantitated in terms of nuclear disintegrations per second (dps, where 1 dps = 1 Becquerel or Bq) in experimental samples by liquid scintillation spectrometry; this method does not require major sample preparation unless solid or highly-coloured material is involved. Both [^{3}H] and [^{14}C] are low-energy β^--emitters with long (> 10 years) half-lives. [^{11}C]- or [^{13}N]-labelled AAs may also be used, but both these radioisotopes are relatively high-energy β^+-emitters with short (< 30 minute) half-lives; their use requires both specialised on-site facilities for tracer preparation, and rapid post-experimental analysis.[18,19] Advantages of using [^{11}C]- or [^{13}N]-tracers are that they can be prepared at extremely high-specific activity, and are detectable *in situ* (using solid scintillation counter or imaging methods) without sample removal or processing.[18] Stable-isotope (e.g., [^{13}C], [^{15}N]) labelled tracers may require substantial modification (derivatisation) of the sample prior to quantitation by mass spectrometry.[3,4,20]

　　AA flux (i.e., the quantity of substrate that crosses a membrane per unit time) measured by tracer methods generally assumes[13,14,21] that (a) the experimental system consists of two well-stirred compartments separated by a single membrane barrier;

(b) the tracer is chemically indistinguishable from the unlabelled (bulk) substrate and is not metabolised over the measurement period; and (c) the substrate under consideration is distributed in a steady state, i.e., there is no overall net flux within the system (although there are unidirectional fluxes which balance across the membrane). Diffusional equilibration of tracer within the compartments is usually rapid compared with transport across the membrane, so the problems of poor mixing are usually not of great significance. Unidirectional influx of AA into tissues, cells or membrane vesicles is measured from the initial rate of uptake of a tracer added to the external medium. Initial rate refers to uptake measured over a time period which is sufficiently short so that increase in tracer activity is linear with time, although the period should be sufficiently long to maximize the amount of tracer internalized (hence, minimizing errors associated with tracer quantitation). Initial-rate conditions should apply over the full range of substrate concentrations used. Fluxes are calculated from the initial rate of change in internal tracer activity divided by the *specific-activity* (for radiotracers, the quantity of radioactivity produced by a known amount of radioactive substance, expressed as Bq/mole*) of substrate in the external compartment. Tracer equilibrium is ultimately achieved when the specific activity approaches equality on the two sides of the membrane barrier. Unidirectional flux may also be estimated from fractional extraction of tracer during tissue perfusion (see Section 1.5.2). Efflux from tracer-preloaded experimental preparations is measured as a decrease in intracellular tracer activity (often indirectly from the increase in extracellular tracer activity), and may be quantitated in terms of the rate constant(s) for efflux:

$$Q_t = Q_0 \, e^{-kt} \qquad (4)$$

where Q_t = intracellular tracer activity at time t (e.g., in Bq for radiotracer), Q_0 = initial intracellular tracer activity (Bq), t = time, k = efflux rate constant (units of time^{-1}). Values of k are estimated as the slope of a plot of $\ln(Q_t/Q_0)$ against time, which will be linear if tracer effluxes from a single homogeneous intracellular pool.[12,13,22] Efflux may be calculated from k if the size of the intracellular (or intravesicular) substrate pool is known; e.g., mmol AA/cell x k (h^{-1}) = efflux (mmol/cell . h).

In order to follow the movements of a tracer in an experimental system, it may be necessary to use an extracellular marker which will distribute throughout the extracellular space, but be excluded from the cell or intracellular compartment. The difference in distribution of experimental tracer and extracellular marker will represent uptake into the cellular compartment under study.[17,21] In addition, special care must be taken when using small cells or isolated plasma membrane vesicles (where there is a relatively high surface area to volume ratio) to ensure that the measured uptake of tracer associated with the cell or vesicle actually reflects flux into the intravesicular or intracellular space, and not simply binding to the surface membrane (thus overestimating rate of transfer). This is most likely to cause significant error

---

* Alternatively, tracer-tracee ratio may be used when chemical concentration of tracer is significant, as in many stable-isotope studies[3,4,22]

when using relatively hydrophobic substrates (e.g., aromatic AAs) in experiments with membrane vesicles. (Methods used to assess binding are considered in Section 1.5.4.)

It is advisable, at least in preliminary experiments, to check the fate of tracer over the period of an experiment. The use of synthetic, non-metabolizable AA analogues can circumvent the problems of tracer metabolism as long as information gained is extrapolated to the situation of natural AAs with due care.[1,2,12] Alternatively, the initial steps in substrate catabolism may be inhibited (e.g., by using amino-oxyacetate to inhibit transaminases) in *ex vivo* studies.[21] The problem of tracer metabolism can be alleviated if the chemical identity of labelled molecules is con-firmed using analytical separation techniques such as HPLC or gas chromatography (GC), followed by tracer quantitation using mass spectrometry (MS) or radioactive scintillation counting. This allows the true specific activity of the tracer under study to be measured.[3,4,12] The use of GC-MS has the advantage that several tracers may be studied simultaneously if MS signatures are suitably distinct (concentrations of unlabelled substrates are also measured if appropriate internal standards analysis is performed),[3,4] whereas use of scintillation spectrometry to detect radioactive labels in practice usually limits study to two (^{3}H- and ^{14}C-labelled) tracers simultaneously. The latter technique, however, has advantages of greater sensitivity, greater speed of sample analysis and lower cost, assuming any ethical questions posed by use of radioactive materials can be addressed satisfactorily.

1.4.3 ANALYSIS AND INTERPRETATION OF FLUX DATA

The kinetic data acquired from AA transport investigations is conventionally described in terms of characteristic constants such as V_{max} and K_m. To calculate these values, the data must include fluxes measured over a range of substrate concentra-tions*, ideally with equal numbers of measurements above and below K_m. It is also important to assess the extent of saturability of the measured flux, given that non-saturable processes such as simple diffusion will also contribute to tracer move-ment.[12,21] Non-saturable uptake can be estimated from the residual tracer uptake in the presence of a high (nominally fully-saturating) unlabelled substrate concentra-tion, and this component may be subtracted from the uptake data to give the saturable transport component(s). Non-saturable uptake is usually small when considering polar AAs, but can become significant when looking at transport of hydrophobic AAs, particularly when using artificial phospholipid membranes.[21,23,24]

Kinetic analysis of flux data is facilitated by use of non-linear regression pro-grammes (featured in most computer-based statistics packages), which allow itera-tive fitting of the Michaelis-Menten equation (Equation 3) to experimental data. The curve equation may be adapted (e.g., as in Figure 1.1A) to include a diffusional component of flux and/or multiple transport components (arithmetical sum of two or more Michaelis-Menten relationships). Computer-based kinetic analysis should be performed in parallel with more direct and "visual" methods, such as linear

---

* In tracer-dilution experiments, K_m values may be estimated from comparative analysis of extrac-tion/dilution profiles of simultaneously introduced tracer/bulk substrate, respectively; see Section 1.5.2.

transformation of the Michaelis-Menten equation (Equation 3) to derive K_m and V_{max} values. These transformations should be interpreted with care, however, as they are prone to introduce large non-systematic errors; this is a particular problem with the conventional Lineweaver-Burk plot ($1/v$ against $1/[S]$), due to irregular weighting of data points. We prefer the Hanes plot ($[S]/v$ against $[S]$) for rapid data analysis as it offers more regular weighting plus simple visual assessment of inhibitor effects (see example in Section 1.5.4). Very high apparent K_m values (of the order of tens or hundreds of mmol/litre) generated by any analytical procedure may, in fact, reflect simple diffusion. Multiple pathways for transport of a particular AA can be identified from raw flux data only if the K_m values for the different transporters involved vary considerably (usually by orders of magnitude). This is frequently not the case, and transport systems are often distinguished on the basis of their substrate (including ionic co-substrate) specificity.[1,2,5,8,12] Here, the uptake of a particular AA is measured in the presence of potential competitors, and the extent and pattern of inhibition of uptake can be used to distinguish different transport mechanisms.[2,13,21] Manipulations such as removal of co-substrate (e.g., Na⁺) or addition of excess carrier-specific AA analogue (to block transport of tracer by that system) are also used to reduce the number of pathways contributing to a measured AA tracer flux, facilitating dissection of the transport features of individual systems.[2,21,25] Such experiments require considerable manipulation of the solute composition of fluid bathing at least one face of a membrane, and are therefore performed in isolated preparations of tissue, cells or membranes (see Section 1.5).

The specificity of a transport system can be defined in that all substrate AAs should show mutual *competitive inhibition* ($\uparrow K_m$, unchanged V_{max} for substrate in presence of inhibitor). AAs which either fail to show mutual inhibition of transport or display non-competitive inhibition ($\downarrow V_{max}$, unchanged K_m for substrate in presence of inhibitor) are deemed to be transported by separate systems.[1,21] Non-competitive inhibition of AA transport by other AAs has been reported frequently in the literature, thus simple inhibition studies are insufficient to firmly establish substrate specificity. The strongest kinetic evidence that two (or more) AAs share a transport system is when it can be shown that the concentration at which an inhibitor AA (AA1) exerts half-maximal effect on uptake of tracer AA2 (termed K_i, or "inhibitor constant") equals the transport K_m of AA1.[1,2,21] Effective inhibition analysis requires that experiments are performed using an appropriate range of concentrations of substrate and inhibitor AA (based on estimated K_i and K_m values). K_i values can be estimated from Dixon plots, following measurement of initial-rate uptake of at least three concentrations of substrate in the presence of a variety of fixed concentrations of putative inhibitor.[21,26] A plot of $1/v$ against inhibitor concentration produces a series of lines, which should intersect at a point above the x-axis showing -K_i (lines converging on the x-axis indicate non-competitive inhibition). Ideally, the analysis of mutual competitive inhibition should be carried out for three putative substrate AAs of a carrier, the so-called ABC test.[1,2]

The interpretation of observed changes in AA transport (e.g., after hormone treatment, fasting, exercise or pathophysiological intervention) require consideration of the various ways by which transport activities may be modulated. These include[2,5,8,12,21,27] (a) change in activity or number of carrier proteins (by phosphorylation, synthesis/breakdown or movement between intracellular depots and the cell membrane); (b) altered substrate concentrations; and (c) change in membrane-potential (affecting rheogenic systems). Note that systemic effects of disease and injury include generalized depolarization/reduced Na^+-gradient across cell membranes (the resultant *reduction in concentrating power* of transporters leads to loss of "stored" AAs from cells, notably glutamine from muscle).[28]

1.5 EXPERIMENTAL PREPARATIONS

1.5.1 *IN VIVO* TECHNIQUES

Measurement of AA fluxes *in vivo* is the optimum approach to adopt for many physiological investigations, if technically and ethically feasible. Unfortunately, *in vivo* techniques are not well suited to detailed studies of transport mechanism and kinetics at cellular or molecular level, due both to structural and functional heterogeneity of the experimental system, and to severe limitations on the type and extent of feasible experimental manipulations. The techniques used usually require sampling of blood (at minimum), and great care should be taken to ensure that (a) cannulations minimise disturbances to normal blood flow, and (b) blood sampling does not significantly deplete the circulatory volume (use volume replacement, e.g., donor blood, plasma or saline, if necessary). The likely effects of anaesthetic/operative procedure on variables (including blood flow) under study should also be considered. Measurement of blood flow is an important part of many protocols, and several different techniques for this measurement are available. Peripheral blood flow may be measured using plethysmography.[29] Blood flow through an artery or vein may be measured using a flow probe (Doppler, transit-time) placed around the vessel.[20,30] Such probes are most useful for vessels of > 1mm diameter and flow > 2 ml/min, and may be used in tandem with chronic indwelling cannulae.[30] Indicator dilution (e.g., using p-aminohippurate (PAH) or indocyanine green) can be used to measure tissue plasma flow, and blood flow is calculated from haematocrit.[4] In terminal studies using animals, tissue trapping of labelled microspheres injected into the arterial circulation may be used to measure regional and tissue blood flows (microspheres used are of 15 µm diameter and become trapped in capillaries).[31] This method needs a reference arterial blood sample, and is not appropriate for measuring flow to tissues through portal vessels such as the hepatic portal vein.

1.5.1.1 Whole-Body Investigations

The fate of AA tracer introduced (either orally, by bolus injection or infusion) into the plasma pool may be followed in one of two major ways (both protocols require sequential sampling of blood, preferably via a cannulated vein) :

(a) time-course of disappearence of bolus tracer load from plasma into exchangeable tissue pool(s).[32] Most AAs in the body are chemically combined into protein; the free AA pool, therefore, constitutes only a small proportion of the total, although it is this pool which turns over the most rapidly and is responsible for inter-organ transfer of amino nitrogen and AA carbon.[32] Linear kinetic modelling of tracer disappearance is likely to reveal both rapidly and slowly exchanging free solute pools (compartments) for which size (distribution volume) and exchange rate constant can be estimated.[32,33] Such multi-compartmental analysis is useful for studying turnover but gives no information as to which tissues represent particular compartments (although reasonable guesses can be made in most cases, e.g., rapidly exchanging: lymph, liver, kidney; slowly exchanging: muscle, brain).[33] Radiotracers labelled with ^{11}C or ^{13}N may be used to non-invasively measure (or visualise by imaging) the accumulation of tracers within tissues.[18]

(b) constant infusion (usually after a priming dose) of tracer into plasma to achieve a steady state.[22,34] This can be used to estimate whole-body appearance of AA into the plasma (i.e., net AA efflux from cells to plasma); e.g., for a stable-isotope labelled AA tracer:

$$R_a = i[(E_i/E_p) - 1] \tag{5}$$

where R_a is appearance rate, i is tracer infusion rate (both in mol/kg.h) and E_i and E_p (mole % excess) are the enrichments of the infused tracer and in plasma. In the fasted state, plasma appearance of essential AAs reflects their release by protein breakdown, whereas for non-essential AAs both *de novo* synthesis and protein breakdown contribute to the overall appearance rate.[22,34]

1.5.1.2 Regional and Tissue Studies

The combination of arterio-venous concentration difference and blood flow measurements for tissues with accessible venous drainage *in vivo* provides useful information on net AA fluxes (calculated as flow x ([substrate]$_{art}$ - [substrate]$_{ven}$). Plasma flow should be used if the AA under study is effectively excluded from blood cells over the time course of the experiment, or if plasma AA concentrations were obtained.[1,4] Plasma and whole blood concentrations of certain AAs (notably glutamate and aspartate) differ significantly from one another, but the overall importance of blood cells in AA carriage is likely to be relatively minor under most experimental circumstances.[1,35]

More detailed quantitative information on transport steps may be obtained if tracer is added at the arterial side of a tissue vascular bed, and the venous blood is sampled during the first pass of tracer in the circulation. The paired tracer dilution method (described in Section 1.5.2) has been used *in vivo* (e.g., in the human forearm[15]) by examining tracer profiles in the effluent venous blood.

The inclusion of tissue biopsies (or terminal tissue samples) increases the amount of information which can be obtained. Tissue-blood distribution ratios of AAs *in vivo* may be measured from chemical analysis of biopsy material, or from steady-state distribution of injected AA tracers.[1,2] Transportable tracer plus extracellular marker may be bolus-injected into an arterial circulation and tissue freeze-clamped within 5 to 8 seconds (i.e., less than the circulation time), in which case the tissue retention of tracer relative to extracellular marker can be used as an index of cellular extraction of tracer.[36] AA flux may be calculated from this *unidirectional* extraction value, if both tissue blood flow and plasma AA concentration are known. Alternatively, if constant infusion of tracer is used, a tissue biopsy at plasma steady state may be obtained from which tracer enrichment values may be measured.[3,4] A three-compartment model described recently by Wolfe and colleagues (see Figure 1.1B) allows the quantitation of intracellular AA kinetics, including transmembrane AA transport.[3,4] The model is applicable *in vivo* (given access to the venous circulation draining the tissue of interest and a suitable method for measurement of tissue blood flow) and can be extended to include additional flux components representing appearance or removal of tissue AA due to cell metabolism (proteolysis/*de novo* AA synthesis or protein synthesis, respectively).

1.5.2 ISOLATED ORGANS AND TISSUES

The experimental approaches used in isolated tissue preparations are broadly similar to those used for regional studies *in vivo*, and many common limitations and analytical difficulties apply. Isolated tissues usually consist of more than one cell type with differing transport activities, and measured fluxes will reflect the combination of these processes unless certain cell-types are selectively ablated (e.g., [15]). Isolated, perfused preparations offer the significant advantage over *in vivo* studies that perfusate flow and composition can be manipulated to the experimenter's requirements, whilst retaining tissue integrity; methods to perfuse many tissues have been described.[17,37,38] The preferred method for measurement of AA uptake here is the paired- (or multiple-) tracer dilution technique.[17,39] The preparation is perfused with a medium containing a transportable AA tracer (usually having a radioactive label), together with a suitable extracellular-space marker (a compound, e.g., labelled sucrose, inulin or mannitol, which is largely impermeant to the plasma membrane). The relative dilution of transportable and extracellular tracers in the effluent perfusate (Figure 1.2A) is used to estimate the unidirectional extraction of tracer amino acid from the extracellular fluid (Figure 1.2B). Maximum fractional extraction (U_{max}) and plasma flow are related to permeability-surface area Product (PS) of the perfusate-tissue barrier,[17] where:

$$PS = flow \ x \ -ln(1 - U_{max}).\qquad(6)$$

Unidirectional flux = PS x perfusate [AA]. Extraction is measured over a single pass through the perfused circulation, this short duration minimising problems of tracer metabolism. The technique can also be used to study efflux by following the washout of tracer extracted by the tissue,[38,39] but this poses severe technical difficulties (e.g., tracer dilution within whole tissues is difficult to model, tracer metabolism over a prolonged period). Net AA flux across perfused tissues may be calculated after chemical analysis of influent and effluent perfusates. Limitations of the paired-tracer technique are (a) flow rate must be sufficiently high to maintain adequate tissue oxygenation (unfortunately the measured parameter of extraction is inversely

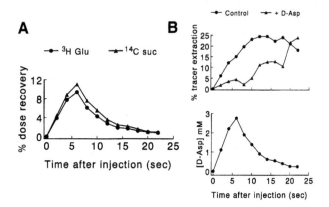

FIGURE 1.2A   Paired-tracer dilution profiles of L-[³H]glutamate and [¹⁴C]sucrose (extra-cellular marker) in venous effluent from perfused rat liver. 0.1ml tracer bolus was injected into arterial inflow (flow rate 1.6 ml/g liver.min [11]) at zero time. **FIGURE 1.2B**   The top graph (control) shows the % extraction of L-glutamate tracer, relative to sucrose, during single-pass through perfused liver. Maximum fractional extraction (U_{max}) is 0.25. The lower line shows the effect of co-injecting 50 mM D-aspartate with L-glutamate on tracer extraction (D-Asp and L-Glu are both substrates of System X^-_{ag}.). The bottom graph shows the calculated D-aspartate concentration at the liver sinusoidal membrane, based on recovery of extracellular marker in venous effluent. D-aspartate inhibits tracer extraction in a concentration-dependent manner (reflected here by time-course of L-Glu extraction as D-Asp is diluted by perfusate; this type of interaction can be analysed using mathematical models[38,39]).

proportional to the flow rate); (b) certain tissues are extremely difficult to perfuse; (c) the composition of the perfusing medium can only be varied within certain limits compatible with tissue viability; and (d) uptake and release of substances such as ions, hormones and unlabelled AAs within the perfused circulation significantly alter perfusate composition within the tissue itself. A net flux of substrate AA results in a gradient of [AA] between arterial and venous compartments; mathematical models are available, if necessary, to account for this factor when calculating fluxes from PS data.[38,40] Additional studies with reversed perfusate flow may reveal important intra-tissue AA fluxes.[41]

AA fluxes may be measured in unperfused isolated tissues (e.g., single muscles, intestinal rings, tissue slices), but problems arise due both to build-up of unstirred layers within the tissue (affecting tracer fluxes) and to diffusional limitations at the "core" of the preparation which may affect both substrate exchanges and oxygen delivery, even with well-oxygenated perfusate and small, thin tissue preparations.[12,36,37] Certain tissues (notably the intestine) lend themselves well to study in Ussing* chambers,[42-45] enabling simultaneous measurement of both trans-cellular ("trans-epithelial") AA flux and associated ionic movements (the latter studied by electro-physiological measurement of either trans-membrane/trans-tissue membrane

---

* Apparatus in which a tissue layer is mounted as a dividing partition between two chambers containing the same or different experimental solutions[42]

potential[45] or short-circuit current[43]). Here, the measured variables reflect the sum of events at two membranes in series plus a paracellular shunt pathway (unless intracellular electrodes are used[45] or tracer flux into the tissue layer from only one membrane face is measured[44]), complicating analysis in terms of events at individual membranes.

1.5.3 SINGLE CELLS

Problems of tissue heterogeneity are circumvented by using isolated cells. Studies of AA transport in single cells are technically and analytically simpler than those in intact tissues, and are extensively used. Other advantages of isolated cells for transport studies are that the external medium can be carefully defined to contain a wide variety of substrates, hormones and co-factors. Since this medium is in direct contact with the cell membrane (intervening barriers such as capillary endothelium being absent), the possibility of unstirred-layer effects can be minimised. Very few cell types are large enough for transport measurements to be made in an individual cell (even using the most sensitive tracer methods), and AA fluxes are usually measured in a large number of functionally identical cells, either in suspension or attached to a culture dish as a confluent cell monolayer. Cells are usually isolated from tissues by a combination of enzymatic (e.g., collagenase or elastase) treatment and mechanical disruption designed to dissociate cells from each other and from the extracellular matrix.[12,21,25,46] Isolation procedures are optimized to preserve the biochemical feature of the original cells as much as possible. Certain cell types isolated from adult tissue (e.g., adipocytes) do not survive in culture and are used immediately after isolation, although others can be readily cultured as monolayers and retained under appropriate conditions for several days. These primary cell cultures usually retain more of the characteristics of cells in the parent tissue than do permanent "transformed" cell lines (derived usually from tumours or fetal tissue). Transformed cell lines offer the advantage that they can be cultured almost indefinitely from deep frozen seed stock, although biochemical characteristics of the cells may change as the number of passages is increased. Cells in culture are usually equilibrated with a gas phase of 95% oxygen, 5% CO_2 to generate a pH of 7.4 in a bicarbonate-based buffer; serum and embryo extract may be added to maintain or reattain original phenotype after tissue dissociation.[21,25] For transport studies of short duration (i.e., < 5 minutes) the experimental medium may use buffers other than bicarbonate. Unidirectional AA influx into cells is measured from the initial rate of uptake of tracer added to the external medium, the uptake reaction being terminated by separating cells from the labelled extracellular medium (be aware of the possibility of significant rapid tracer binding to membranes; see Section 1.5.4). This separation process is an extremely important step determining the accuracy and viability of the method and may involve centrifugal pelleting of cells (ideally through a layer of oil[46]) or washes of cell monolayers in unlabelled medium.[25] The separation method should be rapid to limit any tracer backflux, should not disrupt the cell and should effectively remove all extracellular radioactivity (although use of an appropriate extracellular marker can correct for the latter problem).[21,25,46] If intracellular concentrations of substrates need to be measured, the intracellular volume can be estimated by the volume of distribution of an intracellular marker such as tritiated water[46] or ^{14}C-labelled urea, two substances which rapidly permeate cell membranes and will rapidly equilibrate between intra- and extracellular fluids. Unidirectional efflux can be measured by preloading cells with a known amount of radioactive tracer, washing then measuring the rate of tracer appearance into unlabelled medium.

Measurement of transport in polarized cells poses a particular problem, because it is important to be able to distinguish between transport across apical and basolateral membrane surfaces. Epithelial cells (usually cell lines) will form confluent monolayers, which polarize with the basolateral membranes attached to the base of the culture dish. AA transport measured in these monolayers mainly represents transport across the apical membrane, which protrudes directly into the incubating medium.[21] It is now possible to grow cells on permeable membrane supports, which enable both sides of the confluent monolayer to be in contact with experimental medium. The supports may be placed into Ussing chambers for transport studies.[47] Equally, the net rate of solute movement across the monolayer can be determined. This type of preparation is also suitable for using electrophysiological methods to estimate rheogenic AA transporter fluxes.

1.5.4 PLASMA MEMBRANE VESICLES

The use of plasma membrane vesicles for AA transport studies has major advantages because (a) they contain no intracellular enzymes, so the problems of substrate metabolism are minimized; (b) it is possible to define the solute composition at both surfaces of the cell membrane by careful experimental design; (c) membrane vesicles from polarized cells can be prepared from either or both basolateral and apical cell membranes, allowing the localization of particular transport systems to be determined (although contamination from intracellular membranes is always a potential problem); and (d) many experiments can be performed using membrane vesicles prepared from a single tissue sample.[1,2,48,49] Measured AA flux reflects the stable expression of transport proteins in a membrane at the time of isolation. The major drawback of the method is that loss of cellular integrity largely precludes studies of transporter regulation and "physiological" mode of operation, as well as preventing maintenance of transmembrane ionic gradients.

Membrane vesicles (e.g., Figure 1.3A) are prepared by homogenization of tissue, followed by sub-cellular fractionation using centrifugation techniques, which may include pelleting of $MgCl_2$ precipitatable membrane (e.g., brush-border membrane from polarized cells) or density-gradient fractionation procedures (using compounds such as sucrose to modify solvent density). Yield and purity of membrane (which vary, depending upon the preparation and the technique employed) are estimated from the amount of membrane protein recovered (measured using standard protein quantitation methods) and assay of membrane-specific marker enzymes (e.g., Na^+K^+-ATPase for basolateral membrane, 5′-nucleotidase or gamma-glutamyltransferase for brush border membrane), respectively.[21,48] The extent of contamination from intracellular membranes is assessed from measurements of appropriate marker enzymes, such as succinate dehydrogenase, glucose-6-phosphatase or Ca^{2+}-ATPase. Increasingly, Western blotting is used as an additional tool to determine the protein complement of isolated membrane fractions. The sidedness of membrane vesicles

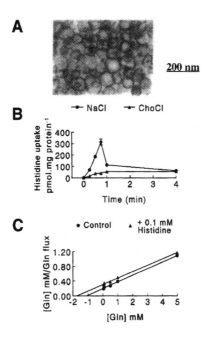

FIGURE 1.3A   Purified sinusoidal membrane vesicles (SMVs) from rat liver. Note relatively homogeneous size (70 nm diameter). **FIGURE 1.3B**   Time course of uptake of L-[³H]histidine into liver SMVs. Note the overshoot, characteristic of Na⁺-dependent processes, prior to collapse of imposed Na⁺ gradient. Equilibrium uptake values are similar +/- Na⁺. Intravesicular volume may be estimated from equilibrium uptake (usually 0.5 to 2.0 µl/mg membrane protein). **FIGURE 1.3C** Hanes plot (line slope = $1/V_{max}$, x-intercept = $-K_m$) showing competitive inhibition of MeAIB-resistant, Na+-dependent glutamine uptake by histidine in liver SMVs (a characteristic feature of System N[12,49]). The K_m for glutamine uptake increased from 1.02 mM to 1.75 mM in the presence of 0.1 mM L-histidine, whereas V_{max} (line slope) was unchanged.

(i.e., whether the extracellular face is located on the inside or outside) is an important factor to be considered when trying to interpret vesicle transport data; it is a difficult parameter to measure accurately, but is usually estimated by assaying marker enzyme activity in the presence and absence of a detergent or pore-forming drug, which allows enzymatic substrates to enter the intravesicular space for measurement of total (rather than simply exofacial) marker enzyme activity.[48,49] Isolated membrane vesicles are usually resuspended by homogenization in a non-ionic medium, such as 0.4 M sucrose buffer, and AA uptake is measured by adding tracer to this suspension in a diluting solution containing ions and other substrates usually made iso-osmotic to the resuspension medium. By varying the composition of the tracer-containing solution, the final ionic composition of the uptake medium can be altered in a defined way. Transport measurements are terminated by the addition of a large excess of ice-cold medium containing no tracer, and the vesicle suspension is then filtered rapidly either on a nitrocellulose filter under negative pressure[21,50] or through a Sephadex* or other ion-exchange column.[49,50] Filters are subsequently washed with further aliquots of ice-cold medium to remove adhering extravesicular radioactivity (without loss of intravesicular radioactivity, if performed rapidly). It is possible to perform uptake experiments over periods of the order of 5 seconds or less using these procedures; indeed, short durations are to be recommended because a major problem with membrane vesicle experiments is that solute gradients imposed across the vesicle membrane at the beginning of an experiment rapidly degrade to equilibrium.[48-50] The time course of tracer uptake in membrane vesicle experiments is very dependent on the permeability of the membrane to ions such as Na^+, because the rapidity with which these ions equilibrate across the membrane will dictate the period over which the initial defined ion and electrical gradients are effectively maintained (Figure 1.3B,C).[21,48] Ion-coupled AA transport processes are dependent on the membrane potential, and typical Na^+-dependent transporters will be most active in the presence of an imposed inside negative membrane potential. This can be created artificially in membrane vesicles by including a permeant anion, such as thiocyanate or nitrate as the Na^+ salt in the external medium.[21,48] Alternatively, the K^+ ionophore valinomycin may be included in the experimental medium and an imposed outwardly directed K^+ gradient will then produce an inside-negative membrane potential over a short period.[48,50]

It is important to confirm the tracer associated with membrane vesicles has been internalized and is not simply binding to the membrane surface. Binding is usually investigated either by (a) extrapolation of a time course of uptake over the linear phase back to zero time (any "instantaneous" uptake component is assumed to reflect rapid binding rather than transport, a method also applicable to isolated cells[21,48]) or (b) measuring equilibrium tracer uptake at a range of external osmolarities. In the latter case, the intravesicular space shrinks with increasing osmolarity, the amount of substrate equilibrating within the vesicles decreases, and a graph of equilibrium uptake against the reciprocal of osmolarity should produce a line which will extrapolate back to zero (i.e., zero intravesicular volume at "infinite" external osmolarity); residual tracer uptake under these circumstances is generally ascribed to surface binding.[48,49,51] Ideally, binding assessed by these two methods should produce similar results.[48,51]

When using membrane vesicles to study the effects of drugs, protein-modifying reagents or other compounds on transport activities, it is important to assess their effects on vesicle integrity (e.g., intravesicular volume) when evaluating experimental data.

1.5.5 RECONSTITUTION/OVEREXPRESSION OF AMINO ACID TRANSPORTERS

Transport activities can be reconstituted into artificial phospholipid membranes, using membrane proteins isolated from various subfractions of cell membranes.[12,21,23,24] Specific transporter proteins may be at least partially purified before reconstitution by fractionation techniques, including electrophoresis, column and

---

* Registered trademark of Pharmacia Biotech AB, Uppsala, Sweden

affinity chromatography.[23,24] A variety of methods exist for reconstituting proteins into artificial membranes, subsequent measurements of AA flux involving methods similar to those employed for native membrane vesicle studies (see Section 1.5.4). Transporter proteins may also be studied after overexpression in a suitable expression system (e.g., *Xenopus* oocyte, mammalian cell line) either from a mixture of nucleic acids or from a single cloned transporter DNA.[5,8,9] Detailed molecular studies of the mechanisms of several AA transport proteins are now being undertaken using the methods described above, in combination with molecular biological techniques such as *in vitro* mutagenesis.[5,8,9]

ACKNOWLEDGMENTS

We are grateful to Dr. K. Smith for useful discussions and Mrs. D. Watt for secretarial assistance. Work from our laboratory was supported by the Wellcome Trust, Medical Research Council and University of Dundee.

REFERENCES

1. Christensen, H. N., Interorgan amino acid nutrition, *Physiol. Rev.*, 62, 1193, 1982.
2. Christensen, H. N., Role of amino acid transport and counter transport in nutrition and metabolism, *Physiol. Rev.*, 70, 43, 1990.
3. Biolo, G., Zhang, X-J. and Wolfe, R. R., Role of membrane transport in interorgan amino acid flow between muscle and small intestine, *Metabolism*, 44, 719, 1995.
4. Biolo, G., Maggi, S. P., Williams, B. D., Tipton, K. D., and Wolfe, R. R., Increased rates of muscle protein turnover and amino acid transport after resistance exercise in humans, *Am. J. Physiol.*, 268, E514, 1995.
5. Malandro, M. S. and Kilberg, M. S., Molecular biology of mammalian amino acid transporters, *Annu. Rev. Biochem.*, 65, 305, 1996.
6. Stevens, B. R., Amino acid transport in intestine, in *Mammalian Amino Acid Transport. Mechanisms and Control*, Kilberg, M. S. and Häussinger, D., Eds., Plenum Press, New York and London, 1992, 149.
7. Schwegler, J. S., Sibernagl, S., Tamarappoo, B. K., and Welbourne, T. C., Amino acid transport in the kidney, in *Mammalian Amino Acid Transport. Mechanisms and Control*, Kilberg, M. S. and Häussinger, D., Eds., Plenum Press, New York and London, 1992, 233.
8. Bertran, J., Testar, X., Zorzano, A., and Palacín, M., A new age for mammalian plasma membrane amino acid transporters, *Cell. Physiol. Biochem.*, 4, 217, 1994.
9. Kanai, Y., Family of neutral and acidic amino acid transporters: molecular biology, physiology and medical implications, *Curr. Op. Cell Biol.*, 9, 565, 1997.
10. Smith, Q. R. and Cooper, A. J. L., Amino acid transport in brain, in *Mammalian Amino Acid Transport. Mechanisms and Control*, Kilberg, M. S. and Häussinger, D., Eds., Plenum Press, New York and London, 1992, 165.
11. Kilberg, M. S. and Häussinger, D., Amino acid transport in the liver, in *Mammalian Amino Acid Transport. Mechanisms and Control*, Kilberg, M. S. and Häussinger, D., Eds., Plenum Press, New York and London, 1992, 133.
12. Kilberg, M. S. and Häussinger, D. Eds., *Mammalian Amino Acid Transport. Mechanisms and Control*, Plenum Press, New York and London, 1992.

13. Stein, W. D., *Channels, Carriers and Pumps*, Academic Press, New York and London, 1990.

14. Macey, R. I. and Moura, T. F., Basic principles of transport, in *Handbook of Physiology*, Hoffman J. F. and Jamieson, J. D., Eds., Oxford University Press, Oxford, 181, 1997.

15. Bonadonna, R. C., Saccomani, M. P., Cobelli, C., and DeFronzo, R. A., Effect of insulin on system A amino acid transport in human skeletal muscle, *J. Clin. Invest.*, 91, 514, 1993.

16. Taylor, P. M. and Rennie, M. J., Perivenous localisation of Na-dependent glutamate transport in perfused rat liver, *FEBS Lett.*, 221, 370, 1987.

17. Yudilevich, D. L. and Mann, G. E., Unidirectional uptake of substrates at the blood side of secretory epithelia: stomach, salivary gland, pancreas, *Fed. Proc.*, 41, 3045, 1982.

18. Conti, P. S., Sordillo, P. P., Schmall, B., Benua, R. S., Bading, J. R., Bigler, R. E., and Laughlin, J. S., Tumor imaging with carbon-11 labelled a-aminoisobutyric acid (AIB) in a patient with advanced malignant melanoma, *Eur. J. Nuclear Med.*, 12, 353, 1996.

19. Conlon, K. C., Bading, J. R., DiResta, G. R., Corbally, M. T., Gelbard, A. S., and Brennan, M. F., Validation of transport measurements in skeletal muscle with N^{13} amino acids using a rabbit isolated hindlimb model, *Life Sci.*, 44, 847, 1989.

20. Watt, P. W., Corbett, M. E., and Rennie, M. J., Stimulation of protein synthesis in pig skeletal muscle by infusion of amino acids during constant insulin availability, *Am. J. Physiol.*, 263, E453, 1992.

21. McGivan, J. D., Techniques used in the study of plasma membrane amino acid transport, in *Mammalian Amino Acid Transport. Mechanisms and Control.* Kilberg, M. S. and Häussinger, D., Eds., Plenum Press, New York and London, 1992, 51.

22. Williams, B. D., Wolfe, R. R., Bracy, D. P., and Wasserman, D. H., Gut proteolysis contributes essential amino acids during exercise, *Am. J. Physiol.*, 270, E85, 1996.

23. Quaesda, A. R. and McGivan, J. D., A rapid method for the functional reconstitution of amino acid transport System A from rat liver plasma membranes; Partial purification of System A, *Biochem. J.*, 255, 963, 1988.

24. Tamarappoo, B. K., Handlogten, M. E., Laine, R. O., Serrano, M. A., Dugan, M. A., and Kilberg, M. S., Identification of the protein responsible for hepatic system N amino acid transport activity, *J. Biol. Chem.*, 267, 2370, 1992.

25. Tadros, L. B., Taylor, P. M., and Rennie, M. J., Characteristics of glutamine transport in primary tissue culture of rat skeletal muscle, *Am. J. Physiol.*, 265, E135, 1993.

26. Taylor, P. M., Mackenzie, B., Hundal, H. S., Robertson, E., and Rennie, M. J., Transport and membrane binding of the glutamine analogue 6-diazo-5-oxo-L-norleu-cine (DON) in *Xenopus laevis* oocytes, *J. Membr. Biol.*, 128, 181, 1992.

27. Low, S. Y., Rennie, M. J., and Taylor, P. M., Signalling elements involved in amino acid transport responses to altered muscle cell volume, *FASEB J.*, 11, 1111, 1997.

28. Rennie, M. J., Khogali, S. E. O., Low, S. Y., McDowell, H. E., Hundal, H. S., Ahmed, A., and Taylor, P. M., Amino acid transport in heart and skeletal muscle and the functional consequences, *Biochem. Soc. Trans.*, 24, 869, 1996.

29. Roberts, D. H., Tsao, Y., and Breckenridge, A. M., The reproducibility of limb blood flow measurements in human volunteers at rest and after exercise by using mercury-in-Silastic strain gauge plethysmography under standardized conditions, *Clin. Sci.*, 70, 635, 1986.

30. Blanchet, L. and Lebrec, D., Changes in splanchnic blood flow in portal hypertensive rats, *Eur. J. Clin. Invest.*, 12, 327, 1982.

31. Waterlow, J. C., Garlick, P. J., and Millward, D. J., *Protein Turnover in Mammalian Tissues and in the Whole Body*, Elsevier North-Holland, Amsterdam, 1978.
32. Gastaldelli, A., Schwarz, J. M., Caveggion, E., Traber, L. D., Traber, D. L., Rosenblatt, J., Toffolo, G., Cobelli, C., and Wolfe, R. R., Glucose kinetics in interstitial fluid can be predicted by compartmental modeling, *Am. J. Physiol.*, 272, E494, 1997.
33. Darmaun, D. and Dechelotte, P., Role of leucine as a precursor of glutamine α-amino nitrogen *in vivo* in humans, *Am. J. Physiol.*, 260, E326, 1991.
34. Felig, P., Wahren, J., and Räf, L., Evidence of inter-organ amino-acid transport by blood cells in humans, *Proc. Natl. Acad. Sci., U.S.A.*, 70, 1775, 1973.
35. Pardridge, W. M., Unidirectional influx of glutamine and other neutral amino acids into liver of fed and fasted rats in vivo, *Am. J. Physiol.*, 232, E492, 1977.
36. Ross, B. D., Perfusion Techniques in Biochemistry, Claredon Press, Oxford, 1972.
37. Hundal, H. S., Rennie, M. J., and Watt, P. W., Characteristics of L-glutamine transport in perfused rat skeletal muscle, *J. Physiol.*, 393, 283, 1987.
38. Goresky, C. A., Bach, G. G., Wolkoff, A. W., Rose, C. P., and Cousineau, D., Sequestered tracer outflow recovery in multiple indicator dilution experiments, *Hepatology*, 5, 805, 1985.
39. Nakai, M., Computation of transport function using multiple regression analysis, *Am. J. Physiol.*, 240, H133, 1981.
40. Sacca, L., Toffolo, G., and Cobelli, C., V-A and A-V modes in whole body and regional kinetics: domain of validity from a physiological model, *Am. J. Physiol.*, 263, E597, 1992.
41. Häussinger, D., Nitrogen metabolism in liver: structural and functional organization and physiological relevance, *Biochem. J.*, 267, 281, 1990.
42. Ussing, H. H. and Zerahn, K., Active transport of sodium as the source of electric current in the short-circuited isolated frog skin, *Acta. Physiol. Scand.*, 23, 1951.
43. Munck, B. G. and Schultz, S. G., Lysine transport across isolated rabbit ileum., *J. Gen. Physiol.*, 53, 157, 1969.
44. Munck, B. G. and Munck, L. K., Phenylalanine transport in rabbit small intestine, *J. Physiol.*, 480, 99, 1994.
45. Okada, Y., Tsuchiya, W., Irimajiri, A., and Inouye, A., Electrical properties and active solute transport in rat small intestine, *J. Membr. Biol.*, 31, 205, 1977.
46. Low, S. Y., Salter, M., Knowles, R. G., Pogson, C. I., and Rennie, M. J., A quantitative analysis of the control of glutamine catabolism in rat liver cells. Use of selective inhibitors, *Biochem. J.*, 295, 617, 1993.
47. Thwaites, D. T., Markovich, D., Murer, H., and Simmons, N. L., Na^+-dependent lysine transport in human intestinal Caco-2 cells, *J. Membr. Biol.*, 151, 215, 1996.
48. Hopfer, U., Tracer studies with isolated membrane vesicles, *Methods in Enzymology*, 172, 313, 1989.
49. Low, S. Y., Taylor, P. M., Ahmed, A., Pogson, C. I., and Rennie, M. J., Substrate-specificity of glutamine transporters in membrane vesicles from rat liver and skeletal muscle investigated using amino acid analogues, *Biochem. J.*, 278, 105, 1991.
50. Ahmed, A., Maxwell, D. L., Taylor, P. M., and Rennie, M. J., Glutamine transport in human skeletal muscle, *Am. J. Physiol.*, 264, E993, 1993.
51. Kemp, H. F. and Taylor, P. M., Interactions between thyroid hormone and tryptophan transport in rat liver are modulated by thyroid status, *Am. J. Physiol.*, 272, E809, 1997.

2 Whole-Body Protein Turnover in Humans: Past and New Applications Using Stable Isotopes

Antoine E. El-Khoury, M.D.

CONTENTS

0-8493-9612-3/99/$0.00+$.5
© 1998 by CRC Press LLC

I cannot give any scientist of any age better advice than this: the intensity of the conviction that a hypothesis is true has no bearing on whether it is true or not .

— Sir Peter B. Medawar[1]

2.1. INTRODUCTION

Protein metabolism is a major area of research in human nutrition because of the functions of proteins that are essential to life. The roles of proteins in muscle structure, enzymes, receptors, transport of other molecules across membranes, plasma oncotic pressure, and immune function make the investigation of protein metabolism in the whole body (this chapter) and in organs and tissues (Chapter 3 by Davis et al.) fundamental to our understanding the role of nutritional physiology and metabolic regulation in health and disease.

For the whole body, protein turnover (PT) is the rate at which protein is synthesized or degraded. It is the sum of turnovers of all the individual proteins of the body. PT is very different among organs, tissues, and individual proteins. Further, in many situations, the responses of protein synthesis (PS) and protein degradation or breakdown (PB) to physiological state, nutritional, or pharmacological interventions, are different from one organ or tissue to the other. The dynamic changes of whole-body PS and PB are the determinants of *endogenous* protein balance (when PS = PB, this balance is neutral or zero) which would be equivalent to *exogenous* protein balance, i.e., protein dietary intake (I) minus Irreversible Protein Nitrogen Loss (IPNL). The latter estimate is essentially derived from amino acid oxidation or nitrogen excretion.

In man, considering a 75 kg subject ingesting 1 g protein per kg Body Weight (BW) per day (75 g of protein), the value for daily whole-body protein synthesis would approximate 270 g of protein that is 3.6 times the dietary intake. PT allows for the regulation of the entire body protein mass. In a stable non-growing adult, daily PS and PB are in equilibrium (PS - PB = 0) over a 24-h period. Small daily changes in one direction or the other may not be detectable using the techniques and methods described below, but different groups of subjects (e.g., different genetic and ethnic backgrounds, different experimental diets, different treatment, different protein sources), or different treatments within the same subjects, can be compared with respect to whole-body protein dynamics. Further, PT is energy-costly, more particularly PS because of the energy cost of the formation of peptide bonds; this may account for 10 to 15% of Resting Metabolic Rate (RMR). Hence, this must be considered when protein-energy interactions are investigated in human subjects.

In this chapter, we focus on the classical approaches to estimate PS and PB: end-product methods using primarily stable-isotopically labeled glycine (^{15}N-glycine) and precursor methods using stable carbon-labeled leucine (L-[1-^{13}C]leucine). We discuss some applications of these approaches. Because of space restrictions, we will not discuss the use of **radio**-isotopes in this context in humans. The nitrogen balance technique and the urinary 3-methylhistidine method are discussed in Chapter 14 by Albright and Nair. Similarly, models based upon the use of labeled phenylalanine as tracer, with or without arteriovenous studies, are discussed in Chapter 13 by Yu et al., and Chapter 14 by Albright and Nair.

While Schoenheimer was a pioneer in synthesizing and utilizing stable isotopes of amino acids,[2] we do owe these methods to the creative work by Waterlow and colleagues.[3] Their original simple model is still being used and remains the basic source for "steady state" (see Sections 2.1.1 and 2.1.2 below) estimations of PS and PB; however, the applications have become more diverse and some refinements have been introduced over the years.

2.1.1 WATERLOW'S TWO-POOL MODEL

As shown in Figure 2.1, when considering the free amino acid pool (FAAP) in a "steady state," physiological (an unchanging physiological condition) and isotopic (unchanging isotopic enrichment in plasma, urine, and expired CO_2), the rate of amino acids leaving the pool per unit time (PS and amino acid oxidation) equals the rate entering the pool [PB and amino acid (dietary + tracer) intake], and equals the so-called "FLUX." Hence, the flux rate Q is as follows:

$$\text{total } Q = PS + AAox = PB + (I + i) \tag{1}^*$$

where AAox is "amino acid oxidation," as measured using either the estimate of $^{13}CO_2$ production in expired air as well as the ^{13}C isotopic abundance into the precursor pool for amino acid oxidation (in the case of ^{13}C-leucine tracer), or total nitrogen excretion in urine (in the case of ^{15}N-glycine tracer), I is dietary amino acid intake, and i is the tracer intake. This will be detailed in Sections 2.2 and 2.3.

In essence, the same model is used for precursor and end-product approaches: body protein is the second pool (very much larger than the first pool, FAAP) and acts as an isotope sink, since the model assumes that over the period of measurement there is no recycling of label via protein breakdown into the FAAP.

The way this model (Figure 2.1) applies when using an ^{15}N-labeled amino acid tracer such as ^{15}N-glycine is similar, except that amino acid oxidation (AAox) is derived from total nitrogen excretion in urine, and most importantly, the ^{15}N abundance (over baseline) into urinary urea and/or ammonia (the end-products) is assumed to be representative of the ^{15}N abundance (over baseline) into the metabolic alpha-amino-nitrogen pool (see Figure 2.2), hence determining whole-body nitrogen flux.

---

* We are not using, in this chapter, the exact designations/abbreviations originally used by Waterlow,[3] primarily to facilitate the reader's integration of the model's various components.

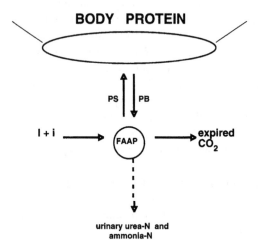

FIGURE 2.1 Simplified model of whole-body amino acid metabolism; the dietary (I) and tracer (i) amino acid intakes enter the free amino acid pool (FAAP). From that pool, amino acids are assumed to have only two fates: oxidation (first carbon to expired air CO_2, and nitrogen primarily to urinary urea and ammonia) and protein synthesis (PS).

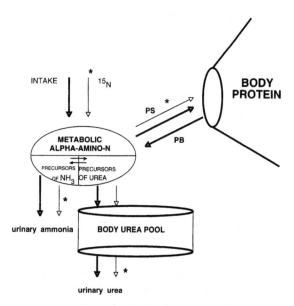

FIGURE 2.2 Application of the Waterlow model to ^{15}N studies; note (a) it is assumed that the tracer does not recycle via protein breakdown into the metabolic alpha-amino-nitrogen pool, over the period of the isotope experiment; (b) the interactions between ammonia and urea precursors, within the metabolic alpha-amino-nitrogen pool, are ignored; and (c) because of the large size of the body urea pool and its elasticity, a correction of urinary urea excretion data must be made for the change in the body urea pool size over the period of the isotope study.

Despite its simplicity and the assumptions involved (see Sections 2.2 and 2.3) the use of the two-pool model has allowed the quantitation of whole-body PS and PB in various physiological and pathological conditions: e.g., the comparison between fasting and feeding states,[4,5,6,7] the study of the role of insulin and substrate (amino acids) availability in the modulation of protein synthesis and breakdown, the role of glucagon in increasing protein breakdown,[8] protein metabolism in diabetes (Chapter 5 by Hoffer, and Chapter 14 by Albright and Nair), trauma (Chapter 13 by Yu et al.), and the elderly (Chapter 10 by Fukagawa and Fisher). Further, the use of stable isotopes has the major safety advantage (vs. radio-isotopes) as no irradiation is emitted, allowing repeated use of a particular tracer or the simultaneous use of different tracers in the same human subject.[9]

2.1.2 COMMON ASSUMPTIONS TO PRECURSOR AND END-PRODUCT METHODS

> **(a)** The precursor pool for protein synthesis is homogeneous, and the flux through this pool can be estimated by measurements on blood/plasma, urine, or expired CO_2.
>
> **(b)** The metabolism of the tracer reflects that of the total amino acid mixture in the body.
>
> **(c)** Protein synthesis equals flux minus oxidation. Other metabolic pathways are considered negligible.
>
> **(d)** As mentioned above (Section 2.1.1), recycling of isotope via labeled-protein breakdown into plasma can be ignored over the period of the measurement.
>
> **(e)** The isotope used for labeling the tracer (^{13}C, ^{15}N) behaves in the same way as the corresponding natural compound (^{12}C, ^{14}N).
>
> **(f)** The dose of the labeled tracer (^{15}N-glycine, ^{13}C-leucine) is extremely small (a "tracer" dose), and does not itself affect the measurement of turnover.
>
> **(g)** The metabolic state does not alter during the course of the measurement.

2.2 END-PRODUCT METHODS

2.2.1 URINARY END-PRODUCTS

A landmark study of children, performed by Picou and Taylor-Roberts,[10] involved a continuous intragastric infusion of ^{15}N-glycine with an assessment of the enrichment of urinary urea when a <u>constant</u> labeling has been reached (isotopic "plateau"). However, because of the large size of the urea pool and its slow turnover rate, at least 30 h were required to reach a plateau in urinary ^{15}N-urea. The long infusion meant that a steady physiological state may not have been maintained over 30 h, and that ^{15}N label could have re-entered the free amino acid pool via PB. A modification by Waterlow et al.[11] involved the use of a single oral dose of labeled glycine and the measurement of the total amount of ^{15}N label into urinary ammonia over a much shorter period (a few hours).

Considering both of the above approaches,[10,11] the interconversions between urinary urea precursors and urinary ammonia precursors, within the metabolic alpha-amino-nitrogen pool, are ignored; the metabolic alpha-amino-nitrogen pool is considered a "black box." This was called a "stochastic" approach. Similarly, studies using a single (oral or intravenous) dose of ^{15}N-glycine (or another ^{15}N-amino acid) followed by a 9-h complete urine collection, were performed by Fern et al.[12,13,14]: this helped assess the role of the choice of amino acid tracer, the route of tracer (intravenous or oral), and the specific urinary end-product (urea vs. ammonia vs. both), in determining the estimate of nitrogen flux.

2.2.1.1   Specific Assumptions Related to the Use of ^{15}N-Glycine

Glycine, a dispensable (non-essential) amino acid, has the simplest molecular configuration of all amino acids: [H - CH(NH3)$^+$ - COO$^-$]. It is involved in protein synthesis but is also a precursor in purine, porphyrin and creatine synthesis. Further, it plays a role in conjugation and detoxification of foreign compounds in the liver. Glycine and serine are interconvertible and play a major role as contributors to the one-carbon pool. A short review of the pathways of glycine metabolism is presented by Neuberger.[15] Interestingly, while Matthews et al.[16] have shown that ^{15}N from glycine and serine can enter the transaminating amino acid pool via glutamate and alanine, a different group[17] has found that alanine and glutamate were not labeled by ^{15}N, and the same authors[18] suggested that the direct deamination of glycine in the kidney may well be an important pathway, more particularly when the glycine tracer is given intravenously. Figure 2.3 outlines the overall flow of metabolic nitrogen in the body, incorporating the possible fates of glycine-N. Figure 2.4 illustrates the various hypotheses with respect to how glycine-nitrogen may preferentially label urinary ammonia.

Hence, the specific assumptions:

(a) Most importantly, the partitioning of ^{15}N from glycine, between protein and end-products, is in the same "proportion" as for total amino-N.

(b) Glycine nitrogen does not give rise to quantitatively significant amounts of products other than protein and excretory products. End-products do not derive nitrogen from non-protein sources.

(c) Dietary total N and glycine-N are treated in the same way as N derived from PB.

2.2.1.2   Constant Administration vs. Single Dose of ^{15}N-Glycine

Because of the poor practicality of using a 30- to 36-h intravenous or intragastric infusion of ^{15}N-glycine and a potentially sizeable recycling of nitrogen label via protein breakdown, one would recommend the use of the single dose approach: it

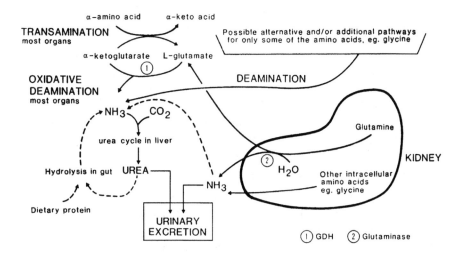

FIGURE 2.3   Simplified representation of the nitrogen metabolic flow in the human body; note (a) the deamination of glycine in the kidney and possibly other tissues, and (b) the scheme herein assumes that all of the ammonia generated by urea hydrolysis in the gut is recycled back into urea.

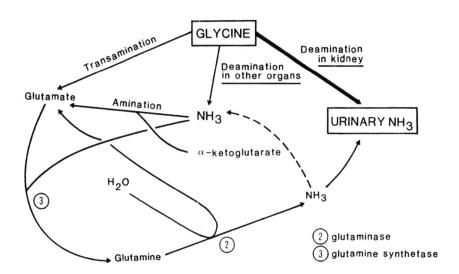

FIGURE 2.4   Illustration of the hypotheses on how ^{15}N-glycine might enrich urinary ammonia-N.

is shorter (about 9-h) and can be repeated easily in the same subject (e.g., fasting vs. feeding state) if about a one/two-week isotope-free period is planned between the two 9-h studies (to allow enough time for the retained label in the body to washout, so that the ^{15}N-<u>baseline</u> abundance in urinary end-products returns to its original value). However, each time, 2 blood samples are required (just before time 0 and just after time 9 h) for the measurement of plasma ureaN concentration and plasma ^{15}N-urea enrichment. Most important is the absolute requirement for collecting a baseline urine sample (prior to giving the isotope) and performing a complete urine collection covering the exact totality of the 9-h period. This approach, using the "average" flux from urinary urea and ammonia ^{15}N enrichments has been extensively used by Garlick and Fern.[19]

Interestingly, a large number of published ^{15}N-glycine studies have been performed in the <u>fed</u> state, and the feeding was usually constant, e.g., enteral intragastric, parenteral, or as frequent small meals such as in the case of healthy volunteers, in order to maintain a steady physiological state.

2.2.1.2.1   Calculations Related to the Single Dose Technique

We will consider, for calculation purposes, one end-product, e.g., urinary ammonia. About the same would apply for urea; then, if required, the average flux (urea and ammonia) can be calculated and used in the computations below (b).
(a) The formula for nitrogen flux (Q) is the following:

$$Q = \text{total N excreted in ammonia} \times (i \text{ / total } ^{15}\text{N excreted in ammonia}) \quad (2)$$

(all units in g N/9 h or g ^{15}N/9 h as appropriate)
where "i (dose of ^{15}N given)" is derived from the dose of tracer amino acid given, its nitrogen content, and its ^{15}N enrichment;

"total N excreted in ammonia" is the product of the concentration of ammoniaN in urine by the volume of the 9-h urinary collection;

"total ^{15}N excreted in ammonia" is calculated as:

^{15}N abundance over baseline in urinary ammonia x (1/100) x (15/14) x N excreted in ammonia.
(b) When flux is calculated, PS and PB are derived from the formula,

$Q = PS + AAox = PB + I$ (the amount of tracer, i, is ignored because it is extremely small; a "tracer" dose)   (same as Equation 1)

if I and AAox are known.
I is known from the dietary composition (g N/9 h) and is null in the fasted state.
AAox (g N/9 h) is calculated as follows:

$$\text{Total urinary N} = \text{ureaN} + \text{ammoniaN} + \textit{other urinary N}, \quad (3)$$

where the ureaN component is corrected for changes in body urea pool size over the course of the 9-h study, as described by Fern et al.[12]:

ureaN excreted (**corrected**) = total urinary ureaN - [(plasma ureaN concentration at time 0 - plasma ureaN concentration at time 9 h) x (Total Body Water/0.92)]   (4)

Here, plasma ureaN concentrations are expressed in g ureaN/L, and the difference between the value at time 0 and that at time 9 h may be positive or negative. Total Body Water (TBW) in liters (L) can be computed, in normal adult subjects, by using the anthropometrics-based equations by Watson et al.[20] This calculation (Equation 4) is based upon the following: the urea volume of distribution is TBW, and the water content of plasma (in which the plasma ureaN concentration is measured) is assumed to represent 92% of plasma volume.

All the results would then be expressed in g protein. kg body weight^{-1}. 12 h^{-1} using a 6.25 conversion factor from nitrogen to protein.

2.2.1.3 Choice of Urinary End-Product: Urea, Ammonia, or Both

It has been demonstrated that when using ^{15}N-glycine as a single dose in the fed state, the oral route generated a small difference in PS, between end-products (PSurea slightly lower than PSammonia); this suggests that slightly more ^{15}N was transferred to urea (vs. ammonia). This small difference would become much larger when the intravenous (IV) route is used, and in the opposite direction (PSammonia < PSurea), because more ^{15}N label would be found into urinary ammonia (vs. urea).[13,19] Indirectly, these findings support the possibility of more significant deamination of glycine in the kidney liberating labeled ammonia directly in urine, with the use of the IV route.

When the oral route is not possible, the IV route may be used. Much less variation of PS between routes of tracer (oral vs. IV) are found when the "average" flux (urea and ammonia) is used in the computations. As a consequence, one would be tempted to use, with any route of tracer, the "average" flux.

2.2.1.4 ^{15}N-Glycine, a Tracer Among Many Others: Advantages and Pitfalls

Because of compartmentation within the alpha-amino-nitrogen pool,[13,19] the estimate of whole-body protein synthesis critically depends upon the specific amino acid used as tracer, the route of single dose tracer, and the end-product chosen. Figure 2.5 illustrates some PS values, in the fed state, in one healthy adult male[13] who received different ^{15}N-amino acids orally (single dose each time) at separate occasions, and contrast these values (using ^{15}N-urea or ^{15}N-ammonia as end-product) with the estimate obtained from a 24-h tracer protocol[7] (over the 12-h fed phase of the 24-h tracer protocol) using the precursor approach (^{13}C-leucine IV infusion). We note that the use of ^{15}N-glycine (oral single dose in fed state) with any of the end-products (most particularly, ammonia) for flux calculation generates PS estimates that are almost identical to the mean value observed in our ^{13}C-leucine study (1.9 g protein. kg^{-1}. 12 h^{-1}).[7]

In addition, Figure 2.5 outlines the following:

Using urinary urea as end-product, the PS rate observed with ^{15}N-leucine is about 3 to 4 times the rate observed with the use of a highly transaminating amino acid such as alanine.[13,19] Using urinary ammonia as end-product, the PS rate observed

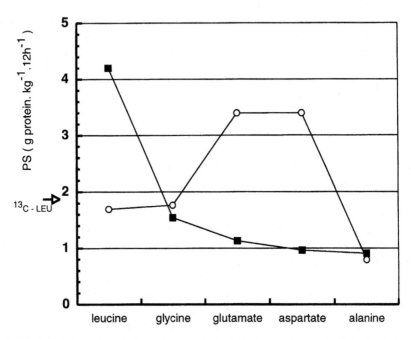

FIGURE 2.5 Illustration of the estimates of whole-body protein synthesis in the fed state when using different ^{15}N-labeled amino acids as tracers, sequentially, in the same subject, and by the single dose approach; clear circles correspond to the use of urinary ammonia as end-product, and dark squares correspond to the use of urinary urea as end-product (developed from result data in reference[13]). In addition, we compare all ^{15}N-derived fed state PS data to our mean fed state PS that was obtained via our 24-h ^{13}C-leucine tracer protocol (see arrow on Y axis) (see our results in Reference 7). Only if the latter approach is considered a standard, the use of ^{15}N-alanine would possibly underestimate the fed state PS by one half.

with ^{15}N-leucine is close to that observed with ^{15}N-glycine, and to the estimate derived from our 24-h ^{13}C-leucine protocol.[7] One could predict from Figure 2.5 that with the use of ^{15}N-glutamate or ^{15}N-aspartate, and averaging the ammonia-derived N flux with that derived from urea as end-product, PS estimates would become closer to those from ^{15}N-glycine.

In sum, the use of ^{15}N-glycine as a tracer, with the single oral dose approach as described above, has many advantages: (a) the method is simple and non-invasive; (b) the tracer is relatively cheap and available in a pure state: 1 gram of 99% labeled ^{15}N-glycine is sufficient to conduct 10 single dose tracer studies; (c) taste and smell are almost absent; and (d) the "precision" (reproducibility) of PS estimates, as tested in the same subject, is within 5 to 7% — quite good for a method of this kind.[21]

However, some pitfalls are noted: (a) the uncertainty about how the partitioning of glycine-N between end-products and protein synthesis may change in disease states, and if it would still reflect the partitioning of the amino-N pool; (b) even when glycine-tracer-based PS data agrees with that from the precursor approach, this would not necessarily indicate that the "accuracy" (how close the measured estimate is to the real true value) is appropriate (and this is an issue with both precursor and end-product methods; see Section 2.3); and (c) background of ^{15}N (i.e., the ^{15}N content in the baseline samples) is relatively high when compared to the enriched samples; hence, the enrichments above baseline are very low [in the order of 0.01 to 0.1 Atom Percent Excess (APE)], and this will require very tedious sample processing and analysis techniques (see Section 2.5).

2.2.1.5 Do ^{15}N-Proteins as Tracers Improve Upon the Use of ^{15}N-Amino Acids?

While several uniformly-labeled ^{15}N-proteins have been used as oral tracers in order to more uniformly label the amino-nitrogen pool, and the estimated N flux data contrasted to that from ^{15}N-glycine, the conclusion was that N flux rates observed when using an ^{15}N-protein could be predicted from the proportion of each of several amino acids in the ^{15}N-protein together with the fluxes obtained from the use of each of these amino acids independently (such as alanine, aspartate, glutamate, glycine, leucine, lysine, and glutamine). We cite as examples the use of ^{15}N-egg-protein,[10] ^{15}N-wheat,[13,22] and ^{15}N-yeast.[13,23] A significant determinant (not the only one, however) of N flux rates is the lysine content of the ^{15}N-protein. The use of ^{15}N-lysine alone[13] generates extremely high values for N flux and PS, at least five-fold higher than those obtained with ^{15}N-glycine, essentially because lysine-amino-N transfer to urinary end-products is very low, thereby overestimating N flux and PS. Hence, a high lysine content of the tracer protein would be often associated with higher N flux and PS estimates when using the ^{15}N-protein as tracer; for example, with ^{15}N-soybean protein[24] as tracer [containing about 6.4% (w/w) ^{15}N-lysine], PS and PB rates were about two-fold higher than those observed with ^{15}N-glycine, in the fast and fed states. However, with any of the two tracers (glycine and soybean), PS was shown to increase with feeding.[24]

2.2.2 $^{13}CO_2$ AS END-PRODUCT

Originally, this approach was used by Golden and Waterlow.[25] It involved a constant administration of radioactive leucine tracer (1-^{14}C-leucine) and the measurement of $^{14}CO_2$ production in elderly human subjects; no blood samples were required for measurement of ^{14}C-labeling in the free amino acid pool. The method was later extensively used by Imura and Walser[26] in the rat, and this was followed by several studies from this group. There is no reason why this method could not be applied further in humans by using a constant infusion protocol with stable isotopically labeled leucine (1-^{13}C-leucine).

This method is very attractive because it is much less invasive (vs. precursor methods) since it does not require blood drawing for measurement of ^{13}C-labeling in the precursor amino acid pool. Further, time-consuming laboratory isotopic analyses of plasma would not be required, dispensing the investigator from the need for Gas Chromatography-Mass Spectrometry (GC-MS) equipment (see Section 2.5). For this method, only Isotope Ratio Mass Spectrometry (IRMS) analysis would be required (for the measure of expired air $^{13}CO_2$ enrichment), in addition to an indirect calorimeter [for the measure of total CO_2 production (VCO_2)]. The assumption is:

the amino acid <u>precursor</u> pool isotopic enrichment (over baseline) is the "same" for amino acid oxidation and for protein synthesis. The computations are based upon the knowledge of the "fraction" $(1 - F)$ of given ^{13}C-label (via ^{13}C-leucine constant infusion) that appears in expired air CO_2 [e.g., $(1 - F) = 0.25$]. This requires an exact estimate of $^{13}CO_2$ production (see Section 2.3) as for precursor methods. F is the fraction of ^{13}C-label that is disposed of via protein synthesis, computed from $(1 - F)$ (e.g., $F = 0.75$). Hence, to derive PS with this approach, the following equation is used:

$$PS = AAox \times [F / (1 - F)] \qquad (5)$$

where PS and AAox are expressed in g protein. kg^{-1}. time $period^{-1}$, and AAox is calculated as described above for the urinary end-product methods (Equations 3 and 4).

As long as AAox can be estimated reliably from urinary N (x 6.25), the method would be as valid as the precursor methods described below (Section 2.3). We found[7] that over a complete time period of 6 h of small meal hourly feeding, there was a moderate mismatch between the direct estimate of AAox (precursor approach) and the AAox estimate from total urinary N excretion, probably because of the time-delay in N excretion (as compared to the leucine oxidation rate).[7] However, in the fasting state, and other feeding states where the time period of interest comprises a few hours of fasting following feeding, and when using a more prolonged tracer protocol (e.g., 12 h and longer), we have not observed the latter mismatch. Hence, with an appropriate protocol design, this method would be recommended, more particularly in situations where blood sampling is not readily feasible, or where GC-MS equipment and expertise are not available.

2.3   PRECURSOR METHODS

2.3.1   Specific Assumptions Related to the Use of L-[1-^{13}C]Leucine

This tracer, an Indispensable Amino Acid (IAA) and a branched-chain amino acid (together with valine and isoleucine), is by far the most widely used tracer for the investigation of whole-body protein turnover in humans. Also, it is relatively cheap compared to other ^{13}C-amino acids, and available from many manufacturers of stable isotope compounds. In addition to the assumptions noted in Section 2.1.2, we discuss below some specific important assumptions to be considered in the application of the ^{13}C-leucine approach:

> **(a)** In physiological and isotopic "steady state," the amount of ^{13}C label entering the FAAP equals the amount of label leaving this pool. Hence, if total leucine flux (Q_{LEU}) through the FAAP and leucine oxidation (OX_{LEU}) are measured, leucine disappearance into protein synthesis (PS_{LEU}) can be estimated (see Figure 2.1 and Equation 1). Leucine appearance from protein breakdown (PB_{LEU}) can be estimated in the fasted state as $(Q_{LEU} - i)$, and in the fed state as $[Q_{LEU} - (I_{LEU} + i)]$.

(b) Leucine kinetics (flux, disappearance into protein synthesis, appearance from protein breakdown, oxidation) are representative of whole-body protein kinetics which can be estimated by extrapolation, using a value for the leucine content (e.g., weight/weight) in total body mixed protein. As will be discussed below (Section 2.3.3) this is not always directly feasible.

(c) Changes of $^{13}CO_2$ <u>background</u> abundance over the time period of the tracer protocol can be determined using a tracer-free protocol (so-called "sham" study), in the same subjects if possible, but certainly using the same experimental design and diet. Examples are shown in some of our publications.[27,28] Only with a very large tracer infusion rate where the expired air $^{13}CO_2$ enrichment over baseline would become very elevated, the temporal changes of $^{13}CO_2$ background over the time frame of the protocol can be ignored, because their amplitude would become relatively too small as compared to the $^{13}CO_2$ enrichment over baseline at "plateau" (the level at which the enrichment is steady). However, in this case, because of a very large tracer dose, the assumption of "tracer" dose (a very small dose of tracer that does not affect its own kinetics) may become invalid. Although Tessari et al.[29] demonstrated that the infusion of a stable-isotopically labeled leucine at a rate below 10% of the ^{13}C-leucine flux did not significantly affect leucine kinetics, one would recommend, with the use of any rate of ^{13}C-leucine infusion, to account for the mass of ^{13}C-leucine given, where possible (see Calculations, Section 2.3.2.4). This would be feasible when the total leucine dietary intake is in the range of clearly adequate-to-generous.

(d) Because the estimate of $^{13}CO_2$ production rate requires the use of correction factors for body retention of $^{13}CO_2$ under the exact experimental conditions of the study, if these correction factors cannot be determined (for practical reasons) for each of the subjects participating in a research study, it is assumed that these correction factors are similar to those determined in a similar group of other subjects and under the same experimental conditions.

The knowledge of the behavior of $^{13}CO_2$ in terms of recovery (%) in expired air is **absolutely fundamental** for appropriately estimating $^{13}CO_2$ production. Indeed, recovery is very much incomplete under the majority of experimental situations (between about 50% and 100%) because CO_2 recovery in breath, from a bicarbonate infusion, is delayed by stagnation of CO_2 in very slowly turning over pools, such as the bone mass; ideally, a ^{13}C-bicarbonate-sodium tracer study is conducted under the same experimental conditions, as a necessary additional study within the overall research protocol, unless these recoveries have been firmly established in similar subjects and under very identical experimental conditions.

We quote some references,[27,28,30] and a detailed list of bicarbonate recovery studies is found in Table 8 of Reference 31, as well as a discussion of some factors influencing bicarbonate recoveries[31] such as VCO_2, feeding, length of bicarbonate infusion and modality of tracer administration (single dose vs. primed or unprimed constant infusion). The labeled bicarbonate priming dose can be given over 1 min, just before starting the constant infusion, in order to speed up the reaching of steady isotopic state in breath $^{13}CO_2$ (typically, a bicarbonate prime dose is equivalent to an 80-min infusion dose). Without a prime, about 6 h of bicarbonate infusion are needed to reach plateau. It appears that the use of the oral route (vs. IV) of bicarbonate tracer does not significantly affect recovery in breath.[30] Interestingly, at the beginning of exercise, it was found that $^{13}CO_2$ recovery can exceed 100%, probably because of the acute flushout of $^{13}CO_2$ from the rapidly exchangeable bicarbonate pool.[28]

Further, there are many sources of error in estimating $^{13}CO_2$ recovery in breath from infused (usually IV) labeled bicarbonate. Some of these are related to the technique of tracer solution preparation, pumping rate, and possible losses of $^{13}CO_2$ from the solution and infusion tubes, before, during, and after the infusion. An extensive discussion of all possible sources of error and factors directly and/or indirectly affecting the estimates of CO_2 recoveries is presented in an excellent publication by Leijssen and Elia.[32]

Despite the potential problems associated with the need for accuracy and precision of the estimates of labeled CO_2 recovery, the ^{13}C-leucine technique survived more than 20 years of scrutiny,[33] primarily because of the model's simplicity and its straightforward mathematics. Further, the confidence in using plasma ^{13}C-alpha-ketoisocaproate (^{13}C-KIC, a direct transamination product of ^{13}C-leucine) as an indicator of the enrichment of the leucine precursor pool for oxidation as well as for protein synthesis, helped confirm the ^{13}C-leucine method as a reference standard for the evaluation of whole-body protein turnover in humans. Aspects related to the precursor enrichment are discussed herein.

(e) Originally, the precursor enrichment used was that of plasma ^{13}C-leucine.[34] It was then demonstrated that it was higher than the intracellular precursor enrichment. Because KIC (intracellular and in plasma) is only derived from intracellular transamination of leucine (reversible transamination) and since this process is extremely fast within cells, Matthews et al.[35] have suggested the use of plasma ^{13}C-KIC as a precursor enrichment for oxidation and for protein synthesis. Naturally, because the ^{13}C label in KIC is almost a direct precursor to $^{13}CO_2$, it was expected that the ^{13}C-KIC based estimates of <u>leucine oxidation</u> would be accurate. By applying a complex 24-h IV ^{13}C-leucine protocol (12 h fasting, 12 h feeding) where leucine dietary intake was generous and where a neutral (zero) 24-h leucine balance (input - output) was to be expected, we validated the reliability of using ^{13}C-KIC as the precursor enrichment for leucine oxidation by finding a neutral 24-h body leucine balance.[27] Further, 24-h leucine oxidation compared well with 24 h N excretion (see Table 5 in Reference 27).

With respect to PS_{LEU}, based on theoretical grounds, two different pools may be involved as precursors to various degrees: plasma free leucine and intracellular leucine. Because of the uncertainty about the contribution of each of these pools, and about how these contributions may change from one organ or tissue to another, some research investigators were originally skeptical with respect to the use of plasma ^{13}C-KIC as a precursor enrichment in the computation of Q_{LEU} and PS_{LEU}. However, some years later, at least two studies offered support for the use of plasma ^{13}C-KIC as a precursor enrichment for estimation of PS_{LEU}. In post-absorptive dogs, the plasma "enrichment" [or "specific activity" (SA); term used in radioisotope studies] of the transaminated product of infused labeled KIC or leucine, was shown to be an excellent predictor of the intracellular leucine SA in most tissues, except in the kidney.[36] In healthy humans, plasma KIC SA reflected the precursor pool for pancreatic PS.[37] However, in one recent study with respect to human *muscle* PS, it was shown that plasma ^{13}C-KIC enrichment was well above that of leucyl-tRNA, suggesting that the use of ^{13}C-KIC as a precursor enrichment for the estimation of *muscle* PS may lead to an underestimation of that rate.[38] More studies are needed to resolve this issue.

2.3.2 TRACER STUDY DESIGN

2.3.2.1 Physiological States: Fasting and Feeding

In contrast to end-product methods where many studies were conducted in feeding, most of the original early studies using the precursor approach were conducted in fasting, classically over the morning hours after an overnight fast. However, it was soon realized that in order to obtain data which would reflect the whole 24-h day, a protocol that combines the study of leucine kinetics in the fasting state and in the fed state was necessary; one additional assumption was that extrapolation of leucine kinetic data from a short protocol (e.g., last h of 3-h fasting + last h of 5-h feeding) to a 24-h period, e.g., [(last h of fast x 12) + (last h of fed x 12)] is appropriate. We quote two studies as examples of short duration protocols.[5,39] The majority of published studies to date have also used short protocols.

More recently, because we were interested in the assessment of 24-h leucine oxidation and balance, we have developed a 24-h tracer protocol (12-h fasting and 12-h feeding).[27] This study demonstrated that, at rest, under the specific dietary conditions where energy was sufficient and protein was given at 1 g protein. kg^{-1}. d^{-1}, extrapolations of leucine oxidation data from the 12th or 15th h of fasting (x 12) and the 5th h of feeding (x 12) were valid. A different 24-h protocol was applied to the study of the effect of diet and exercise on leucine kinetics.[28]

As shown in Figure 2.6, the ratio (leucine oxidation/leucine flux), in both the fasted and fed states, correlates with dietary protein intake. Hence, in order to study the effect of various dietary protein intake levels on leucine kinetics, the tracer protocol must incorporate both the fasting and feeding periods. A typical 9-h tracer protocol is depicted in Figure 2.7. The IV ^{13}C-leucine infusion is primed in order to reduce the time required to reach isotopic plateau in plasma ^{13}C-KIC. Further, the bicarbonate pool can be primed in order to shorten the time required to reach isotopic plateau in expired $^{13}CO_2$.

The rate of intravenous infusion of ^{13}C-leucine should be as low as possible but should be sufficient for good detection of $^{13}CO_2$ enrichment over baseline in expired air. We have used 2.8 µmol ^{13}C-leucine. kg^{-1}. h^{-1} in standard conditions where the diet was adequate in energy, provided 1 g protein. kg^{-1}. d^{-1}, and where the subjects

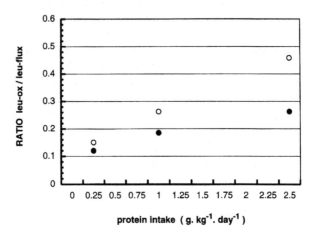

FIGURE 2.6   The relationship between protein intake in the fed state and the mean fraction of leucine flux that is oxidized in the fasting (dark circles) and the feeding (clear circles) states. Note the stronger relationship during feeding (vs. fasting). Data cumulated from results in References [7,27,28,41] for the 1 g level, Reference [41] for the 2.5 g level, and personal yet unpublished data for the 0.25 g level.

were at rest.[7,27] In contrast, for studies involving exercise (e.g., [28]), and because exercise increases VCO_2 by as much as six-fold (thereby diluting $^{13}CO_2$), a much higher ^{13}C-leucine infusion rate was necessary (8 μmol. kg⁻¹. h⁻¹).

2.3.2.2   Route of Tracer: Intravenous or Intragastric

While the IV route is probably appropriate for studies in the fasting state, it is not the ideal tracer route for the investigation of leucine and protein kinetics in the fed state. In the latter, on theoretical grounds, the oral or intragastric (IG) route of tracer (i.e., same route as food) would be more appropriate, because with this route the first-pass splanchnic extraction and metabolism of leucine would be better reflected as part of whole-body leucine kinetics. Following the same reasoning (i.e., same route as food) in patients receiving continuous total parenteral nutrition, and in order to investigate leucine kinetics in such patients, the IV ^{13}C-leucine route would be used.[40]

However, it happens that fed-state leucine kinetics with the IV vs. IG route are not dramatically different, at least when this is compared to phenylalanine kinetics where the difference (IV vs. IG) is large, essentially because the primary organ of phenylalanine metabolism is the liver. Also, there are some approaches for estimating and/or accounting for the first-pass splanchnic extraction of leucine, as well as splanchnic leucine oxidation in the fed state: this will be described below (Section 2.3.4).

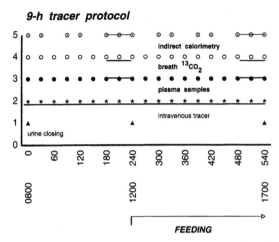

FIGURE 2.7   A representation of a standard 9-h stable isotope-based research protocol. The duration of the overnight fasting would depend upon the investigator's instructions to the volunteer subjects with respect to the time of the last meal on the evening prior to the isotope study. Time is indicated as experimental time (0 min to 540 min) and real time (0800 to 1700). Feeding frequent small meals over 5 h (240 min to 540 min) follows the fasting period, and would represent 5/12 of the total daily dietary intake. (1) Urine is collected separately for the fasted (4-h) and fed (5-h) phases of the protocol, in order to measure urinary N excretion if necessary. (2) The constant intravenous infusion of tracer such as ^{13}C-leucine (for priming doses, see text). (3) Half-hourly blood samples, in order to separate plasma for isotopic analysis of ^{13}C-KIC (and ^{13}C-leucine if required); note that baseline plasma samples must be taken over the few minutes preceding time 0. (4) half-hourly expired air samples for the analysis of ^{13}C abundance into CO_2 ; as described for blood, breath baseline samples are absolutely required prior to time 0. (5) Semi-continuous indirect calorimetry in order to measure oxygen consumption (VO_2) and carbon dioxide production (VCO_2). For (3), (4), and (5), the solid lines indicate the last hour of fasting (180 to 240 min) and the fifth hour of feeding (480 to 540 min); data over these intervals are used to estimate leucine kinetics and for potential data extrapolation from the last hour of fasting to 12 h fasting, and from the fifth hour of feeding to 12 h feeding.

2.3.2.3   Are Steady Physiological and Isotopic States Absolutely Necessary?

Based on theoretical grounds, it would be reasonable to use non-steady state computations (that usually account for changes in plasma leucine concentration) for estimating leucine flux and oxidation (hence, PS) when the physiological and isotopic states are not steady over the time frame of interest. However, many assumptions are involved in non-steady state computations, and it is not certain whether such methods of computation would improve upon the validity of comparisons of PS data among different groups or treatments, for example.

By frequently sampling blood and expired air, and applying semi-continuous indirect calorimetry, e.g., samples every 15 min or less during moderate exercise (see Reference 41), our estimates of leucine oxidation and flux using the steady state model were not significantly different from those generated by the use of a modified Steele equation (non-steady state computations).[42]

The estimate of leucine *oxidation* is possible in most conditions by using frequent measures of plasma ^{13}C-KIC, expired air ^{13}CO$_2$, and VCO$_2$. Further, the recycling of leucine label from protein breakdown into plasma did not significantly affect the estimate of leucine oxidation; this is because (a) both components of the oxidation equation (^{13}CO$_2$ production divided by ^{13}C-KIC) are equally increased by recycling of label, and (b) ^{13}C-KIC is the direct precursor of ^{13}CO$_2$.[27,43] However, with respect to leucine *flux* (considered alone), certainly, recycling would erroneously increase plasma ^{13}C-KIC, thereby underestimating flux.

2.3.2.4 Calculations

In addition to the basic calculations described in Section 2.3.1.a, we present the simplified equations below:

VCO$_2$ (millimoles. kg^{-1}. 30 min^{-1}) = [VCO$_2$ (mL/min) x 30] /
[Weight (kg) x 22.4]   (6)

where 1 millimole of CO$_2$ is assumed to have a volume of 22.4 mL.

^{13}CO$_2$ production (μmol. kg^{-1}. 30 min^{-1}) = [VCO$_2$ (millimoles. kg^{-1}. 30 min^{-1})
x ^{13}CO$_2$ enrichment (APE x 1000)] all divided by % bicarbonate recovery (7)

where ^{13}CO$_2$ enrichment is the average of the values for the two time-points delimiting the 30 min interval, and bicarbonate recovery is the recovery observed under these conditions.

Example: VCO$_2$ = 5, ^{13}CO$_2$ enrichment = (4 + 3.6) / 2 = 3.8, Bicarbonate recovery (%) = 76, then (5 x 3.8) / 76 = 0.25 μmol. kg^{-1}. 30 min^{-1}.

Leucine oxidation (μmol. kg^{-1}. 30 min^{-1}) = [^{13}CO$_2$ production
(μmol. kg^{-1}. 30 min^{-1})/^{13}C-KIC (APE)] x 100   (8)

where ^{13}C-KIC is the average of the values for the two time-points delimiting the 30 min interval. Example: (0.25/2.6) x 100 = 9.6 μmol. kg^{-1}. 30 min^{-1}.

Total leucine flux Q (μmol. kg^{-1}. 30 min^{-1}) =

[i (μmol. kg^{-1}. 30 min^{-1}) / ^{13}C-KIC (APE)] x 100   (9)

where i is the rate of ^{13}C-leucine infusion, and it should be corrected for the enrichment of this isotope. Example: the manufacturer provides a value for ^{13}C abundance in the ^{13}C-leucine isotope powder of 99.4% (or 99.4 atom%), then the "correct i" would be (i x 0.994).

2.3.3 LEUCINE CONTENT IN DIET VS. LEUCINE IN BODY MIXED PROTEINS

2.3.3.1 Can We Extrapolate Data Reliably from Leucine Kinetics to Protein Kinetics?

Because of the partitioning of "protein oxidation" or "irreversible protein nitrogen loss" (IPNL) between the fasting and feeding phases of a 24-h day, it is difficult to predict the exact profile of the amino acids oxidized within <u>one</u> physiological state (fasting or feeding). In contrast, when 24-h leucine and protein balances (input - output) are expected to be neutral (zero), e.g., at normal protein intake and sufficient energy intake, one may predict the amino acid profile of 24 h IPNL: it is that of the dietary protein.

Leucine concentration in whole-body mixed proteins of human fetuses was shown to be about 8% (w/w), and this value did not change with the age and development of the fetus.[44] We assume that this value is applicable to adult humans. Hence, when leucine input (dietary protein + tracer) over 24 h has a concentration of 8% (w/w), it would make the extrapolation from leucine kinetics to protein kinetics a direct calculation. With the above condition:

$$\text{IPNL (mg protein. kg}^{-1}. \text{day}^{-1}) = \text{leucine oxidation}$$
$$\text{(mg leucine. kg}^{-1}. \text{day}^{-1}) \times (100/8) \tag{10}$$

The same would apply for PS and PB because no matter which is the source for the amino acids used for PS and those liberated by PB (e.g., whole-body mixed proteins, the diet, or both) the estimates of protein kinetics would not be affected.

On this basis, we have purposely designed experimental diets where there was a match between leucine concentration in (dietary protein + tracer) and that in whole-body mixed proteins. Further, when the tracer alone was inducing a mismatch, we corrected for it.[27] When both the tracer and diet were inducing the mismatch, we also applied correction factors.[28] However, while these correction factors have been very helpful, we have uncertainty about their validity when the mismatch is dramatic.

2.3.3.2 Applications Using the Estimate of Irreversible Protein Nitrogen Loss (IPNL)

Estimates of IPNL (from leucine oxidation and/or from N excretion) helped us confirm the quantitative agreement between leucine-derived and N-derived estimates of IPNL.[27,28,43]

Recently, we were interested in testing the use of different precursor enrichments for the estimate of **lysine** oxidation. We designed the dietary amino acid mixture and the amount of ^{13}C-lysine tracer so that a match with lysine in whole-body mixed proteins was met (7.7% w/w).[45] Since we were uncertain about the appropriate precursor enrichment and about the best route (IV vs. IG) of tracer delivery, our only reference was the expectation of neutrality (zero) in 24 h protein balance (input-output). Hence, we have used for comparison the mean value of 24 h IPNL, which was obtained via ^{13}C-leucine studies (IPNL$_{leu}$) (under identical conditions); it was identical to 24 h IPNL from N excretion (IPNL$_N$) that was observed in the lysine study. All this meant that the one estimate of 24 h lysine oxidation, which would generate an IPNL (IPNL$_{lys}$) close to IPNL$_{leu}$ and IPNL$_N$, would potentially indicate the most appropriate precursor enrichment for use under these specific experimental conditions.[45] This is an example where IPNL values were used in order to attempt to solve questions related to (a) precursor pool enrichment for use in the estimate of lysine oxidation, and (b) the choice of route of ^{13}C-lysine administration.[45]

2.3.4   ACCOUNTING FOR THE SPLANCHNIC METABOLISM OF LEUCINE IN THE FED STATE

As described in Section 2.3.2.2, the most common design involves oral feeding with the use of an IV ^{13}C-leucine. Hence, some of the dietary leucine may be oxidized in the splanchnic area, and utilized for splanchnic protein synthesis prior to its labeling by the IV ^{13}C-leucine tracer. Some methods have been developed to investigate this problem. First, with the use of two differently labeled leucine tracers (e.g., ^{13}C and ^{2}H$_3$) and by infusing one tracer IV and the other tracer IG (ideally, the same rate of administration for both tracers) one can determine the splanchnic first-pass uptake of leucine that is essentially derived from the difference between leucine Q$_{IG}$ and leucine Q$_{IV}$, and how this difference relates to dietary leucine. For an example, see Matthews et al.[46]

Others[42] have used a slightly different approach but utilized non-steady state equations because the feeding mode was a "one bulk meal," in contrast to the "multiple small frequent meals" as in the case of steady-state studies. Their results revealed a very significant increase of PS with feeding the meal, and no change in PB.[42]

We have attempted to simplify the computation of the correction to flux data. By knowing the approximate leucine splanchnic uptake from our very similar previous studies, the leucine flux measured in the fed state was accordingly corrected upwards. In addition, a small upwards correction to the estimate of whole-body leucine oxidation was made, by assuming that the oxidized fraction of the splanchnic first-pass of leucine is the same as the oxidized fraction of whole-body leucine flux. Because of space limits, we refer the reader to our publications.[7,41] Figure 2.8 compares fed state protein Q, PS, and PB, using (a) the direct uncorrected Q, vs. (b) the corrected flux for a splanchnic uptake of 25% (see Reference 7). For published reviews, we direct the reader to Waterlow[47] and Young et al.[48]

2.4   SOME RECENT APPLICATIONS

Some studies (e.g.,[42]) investigated the effect of the form by which the tracer ^{13}C-leucine is delivered upon whole-body leucine kinetics; e.g., comparing non-steady state leucine kinetic data where ^{13}C-leucine had been incorporated into dietary protein (i.e., intrinsic label) vs. the case where free ^{13}C-leucine had been given orally with the dietary protein (i.e., extrinsic label). These studies suggested that the estimate of whole-body leucine oxidation in the fed state was lower with the use of the

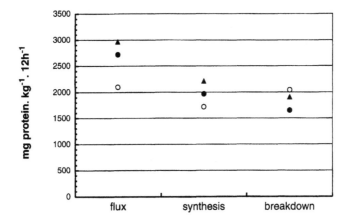

FIGURE 2.8 Illustration of mean values for protein flux, whole-body protein synthesis, and whole-body protein breakdown, over an overnight fast (clear circles) and when feeding a diet containing 1 g protein. kg⁻¹. day⁻¹ and sufficient energy as small hourly meals (dark circles for uncorrected data, dark triangles for corrected data with respect to a 25% splanchnic first-pass uptake of leucine). Note the larger increase of mean PS with feeding when data are corrected for splanchnic first-pass; in contrast, with these corrections, we find a smaller decrease of mean PB with feeding. Figure is developed from results data in Reference 7.

intrinsic label.[42] Metges[49] has recently conducted steady-state comparisons of fed-state leucine kinetics with three different forms of tracer ^{13}C-leucine administration: (a) intrinsic ^{13}C-leucine into goat casein; (b) free ^{13}C-leucine given simultaneously with goat casein; and (c) free ^{13}C-leucine given simultaneously with an amino acid mixture. Preliminary findings suggest that the estimate of whole-body leucine oxidation in the fed state can be influenced by the form of ^{13}C-leucine delivery, and in this case, leucine oxidation values with (a) were lower than with (b), which in turn were lower than with (c).[49]

2.5 ANALYTICAL ASPECTS

Because of space restrictions, we have shortened this section and refer the reader to key publications. With respect to ^{15}N-based methods, a critical issue is the extraction of ammonia and urea, separately, from urine samples. This extraction must be complete (close to 100% recovery) and free from ^{14}N-^{15}N isotope fractionation processes. The original procedure was described by Jackson et al.[50] Any error in this step will directly reflect upon the ^{15}N enrichments of ammonia-N and urea-N, and the estimates of nitrogen kinetics. Primarily, ammonia gas is extracted first using a Leurquin apparatus and an acid trap. Then, urea in the sample is hydrolyzed, and produces ammonia that is trapped similarly but separately. In order to analyze ^{15}NH$_3$ enrichment (originating from one of the end-products, urea or ammonia) nitrogen gas must be liberated from ammonia. The ^{15}N enrichment of the latter is analyzed by IRMS.

With respect to precursor methods, $^{13}CO_2$ in expired air is measured by IRMS. Plasma $^{13}CKIC$ (and if needed, plasma ^{13}C-leucine) requires the use of GC-MS[27] (see Chapter 6 by Patterson). In addition, the use of GC-C-IRMS (see Chapter 7 by Metges and Petzke) offers some advantages, most particularly with respect to the estimates of very low ^{13}C enrichments (over baseline) in several amino acids.

ACKNOWLEDGMENTS

MIT (Cambridge, Massachusetts) studies and Uppsala University (Sweden) collaborative studies were funded by grants from the NIH (RR88, DK.15856) and from a STINT Grant 96/52 (Swedish Foundation for International Cooperation in Research and Higher Education), Swedish Grants SJFR 50.0204/94 and CiF55194.

REFERENCES

1. Medawar, P. B., *Advice to a Young Scientist*, Basic Books Inc. Publishers, New York, 39, 1979.
2. Schoenheimer, R. and Ratner, S., Studies in protein metabolism. III. Synthesis of amino acids containing isotopic nitrogen, *J. Biol. Chem.*, 127, 301, 1939.
3. Waterlow, J. C., Garlick, P. J., and Millward, D. J., *Protein Turnover in Mammalian Tissues and in the Whole Body*, Elsevier/North-Holland, 1978, 804 pages.
4. Garlick, P. J., McNurlan, M. A., and Ballmer, P. E., Influence of dietary protein intake on whole-body protein turnover in humans, *Diabetes Care*, 14, 1189, 1991.
5. Motil, K. J., Matthews, D. E., Bier, D. M., Burke, J. F., Munro, H. N., and Young, V. R., Whole-body leucine and lysine metabolism: response to dietary protein intake in young men, *Am. J. Physiol.*, 240, E712, 1981.
6. Hoffer, L. J., Yang, R. D., Matthews, D. E., Bistrian, B. R., Bier, D. M., and Young, V. R., Effects of a meal consumption on whole body leucine and alanine kinetics in young adult men, *Brit. J. Nutr.*, 53, 31, 1985.
7. El-Khoury, A. E., Sanchez, M., Fukagawa, N. K., and Young, V. R., Whole-body protein synthesis in healthy adult humans: $^{13}CO_2$ technique versus plasma precursor approach, *Am. J. Physiol.*, 268, E174, 1995.
8. Nair, K. S., Halliday, D., Matthews, D. E., and Welle, S. L., Hyperglucagonemia during insulin deficiency accelerates protein catabolism, *Am. J. Physiol.*, 253, E208, 1987.
9. Bier, D. M., The use of stable isotopes in metabolic investigation, in *Techniques for Metabolic Investigation in Man*, Bailliere's Clinical Endocrinology and Metabolism-Vol. 1-No. 4, Bailliere Tindall, 1987, 817.
10. Picou, D. and Taylor-Roberts, T., The measurement of total protein synthesis and catabolism and nitrogen turnover in infants in different nutritional states and receiving different amounts of dietary protein, *Clin. Sci.*, 36, 283, 1969.
11. Waterlow, J. C., Golden, M. H. N., and Garlick, P. J., Protein turnover in man measured with ^{15}N: comparison of end-products and dose regimes, *Am. J. Physiol.*, 235, E165, 1978.
12. Fern, E. B., Garlick, P. J., McNurlan, M. A., and Waterlow, J. C., The excretion of isotope in urea and ammonia for estimating protein turnover in man with (^{15}N)glycine, *Clin. Sci.*, 61, 217, 1981.

13. Fern, E. B., Garlick, P. J., and Waterlow, J. C., Apparent compartmentation of body nitrogen in one human subject: its consequence in measuring the rate of whole-body protein synthesis with ^{15}N, *Clin. Sci.*, 68, 271, 1985.

14. Fern, E. B., Garlick, P. J., and Waterlow, J. C., The concept of the single body pool of metabolic nitrogen in determining the rate of whole-body nitrogen turnover, *Hum. Nutr. Clin. Nutr.*, 39C, 85, 1985.

15. Neuberger, A., Pathways of glycine metabolism, in *Nitrogen Metabolism in Man*, Waterlow, J. C. and Stephen, J. M. L., Eds., Applied Science Publishers, London and New Jersey, 1981, 253.

16. Matthews, D. E., Conway, J. M., Young, V. R., and Bier, D. M., Glycine nitrogen metabolism in man, *Metabolism*, 30, 886, 1981.

17. Jackson, A. A. and Golden, M. H. N., (^{15}N) Glycine metabolism in normal man: the metabolic alpha-amino-nitrogen pool, *Clin. Sci.*, 58, 517, 1980.

18. Golden, M. H. N. and Jackson, A. A., Assumptions and errors in the use of ^{15}N-excretion data to estimate whole-body protein turnover, in *Nitrogen Metabolism in Man*, Waterlow, J. C. and Stephen, J. M. L., Eds., Applied Science Publishers, London and New Jersey, 323, 1981.

19. Garlick, P. J. and Fern, E. B., Whole-body protein turnover: theoretical considerations, in *Substrate and Energy Metabolism*, Garrow, J. S. and Halliday, D., Eds., John Libbey, 7, 1985.

20. Watson, P. E., Watson, I. D., and Batt, R. D., Total body water volumes for adult males and females estimated from simple anthropometric measurements, *Am. J. Clin. Nutr.*, 33, 27, 1980.

21. Fern, E. B., Garlick, P. J., Sheppard, H. G., and Fern, M., The precision of measuring the rate of whole-body nitrogen flux and protein synthesis in man with a single dose of (^{15}N)-glycine, *Hum. Nutr. Clin. Nutr.*, 38C, 63, 1984.

22. Fern, E. B. and Garlick, P. J., The rate of nitrogen metabolism in the whole body of man measured with (^{15}N)-glycine and uniformly labelled (^{15}N)-wheat, *Hum. Nutr. Clin. Nutr.*, 37C, 91, 1983.

23. Wutzke, K., Heine, W., Drescher, U., Richter, I., and Plath, C., ^{15}N-labelled yeast protein — a valid tracer for calculating whole-body protein parameters in infants: a comparison between (^{15}N)-yeast protein and (^{15}N)-glycine, *Hum. Nutr. Clin. Nutr.*, 37C, 317, 1983.

24. McNurlan, M. A., El-Khoury, A. E., Milne, E., and Fern, E. B., Assessment of protein metabolism in man with ^{15}N-labelled soybean, *Proc. Nutr. Soc. (U.K.)*, Vol.50-No.1, 46A, 1991.

25. Golden, M. H. N. and Waterlow, J. C., Total protein synthesis in elderly people: a comparison of results with [^{15}N]glycine and [^{14}C]leucine, *Clin. Sci. Mol. Med.*, 53, 277, 1977.

26. Imura, K. and Walser, M., Rate of whole-body protein synthesis in the rat as calculated from fractional oxidation of leucine, valine or methionine, *Metab. Clin. Exp.*, 37, 591, 1988.

27. El-Khoury, A. E., Fukagawa, N. K., Sanchez, M., Tsay, R. H., Gleason, R. E., Chapman, T. E., and Young, V. R., Validation of the tracer balance concept with reference to leucine: 24h intravenous tracer studies with L-[1-^{13}C]leucine and [^{15}N-^{15}N]urea, *Am. J. Clin. Nutr.*, 59, 1000, 1994.

28. El-Khoury, A. E., Forslund, A., Olsson, R., Branth, S., Sjödin, A., Andersson, A., Atkinson, A., Selvaraj, A., Hambraeus, L., and Young, V. R., Moderate exercise at energy balance does not affect 24-h leucine oxidation or nitrogen retention in healthy men, *Am. J. Physiol.*, 273, E394, 1997.

29. Tessari, P., Tsalikian, E., Schwenk, W. F., Nissen, S. L., and Haymond, M., Effects of [^{15}N]leucine infused at low rates on leucine metabolism in humans, *Am. J. Physiol.*, 249, E121, 1985.

30. Hoerr, R. A., Yu, Y-M., Wagner, D. A., Burke, J. F., and Young, V. R., Recovery of ^{13}C in breath from NaH^{13}CO$_3$ infused by gut and vein: effect of feeding, *Am. J. Physiol.*, 257, E426, 1989.

31. El-Khoury, A. E., Sanchez, M., Fukagawa, N. K., Gleason, R. E., and Young, V. R., Similar 24h pattern and rate of carbon dioxide production, by indirect calorimetry versus stable isotope dilution, in healthy adults under standardized metabolic conditions, *J. Nutr.*, 124, 1615, 1994.

32. Leijssen, D. P. C. and Elia, M., Recovery of ^{13}CO$_2$ and ^{14}CO$_2$ in human bicarbonate studies: a critical review with original data, *Clin. Sci.*, 91, 665, 1996.

33. Abumrad, N. N., Darmaun, D., and Cynober, L. A., Approaches to studying amino acid metabolism: from quantitative assays to flux assessment using stable isotopes, in *Amino Acid Metabolism and Therapy in Health and Nutritional Disease*, Cynober, L. A., Ed., CRC Press, Boca Raton, Florida, 1995, Chapter 1.

34. Matthews, D. E., Motil, K. J., Rohrbaugh, D. K., Burke, J. F., Young, V. R., and Bier, D. M., Measurement of leucine metabolism in man from a primed, continuous infusion of L-(1-^{13}C) leucine, *Am. J. Physiol.*, 238, E473, 1980.

35. Matthews, D. E., Schwarz, H. P., Yang, R. D., Motil, K. J., Young, V. R., and Bier, D. M., Relationship of plasma leucine and alpha-ketoisocaproate during a L-(1-^{13}C)leucine infusion in man: a method for measuring human intracellular leucine tracer enrichment, *Metabolism*, 31, 1105, 1982.

36. Horber, F. F., Horber-Feyder, C. M., Krayer, S., Schwenk, W. F., and Haymond, M. W., Plasma reciprocal pool specific activity predicts that of intracellular free leucine for protein synthesis, *Am. J. Physiol.*, 257, E385, 1989.

37. Bennet, W. M., O'Keefe, S. J. D., and Haymond, M. W., Comparison of precursor pools with leucine alpha-ketoisocaproate and phenylalanine tracers used to measure splanchnic protein synthesis in man, *Metab. Clin. Exp.*, 42, 691, 1993.

38. Ljungqvist, O. H., Persson, M., Ford, G. C., and Nair, K. S., Functional heterogeneity of leucine pools in human skeletal muscle, *Am. J. Physiol.*, 273, E564, 1997.

39. Pacy, P. J., Price, J. M., Halliday, D., Quevedo, M. R., and Millward, D. J., Nitrogen homeostasis in man. 2 . The diurnal responses of protein synthesis, degradation and amino acid oxidation to diets with increasing protein intakes, *Clin. Sci.*, 86, 103, 1994.

40. Goulet, O., DePotter, S., Salas, J., Robert, J-J., Rongier, M., Ben Hariz, M., Koziet, J., Desjeux, J-F., Ricour, C., and Darmaun, D., Leucine metabolism at graded amino acid intake in children receiving parenteral nutrition, *Am. J. Physiol.*, 265, E540, 1993.

41. Forslund, A. H., Hambraeus, L., Olsson, R. M., El-Khoury, A. E., Yu, Y-M., and Young, V. R., The 24-h whole body leucine and urea kinetics at normal and high protein intakes with exercise in healthy adults, *Am. J. Physiol.*, 275, E310, 1998.

42. Boirie, Y., Gachon, P., Corny, S., Fauquant, J., Maubois, J-L., and Beaufrere, B., Acute postprandial changes in leucine metabolism as assessed with an intrinsically labeled milk protein, *Am. J. Physiol.*, 271, E1083, 1996.

43. El-Khoury, A. E., Sanchez, M., Fukagawa, N. K., Gleason, R. E., Tsay, R. H., and Young, V.R., The 24-h kinetics of leucine oxidation in healthy adults receiving a generous leucine intake via three discrete meals, *Am. J. Clin. Nutr.*, 62, 579, 1995.

44. Widdowson, E. M., Southgate, D. A. T., and Hey, E. N., Body composition of the fetus and infant, in *Nutrition and Metabolism of the Fetus and Infant*, Visser, H. K. A., Ed, Nijhoff, London, 1979, 169.

45. El-Khoury, A. E., Basile, A., Beaumier, L., Wang, S. Y., Al-Amiri, H. A., Selvaraj, A., Wong, S., Atkinson, A., Ajami, A. M., and Young, V. R., Twenty-four-hour intravenous and oral tracer studies with L-[1-^{13}C]-2-aminoadipic acid and L-[1-^{13}C]lysine as tracers at generous nitrogen and lysine intakes in healthy adults, *Am. J. Clin. Nutr.*, 68, 827, 1998.
46. Matthews, D. E., Marano, M. A., and Campbell, R. J., Splanchnic bed utilization of leucine and phenylalanine in humans, *Am. J. Physiol.*, 264, E109, 1993.
47. Waterlow, J. C., Whole body protein turnover in humans — past, present, and future, *Annu. Rev. Nutr.*, 15, 57, 1995.
48. Young, V. R., Yu, Y-M., and Krempf, M., Protein and amino acid turnover using the stable isotopes ^{15}N, ^{13}C, and ^{2}H as probes, in *New Techniques in Nutrition Research*, San Diego Academic Press, San Diego, CA, 1991, 17.
49. Metges, C. C., Personal communication.
50. Jackson, A. A., Golden, M. H. N., Jahoor, P. F., and Landman, J. P., The isolation of urea nitrogen and ammonia nitrogen from biological samples for mass spectrometry, *Anal. Biochem.*, 105, 14, 1980.

3 Protein Synthesis in Organs and Tissues: Quantitative Methods in Laboratory Animals

Teresa A. Davis, Marta L. Fiorotto, Douglas G. Burrin, and Rhonda C. Vann

CONTENTS

3.1 INTRODUCTION

The protein mass of the body is regulated by changes in the relative rates of protein synthesis and protein degradation. Whole-body protein synthesis rates represent the compilation of the rates of synthesis of protein in all tissues and organs of the body. Growth, aging, nutrition, hormones, injury, and disease can affect protein synthesis in individual tissues differently, stimulating or suppressing protein synthesis in some tissues, while having little effect in others. Thus, to understand the mechanism by which these phenomena alter protein balance, it is critical that the effects of these factors on protein synthesis be examined on an individual tissue basis rather than in the body as a whole.

The most commonly employed methods for measuring tissue protein synthesis use isotopic tracers to measure the rate of incorporation of a labeled amino acid into tissue protein over time, with adjustment for the level of labeling of the precursor pool at the site of protein synthesis. These methods, referred to as the "constant infusion method" and the "flooding dose method," have been widely used in animal studies to measure rates of tissue protein synthesis. However, methods using arteriovenous differences of amino acids across individual organs and tissue beds and methods to measure the response of individual proteins have also provided important information. This chapter will discuss the principles of these methods, evaluate their advantages and disadvantages, and offer some practical advice on the performance of these methods in the laboratory. A summary of the advantages and disadvantages of the constant infusion, flooding dose, and arteriovenous difference methods is presented in Tables 3.1 and 3.2.

TABLE 3.1
Advantages of the Most Commonly Used Methods for Measuring Tissue Protein Synthesis in Animals

Method	Advantages
Constant Infusion	Measurement can be made from a single tissue sample. Particularly applicable to tissues with slow protein synthesis rates. Synthesis rates are not altered by performance of the method. Tissue and whole-body protein synthesis can be measured concurrently.
Flooding Dose	Measurement can be made from a single tissue sample. Particularly applicable to tissues with rapid protein synthesis rates. Particularly applicable to tissues with secretory proteins. Can be used to measure acute changes in protein synthesis. Most feasible method for use in very small animals.
AV Difference	Does not require tissue biopsy or killing of the animal. Longitudinal measurements can be made in the same animal. Influence of varying treatments can be determined in the same animal. Relative proportion of individual tissue to whole-body protein synthesis can be measured.

TABLE 3.2
Disadvantages of the Most Commonly Used Methods for Measuring Tissue Protein Synthesis in Animals

Method	Disadvantages
Constant Infusion	Animal must be in isotopic and metabolic steady state.
	Recycling of tracer in tissues with high turnover rates.
	Underestimation of synthesis rates in tissues with high proportion of secretory proteins.
	Measurement of acute changes in protein synthesis is difficult.
	Determination of protein synthesis in very small animals is difficult.
Flooding Dose	Large dose of amino acids may directly alter protein synthesis.
	Tissue uptake of amino acids may be influenced by the flooding dose.
	High amino acid concentration may alter hormonal balance.
AV Difference	Variation is introduced by sampling and blood flow error.
	Differences in RBC and plasma pool isotope equilibration may occur.
	Plasma proteins, peptides, and noncovalently bound amino acids may be exchanged during perfusion through a tissue bed.
	Rates represent a mixed population of tissues and cells.

3.2 MEASUREMENT OF TISSUE PROTEIN SYNTHESIS BY DIRECT LABELING

3.2.1 CONSTANT INFUSION METHOD

The constant infusion method has been used by a number of laboratories for measuring protein synthesis in different tissues of a variety of animal species,[1-6] and to explore the effects of numerous factors, including nutrition,[7-9] hormones,[10-14] development,[15] and disease,[10,16] on this process. With the constant infusion method, a labeled tracer amino acid (labeled with either a stable or radioactive isotope) is infused into the animal at a constant rate so as to rapidly achieve steady-state labeling in the free amino acid pool. Protein synthesis can be determined with a single tissue sample, because the kinetics of free pool labeling can be predicted from knowledge of the relative amounts of the tracee amino acid in the protein-bound and free pools.[6,8] Protein synthesis is calculated from the ratio of protein-bound and free amino acid isotopic enrichment or specific radioactivity with the generally applicable formula:

$$\frac{S_b}{S_i} = \frac{R}{(R-1)} \times \frac{(1 - e^{-Kst})}{(1 - e^{-RKst})} - \frac{1}{(R-1)}$$

where S_b is the isotopic enrichment of the protein-bound labeled amino acid, S_i is the isotopic enrichment of the tissue free amino acid, R is the ratio of protein-bound to free amino acid pool size, Ks is the fractional rate of protein synthesis, t is the duration of labeling, and e is the base for natural logarithms.[3]

Because of the prolonged length of the labeling period, typically 4 to 8 hours, the constant infusion method is particularly well suited for slowly turning over proteins in peripheral tissues, such as skeletal muscle. However, recycling of tracer can be a problem in measuring the synthesis rates of rapidly turning over proteins in visceral tissues, such as liver. The intracellular recycling of tracer from protein into the free amino acid pool results in a rise in labeling, thus altering the calculated rate of tissue protein synthesis. Another disadvantage of the prolonged infusions required by the constant infusion method is that total protein synthesis in such tissues as the liver and gut, in which a substantial portion of synthesized proteins is exported, can be underestimated because during the 6-hour period normally required for the constant infusion experiments, the majority of the labeled secretory proteins has been exported. Prolonged infusion can also obscure the determination of the acute effects of hormone manipulations or dietary treatment on protein synthesis.

The constant infusion method assumes that there is both an isotopic and metabolic steady state during the tracer infusion. Although a constant tracer:tracee ratio of the labeled amino acid may be obtained over much of the infusion period, during the initial period of infusion (usually the first hour) the tracer:tracee ratio is rising to plateau. The initial rate of incorporation of label, when the precursor pool enrichment is still rising to plateau, is slower than the final rate of incorporation achieved, when the precursor pool has reached isotopic steady state. Therefore, the true rate of incorporation of labeled amino acid into tissue protein can be slightly underestimated if only one tissue sample is obtained at the end of the tracer infusion period.[9] In addition, if the plasma amino acid concentration changes during the infusion, transient changes in amino acid isotopic enrichment can occur in the extracellular precursor pool, and hence in the incorporation of the tracer, without a change in protein turnover. An additional consideration of the prolonged infusion required by the method is that achievement of a metabolic steady state throughout the infusion may be difficult; for example, in small animals in which the required physical restraint does not allow feeding, the fasting period lengthens as the infusion continues.

To achieve the appropriate level of labeling in the free amino acid pool more rapidly, a priming dose of the isotopically labeled tracer amino acid frequently is given at the initiation of the infusion. The amount of prime that is given as a bolus at the initiation of the infusion is generally equivalent to the amount of label given over one hour of infusion. The tracer infusion rate must be adequate to ensure reliable detection of tracer incorporation into protein pools, particularly in those tissues in which the proteins are synthesized at a very slow rate, e.g., skeletal muscle. If it is anticipated that the protein synthetic rate will be reduced by the treatment given, higher tracer infusion rates and prolonged infusions may be required. For example, in studies in which the isotope L-[5,5,5-D_3]-leucine was infused for eight hours,[9] a priming dose of 30 μmol/kg, followed by a constant infusion of 30 μmol/(kg · h) was administered to control pigs, but a 45 μmol/kg priming dose and constant infusion of 45 μmol/(kg · h) was administered to protein-deficient pigs.

One of the advantages of the constant infusion method is that individual tissue protein synthesis rates and the whole-body protein synthesis rate can be measured at the same time, using the same tracer. This allows direct comparison of the contribution of different tissues to whole-body protein synthesis.[5,15]

3.2.2 FLOODING DOSE METHOD

The flooding dose method has been used extensively to measure the influence of a variety of factors on tissue protein synthesis in large[17-23] and small animals.[24-35] The method involves the relatively rapid injection (usually intravenous) of a large dose of tracee amino acid along with the tracer amino acid. The aim of this method is to "flood" the free amino acid pools, thereby minimizing the differences between extracellular and intracellular free amino acid specific radioactivity (in the case of radioisotopes, or isotopic enrichment in the case of stable isotopes) and the specific radioactivity of the amino acids acylated to tRNA (see below). Following the injection of the flooding dose, the specific radioactivity of the protein-bound amino acid increases linearly. If the dose of tracee amino acid is large enough to achieve "flooding" conditions, the specific radioactivity of the precursor pool will not change appreciably over the period during which the rate of incorporation of the tracer into tissue protein is measured. The fractional rate of protein synthesis (K_S) can then be calculated as:

$$K_S \ (\%/day) = (S_B/S_A) \times (100/t)$$

where S_B is the specific radioactivity of the protein-bound labeled amino acid, S_A is the specific radioactivity of the precursor pool, and t is the duration of labeling in minutes.[24,26]

Because the flooding dose technique allows the determination of acute changes in tissue protein synthesis over a period of 5 to 30 minutes, it is particularly attractive in acute intervention studies such as feeding and short-term hormone infusions in which metabolic nonsteady-state conditions exist. The ability to measure protein synthesis over a short period of time is a specific advantage in tissues with rapid protein synthesis rates, and especially in those with a large secretory component, such as liver and intestine. Moreover, because the flooding dose method requires a single rapid injection of tracer rather than a prolonged constant infusion, the flooding dose method is the most feasible for measuring protein synthesis in very small animals.

Some investigators[36-39] have expressed concerns that the flooding dose may affect protein synthesis directly or indirectly, either through alterations in the tissue uptake of other amino acids or by altering hormonal balance. Although evidence has been presented which suggests that a large dose of leucine stimulates protein synthesis,[38] a reduction in protein synthesis following a flooding dose of leucine has also been reported.[37] There is also evidence to suggest that the protein synthesis rates obtained by the flooding dose and constant infusion method are generally similar, and that the large dose of amino acid does not alter the rate of protein synthesis, at least over periods of 30 minutes or less.[24,40-43] It should be kept in mind that some of the reported differences in protein synthesis values between the two methods may be accounted for by the different populations of proteins whose synthesis rates are measured by the two methods. The flooding dose method measures the synthesis rates of both constitutive and secretory proteins, whereas the values obtained from the constant infusion method primarily reflect the synthesis of constitutive proteins. In addition, measurements with the flooding dose method will be inevitably weighted towards the measurement of the synthesis rates of short-lived proteins, thereby producing higher apparent synthesis rates.

To perform the flooding dose method, small animals such as rats and mice are lightly restrained using a gauze wrap, and injected via a lateral tail vein. If a tail vein cannot be accessed because of the small size of the animal (e.g., rats less than 10 days of age), the injection can be given intraperitoneally, carefully avoiding the puncture of the intestine. Larger animals such as pigs can be placed in a sling or held and injected via a jugular vein catheter. For the flooding dose, labeled amino acid is combined with a large amount of the unlabeled amino acid which approximates 5 to 10 times the body's free pool (150 mM for phenylalanine, 100 mM for leucine, and 62 mM for valine in any species). The amount of label required depends upon the synthesis rate of the tissue (i.e., more label would be required to measure synthesis in a slowly turning over tissue) and the sensitivity of the detection system. If blood can be accessed, such as through a catheter, it can be collected at various times after the injection to determine the time course of the change in the specific radioactivity of the plasma free amino acid pool, although this change should be small. The length of the period of labeling is generally 10 minutes in rodents and up to 30 minutes in larger animals, and must be accurately measured to the fraction of a minute. The flooding dose method was designed for short-term measurement of protein synthesis. Labeling periods longer than 30 minutes are not recommended, due to the decline in the specific radioactivity of the precursor pool as unlabelled amino acid is removed from the pool and the kinetics of the system become more complex and difficult to monitor. The method has been commonly used with radio-isotopes, but more recently, stable isotopes have also been used, particularly when the method is applied to domestic animals.

3.3 MEASUREMENT OF TISSUE PROTEIN SYNTHESIS BY ARTERIOVENOUS DIFFERENCE

The arteriovenous difference (AV) method can be used to measure the rates of protein synthesis in organs and tissue beds when it is not practical or economical to obtain tissue samples by either biopsies or killing the animal. The AV method has been used most frequently in studies with domestic animals such as dogs, pigs, cattle, and sheep, to measure the net mass balance of amino acids across a variety of organs and tissues, including the liver, portal-drained viscera, spleen, kidney, brain, hind-limb, mammary gland, and uteroplacenta.[44-52] The net amino acid balance (μmol/h) calculated using the AV method is based on the Fick principle:

$$\text{Net amino acid balance} = (Ca - Cv) \times F$$

where Ca and Cv represent the amino acid concentrations (μmol/L) in the arterial input and venous drainage, respectively, and F represents the blood flow rate (L/h).

The amino acid balance determined by the AV method, however, only gives an estimate of the net metabolism among various potential pathways within an organ or tissue. These possible metabolic fates may include not only protein synthesis and degradation, but also transamination or complete oxidation to CO_2. Thus, in order to measure the rate of protein synthesis with the AV method, the unidirectional rates of amino acid utilization for these alternative metabolic pathways must be determined using isotopic tracers. To determine unidirectional flux, isotopic tracer amino acids are usually infused into a peripheral vein, and several paired arterial and venous blood samples are collected after four to six hours of infusion, depending on when steady-state conditions are achieved. In situations where the tracer is 1-^{13}C-leucine, its metabolism to ^{13}C-α-keto-isocaproic acid (KIC) and $^{13}CO_2$ can be quantified, and separate rates of protein synthesis, as well as degradation, can be determined for various tissues.[53,54] However, if the rates of amino acid transamination and oxidation by a particular tissue are negligible, then the net amino acid balance equals the difference between protein synthesis and degradation. In the case of phenylalanine and tyrosine metabolism by the hindlimb,[45,55,56] these assumptions are essentially valid; therefore, protein synthesis, as well as degradation, can be estimated from the unidirectional rates of phenylalanine utilization and production, respectively:

$$\text{Phe utilization } (\mu\text{mol/h}) = [((\text{IEa} \bullet \text{Ca}) - (\text{IEv} \bullet \text{Cv}))/(\text{IEa})] \times \text{F}$$

$$\text{Phe production } (\mu\text{mol/h}) = \text{Ca} \times \text{F} \times ((\text{IEa/IEv}) - 1)$$

where IEa and IEv represent the isotopic enrichment (tracer:tracee ratio or mol % excess) of the stable isotope tracer, phenylalanine, in the arterial input and venous output, respectively. These equations are based on the assumption that the isotopic enrichment of the arterial amino acid best reflects that of the tissue aminoacyl-tRNA precursor, a topic that will be addressed subsequently. The rates of protein synthesis and of degradation can be determined from the net amino acid balance. For example, for phenylalanine:

$$\text{Protein synthesis} = \text{Protein degradation} + \text{net phenylalanine balance}$$

$$\text{Protein degradation} = \text{Protein synthesis} - \text{net phenylalanine balance}$$

In order to convert the unidirectional rates of amino acid utilization and production into actual rates of protein synthesized and degraded, one must know the amino acid composition of the organ or tissue protein. Furthermore, the estimates derived from unidirectional rates of amino acid exchange using the AV method represent absolute rates of protein synthesis and degradation and not fractional rates; the fractional rates can only be determined if the tissue protein mass is known.

A consideration with the AV method is the extent to which red blood cells, peptides, and plasma proteins participate in the interorgan transport and exchange of the tracer amino acid. Although a large proportion of the circulating amino acids is transported in plasma,[57] the concentration of some amino acids is higher in erythrocytes.[58] Therefore, it is important to consider whether the flow rates and corresponding amino acid analyses are best estimated with either plasma or whole blood. Despite the evidence of net tissue uptake of some plasma proteins and peptides, the quantitative significance of this phenomenon is uncertain, largely due to the limitations of the analytical methods used to quantify peptides accurately.[59]

A critically important technical consideration when using the AV method is determining the rate of blood flow, since the accuracy of the calculated rates of amino acid utilization and production are dependent on the accuracy of the blood flow measurement. Blood flow can be determined indirectly by using techniques based on the dilution, clearance, or diffusion of marker compounds such as indocyanine green,[60] para-aminohippuric acid,[61] antipyrine,[62] labeled microspheres,[63] or ^3H_2O.[64] Blood flow can also be measured more directly by using commercially available real-time sensing devices that use electromagnetic,[65] ultrasonic,[66] or Doppler shift technology,[67] which are physically attached around the sole arterial supply or venous output. Provided that the probes can be surgically implanted, these real-time flow measurements are more convenient and simpler than marker dilution, but they require an initial investment in the probes and flowmeter.

In order to use the AV method, samples of both venous and arterial blood must be obtained. It is not critical that the arterial sample be obtained from the particular artery supplying blood locally for the tissue organ, under the assumption that substrate concentrations and isotopic enrichments do not change during arterial transport. However, the venous sample must be obtained from the particular vein which drains blood from the tissue bed being studied. For this reason, positioning the location of tips of blood sampling catheters during surgery can be critical. Since catheters are usually surgically implanted in animals one to three weeks before the study, it is also advisable to verify the location of the venous catheter tip by autopsy of the animal.

It is also important to obtain the most accurate determination of arterial and venous amino acid concentrations and isotopic enrichments. Accurate determination of amino acid concentration and isotopic enrichment can be obtained when a series of paired arterial and venous blood samples are collected under steady-state conditions.

3.4 MEASUREMENT OF SYNTHESIS OF SPECIFIC TISSUE PROTEINS

3.4.1 OVERVIEW AND PROTOCOLS

Just as the measurement of whole-body protein synthesis represents the weighted average of the individual tissues, the measurement of protein synthesis of an individual tissue or organ represents the weighted average of the individual proteins synthesized by the cells within that tissue or organ. Thus, to understand the fundamental mechanisms that underlie variations in the protein synthetic response of a tissue, it is essential to measure the response of the individual proteins. For example, as a first step in determining the extent to which increases in protein synthesis are due to a change in transcriptional or translational activity, the changes in synthesis rate of a specific protein and the abundance of its mRNA can be compared.[68] Numerous functionally important proteins are synthesized in precursor forms (e.g., membrane glycoprotein, plasma lipoprotein, collagen), and then are modified post-translationally to the mature, biologically active form, frequently involving cellular translocation. Thus, to determine how factors such as diet, age, or a genetic defect influence the level of expression of the mature protein, it is necessary that variations in the post-translational processing steps be considered in addition to transcriptional and translational events;[69] again, this can only be accomplished effectively at the level of the individual protein.

Measurement of the synthesis rate of an individual protein *in vivo*, in principle, involves four steps: i) labeling the protein *in vivo* by infusing the animal with a labeled amino acid; ii) purification of the protein of interest (quantitatively, if pool size is required to estimate absolute synthesis rates), and subsequent hydrolysis to its constituent amino acids; iii) determination of the specific radioactivity or the enrichment of the amino acid in the protein and in the precursor pool; and iv) calculation of the fractional synthesis rate of the protein and, if applicable, the synthesis rate of any precursors and their rate of processing, using an appropriate compartmental model.

In designing the most suitable tracer infusion protocol, a number of factors must be considered. This requires some *a priori* knowledge of the metabolic characteristics of the molecule of interest, including its approximate rate of turnover, the kinetics of the labeling of the precursor pool, whether the protein is post-translationally modified, and the amino acid composition of the protein.

The duration of the infusion must be such that the protein to be analyzed is sampled during the phase of linear incorporation of the labeled amino acid. Thus, for rapidly turning over proteins, this period must be short, and must occur before the labeled amino acid in the protein reaches isotopic equilibrium with the precursor pool. Ideally, the amino acid precursor must also attain isotopic equilibrium rapidly, relative to its rate of incorporation into protein; this is more likely to be achieved by an amino acid with a relatively small pool size. For slowly synthesized proteins or proteins that are post-translationally modified, the infusion time should be lengthened so long as the labeling of the precursor pool remains constant. The time should be long enough to ensure that the degree of labeling of the protein can be measured accurately, but not so long that recycling of label occurs, the metabolic state of the animal changes, or the cost of the isotope becomes too high. Ideally, at least two tissue samples should be taken during this phase, the first occurring some time into the infusion once the precursor pool has come to steady state. While this may be feasible for the plasma proteins (see Chapter 4 by Jahoor and Reeds), it is less practical for other proteins in that it involves taking at least one biopsy, or using several animals per study. In some instances, the flooding dose approach can obviate this problem because it can be reasonably assumed that there is linear incorporation from time 0. However, for slowly synthesized proteins, the amount of label that can be incorporated during the period when the precursor pool is truly "flooded" may not be sufficient to allow for the accurate determination of the product's specific activity. Moreover, for some proteins, prolonged exposure to the high concentration of amino acid may alter the rate of protein synthesis itself. In these instances, the primed-constant infusion approach is preferable. However, because the plasma and intracellular precursor pools do not equilibrate instantaneously with each other, the fractional synthesis rate will tend to be underestimated (unless a biopsy sample can be obtained). Clearly, the longer the infusion time, and the smaller the tracer amino acid's pool size, the smaller the error.

For proteins that are post-translationally modified, the precursor form is often synthesized rapidly. Some proteins may be degraded directly, as in the case of the procollagens. Other proteins are translocated through the cell, or extracellularly, where the proteins are processed through a variety of steps which may include cross-linking, glycosylation, proteolytic cleavage, and/or modification of constituent amino acids. Thus, there is some delay before the label begins to appear in the final product. A protocol is required, therefore, that samples the labeled precursor protein after a short infusion, and then samples the various products as they are labeled with a more extended infusion. Such a protocol can be accomplished in a number of ways. Multiple animals that are as biologically similar as possible are infused and then killed at different times.[70] In addition to being very laborious, the error in the measurements will be inherently higher when this approach is used. Alternatively, a single animal can be infused, with repeated tissue samples taken over time.[69] This procedure requires that the animal be anesthetized, which, together with the potential for trauma to the tissue, may alter the processes being measured. A further approach, initially developed for the measurement of collagen synthesis,[71] and more recently amplified for the use of intestinal brush-border hydrolases,[72] circumvents the necessity of multiple tissue samples by using multiple amino acid tracers infused at different times.

3.4.2 PROTEIN PURIFICATION

The purification of the protein is dictated by its physiochemical characteristics. Commonly, the tissue is homogenized and a fraction, enriched in the protein of interest, is prepared by differential centrifugation and/or by differential solubilization in buffers of various ionic strengths and compositions. A final purification step is frequently, but not always, necessary:[68] polyacrylamide gel electrophoresis, either preparative[73] or analytical,[74] or an immunoisolation (with or without subsequent electrophoresis, depending on the specificity of the antibody[70,75]). The protein is either electroluted from the gel or the band of interest is identified and excised from the gel. The protein, either free or in a gel slice, is then subjected to acid hydrolysis. The hydrolysis of the polyacrylamide gel yields products that interfere with subsequent chromatography of the amino acids, and which must be removed by ion exchange procedures. Once the intact protein has been isolated, care must be taken not to contaminate the samples with unlabeled amino acids.

When the objective is simply to measure the fractional synthesis rate of a specific protein, the recovery during processing is not critical. However, if absolute synthesis rates are required, the protein's pool size must also be measured. Although this can be determined concurrently by carrying out the isolation procedure quantitatively, this could be technically difficult in practice. Thus, it usually necessitates the measurement of the abundance of the protein in separate tissue samples using, for example, immunological procedures, or, for enzymes, the measurement of enzyme activity.

3.4.3 Post-Translationally Modified Proteins

The accurate determination of the precursor pool specific activity or enrichment is of critical importance for accurate synthesis measurements. This issue is addressed in greater detail later, and the present discussion is limited to the measurement of synthesis of post-translationally processed proteins. The true precursor of the mature protein is the initial translation product. Thus, the infusion protocol ideally should be long enough that the precursor attains plateau enrichment in isotopic equilibrium with the aminoacyl-tRNA pool. Therefore, the most accurate estimate of the fractional synthesis rate of the mature protein is derived using the enrichment or specific activity of the precursor protein,[76] which in some instances can be quite different from the specific radioactivity or enrichment of the tissue or plasma free amino acid.[69]

For a protein that is not post-translationally modified, the calculation of its fractional synthesis rate is the same as for total tissue proteins. If a single terminal sample was obtained and analyzed following the infusion of a single tracer, the assumption is made that the rate of incorporation of tracer into the protein was linear with time, and that the degree of labeling of the precursor pool was known and at plateau for the entire time. It should be evident that the degree of accuracy of such an assumption will depend on the characteristics of the protein and the tissue in which it was found, and could vary from being a reasonably accurate to a totally inaccurate estimate. When multiple samples are obtained, the change in product enrichment over time will yield more accurate estimates of fractional protein synthesis rates.

For post-translationally modified proteins, in which an informative infusion and tissue sampling protocol was used, compartmental modeling allows for the estimation of the fractional synthesis of the primary translation product, the various intermediate products, and the final mature product.[69,72] Importantly, it allows for the determination of the amount of time elapsed from the start of the infusion to when the tracer appears in the protein product. Thus, the true labeling period can be calculated. Failure to account for this delay in the appearance of label can lead to marked underestimations of the true fractional synthesis rate of the protein products downstream from the initial translation product.

3.5 CHOICE OF AMINO ACID TRACER

The ideal amino acid for use as tracer in tissue protein synthesis studies is an essential amino acid which is either not limiting in the diet, or is not extensively metabolized to other compounds.[4] The tracer amino acid should be well distributed in body tissues, and should not (itself) influence protein turnover. Practical matters to be considered in choosing an amino acid tracer are the availability and expense of the tracer and the ease of performing the analysis.

The precision and accuracy of the constant infusion method is greatly increased with the use of an amino acid such as tyrosine or phenylalanine with a large ratio of protein-bound to free amino acid pool size. When this ratio is large, the plateau of amino acid labeling will be attained rapidly, and large inaccuracies in the definition of the rate at which the plateau is obtained will have small effects on the calculated value for K_s.[4,6,8,77]

Leucine was the tracer amino acid in the original application of the flooding dose technique,[24] but most studies now use phenylalanine. Phenylalanine is highly soluble, and hence, a higher multiple of the phenylalanine flux can be injected.[26,40] Phenylalanine has a smaller pool size than that of leucine, which makes a "flooding" condition more easily achievable. In addition, because leucine, as opposed to phenylalanine, has been reported to have a stimulatory effect on protein synthesis in some studies,[78,79] although not in others,[40,80] phenylalanine has a distinct advantage for use as a tracer amino acid.

The most commonly used amino acids with the AV method are leucine, phenylalanine, and tyrosine.[45,53-56] The advantage of using leucine as the tracer amino acid is that its transamination to α-keto-isocaproic acid and oxidation to CO_2 can be easily measured. For measurement of protein synthesis in the hindlimb by AV difference, phenylalanine and tyrosine have distinct advantages because these amino acids are not metabolized or synthesized by skeletal muscle and, therefore, determination of protein synthesis rates is simplified.

When measuring synthesis rates of individual proteins, especially those that turn over slowly, an amino acid of relative abundance in the protein would be advantageous for use as a tracer. It is for this reason that proline is frequently used for the measurement of collagen synthesis. When a multiple amino acid infusion protocol is used, an amino acid with multiple isotopomers is of benefit, provided the necessary mass spectroscopic procedures for their measurement are available.

3.6   MEASUREMENT OF PRECURSOR POOLS

Determination of the rate of tissue protein synthesis requires that the enrichment of the direct precursor for protein synthesis be determined. Although the amino acids acylated to tRNA are the immediate precursors for protein synthesis, only a few *in vivo* studies have measured the labeling of aminoacyl-tRNA due to the technical difficulty of the isolation procedure.[81-85] Because aminoacyl-tRNA is present in low concentration within tissues[86] and is extremely labile, measurement of the specific radioactivity or enrichment of aminoacyl-tRNA is problematic.

Because of the difficulty in measuring aminoacyl-tRNA enrichment, surrogates for the precursor pool specific activity have been used to estimate tissue protein synthesis rates. With the constant infusion method, the enrichment in the plasma of the labeled amino acid or its keto acid, derived by the transamination of the labeled amino acid within the tissues, is generally used as a surrogate of the true precursor pool enrichment.[87-89] Because leucine seems to be the preferred tracer amino acid in most constant infusion studies, the enrichment of circulating KIC is frequently used as a surrogate for the leucyl-tRNA enrichment. However, recent studies which assessed the labeling of aminoacyl-tRNA during constant infusion studies have called into question the use of the enrichment of circulating amino acids, or their keto acids, as indicators of the precursor pool for protein synthesis. Some of these studies suggest that the enrichment of aminoacyl-tRNA is intermediate between that of plasma and the tissue free amino acid pools.[81,83] Tissue free amino acid pool enrichment has also been suggested to be the best predictor of aminoacyl-tRNA enrichment during the constant infusion of labeled amino acids,[82,84] particularly under a different physiological perturbation such as meal feeding, when the ratio of the enrichment values of aminoacyl-tRNA to other surrogate pools changes.[84]

With the flooding dose method, the labeling of the free amino acid pool in the tissue is frequently determined as an indication of the precursor pool enrichment.[26] Because the enrichment of the free amino acid pools in plasma and tissue declines slightly after an initial peak,[40] the tissue free amino acid pool enrichment can be corrected for the time course of the change in the enrichment of the free amino acid in plasma.[20-22] Although numerous studies have demonstrated that there is equilibration between the plasma and tissue free amino acid pools with the flooding dose method,[25,28,90] very few studies have examined whether there is equilibration between these pools and the aminoacyl-tRNA precursor pool.[91,92] Our recent studies have demonstrated that following a flooding dose of phenylalanine, there is equilibration of the enrichment among the three precursor pools in both skeletal muscle and liver, and that neither feeding nor insulin status affects the tRNA enrichment relative to that in the tissue or plasma.[85] These results substantiate the assumption that the tissue free amino acid pool specific radioactivity is a valid measure of the precursor pool enrichment when a flooding dose of phenylalanine is used.

To isolate and purify aminoacyl-tRNA, a large quantity (5 to 10 g) of very fine powdered tissue is homogenized in sodium dodecyl sulfate/cacodylic acid buffer.[82,85] The homogenate is then extracted with phenol. RNA is precipitated from the aqueous phase with ethanol and subsequently dissolved in water. The aminoacyl-tRNA is deacylated with KOH and the amino acids are separated from tRNA by acidification with HCl. The amino acids can be purified by cation exchange and the labeled amino acid separated from other amino acids by high-pressure liquid chromatography. Throughout the procedure, precautions must be taken to eliminate contamination by RNases and amino acids. This procedure is quite tedious and laborious, and is not required for determination of the precursor pool specific activity when a flooding dose of phenylalanine is administered to measure skeletal muscle and liver protein synthesis.

As with direct incorporation methods, the absolute rates of protein synthesis determined using the AV method are also dependent on a number of assumptions regarding the equilibration of the tracer amino acid between the plasma, intracellular, and aminoacyl-tRNA precursor pools. Since tissue biopsies are not usually obtained when using the AV method, the isotopic enrichment of the true precursor for protein synthesis, the aminoacyl-tRNA, cannot be measured directly. As a result, the isotopic enrichment of the tracer amino acid in either the arterial or venous blood is commonly used. However, the observation that the arterial amino acid isotopic enrichment is greater than that of either the tissue free pool or venous plasma amino acid pool indicates that the unidirectional flux based on the arterial pool is likely underesti-mated.[45,54,55] Likewise, calculating the unidirectional flux based on the venous amino acid isotopic enrichment is likely an underestimate of flux, because it includes amino acids that have bypassed the capillary bed, and hence are unaffected by the isotopic dilution arising from intracellular proteolysis. This precursor problem can be minimized to some extent by using the venous isotopic enrichment of the corresponding keto acid, such as KIC for leucine, although not all cells within an organ or tissue generate keto acids.[53]

3.7   CONCLUSIONS

We have outlined the major approaches for measuring tissue protein synthesis in experimental animals, and discussed their advantages and limitations. There has been some controversy among several research groups as to the "best" approach for measuring tissue protein synthesis. However, it should be kept in mind that the experimental approach should be dictated by the question addressed, and the method chosen for measurement of tissue protein synthesis in one study may not be the best method for use in a different study. In addition, most studies examine the effect of some treatment, in comparison to a control group, and obtaining an absolutely "true" value may not be crucial.

ACKNOWLEDGMENTS

We are grateful to P. J. Reeds for review of this chapter and L. Loddeke for editorial assistance. This work is a publication of the USDA/ARS Children's Nutrition Research Center, Department of Pediatrics, Baylor College of Medicine, Houston, TX. This project has been funded in part by National Institute of Arthritis and Musculoskeletal and Skin Diseases Institute Grant R01 AR44474 and the U.S. Department of Agriculture, Agricultural Research Service under Cooperative Agreement number 58-6250-6-001. The contents of this publication do not necessarily reflect the views or policies of the U.S. Department of Agriculture, nor does mention of trade names, commercial products, or organizations imply endorsements by the U.S. Government.

REFERENCES

1. Stephen, J. M. L. and Waterlow, J. C., Protein turnover in the rat measured with ^{14}C-lysine, *J. Physiol. (London)*, 178, 40, 1965.
2. Garlick, P. J., Turnover rate of muscle protein measured by constant intravenous infusion of ^{14}C-glycine, *Nature (London)*, 223, 61, 1969.
3. Garlick, P. J., Millward, D. J., and James, W. P. T., The diurnal response of muscle and liver protein synthesis in vivo in meal-fed rats, *Biochem. J.*, 136, 935, 1973.
4. Waterlow, J. C., Garlick, P. J., and Millward, D. J., *Protein Turnover in Mammalian Tissues and in the Whole Body*, North-Holland, Amsterdam, 1978.
5. Lobley, G. E., Milne, V., Lovie, J., Reeds, P. J., and Pennie, K., Whole body and tissue protein synthesis in cattle, *Br. J. Nutr.*, 43, 491, 1980.

6. Reeds, P. J., Isotopic estimation of protein synthesis and proteolysis in vivo, in *Modern Methods in Protein Nutrition and Metabolism*, Nissen, S., Ed., Academic Press, New York, 1992, chap. 10.

7. Waterlow, J. C. and Stephen, J. M. L., Adaptation of the rat to low-protein diet: the effect of a reduced protein intake on the pattern of incorporation of L-^{14}C-lysine, *Br. J. Nutr.*, 20, 461, 1966.

8. Garlick, P. J., Millward, D. J., James, W. P. T., and Waterlow, J. C., The effect of protein deprivation and starvation on the rate of protein synthesis in tissues of the rat, *Biochim. Biophys. Acta*, 414, 71, 1975.

9. Wykes, L. J., Fiorotto, M., Burrin, D. G., Del Rosario, M., Frazier, M. E., Pond, W. G., and Jahoor, F., Chronic low protein intake reduces tissue protein synthesis in a pig model of protein malnutrition, *J. Nutr.*, 126, 1481, 1996.

10. Odedra, B. R., Dalal, S. S., and Millward, D. J., Muscle protein synthesis in the streptozotocin-diabetic rat, *Biochem. J.*, 202, 363, 1982.

11. Eisemann, J. H., Hammond, A. C., and Rumsey, T. S., Tissue protein synthesis and nucleic acid concentrations in steers treated with somatotropin, *Br. J. Nutr.*, 62, 657, 1989.

12. Douglas, R. G., Gluckman, P. D., Ball, K., Breier, B., and Shaw, J. H. F., The effects of infusion of insulinlike growth factor (IGF) I, IGF-II, and insulin on glucose and protein metabolism in fasted lambs, *J. Clin. Invest.*, 88, 614, 1991.

13. McNulty, P. H., Young, L. H., and Barrett, E. J., Response of rat heart and skeletal muscle protein in vivo to insulin and amino acid infusion, *Am. J. Physiol.*, 264, E958, 1993.

14. Jacob, R., Hu, X., Niederstock, D., Hasan, S., McNulty, P. H., Sherwin, R. S., and Young, L. H., IGF-I stimulation of muscle protein synthesis in the awake rat: permissive role of insulin and amino acids, *Am. J. Physiol.*, 270, E60, 1996.

15. Obled, C. and Arnal, M., Contribution of skin to whole-body protein synthesis in rats at different stages of maturity, *J. Nutr.*, 122, 2167, 1992.

16. Chan, C. P., Hansen, R. J., and Stern, J. S., Protein turnover in insulin-treated, alloxan-diabetic lean and obese Zucker rats, *J. Nutr.*, 115, 959, 1985.

17. Attaix, D., Manghebati, A., Grizard, J., and Arnal, M., Assessment of in vivo protein synthesis in lamb tissues with [3H] valine flooding doses, *Biochim. Biophys. Acta*, 882, 387, 1986.

18. Seve, B., Ballevre, I., Ganier, P., Noblet, J., Prugnaud, J., and Obled, C., Recombinant porcine somatotropin and dietary protein enhance protein synthesis in growing pigs, *J. Nutr.*, 123, 529, 1993.

19. Tauveron, I., Larbaud, D., Champredon, C., Debras, E., Tesseraud, S., Bayle, G., Bonnet, Y., Thieblot, P., and Grizard, J., Effect of hyperinsulinemia and hyperaminoacidemia on muscle and liver protein synthesis in lactating goats, *Am. J. Physiol.*, 267, E877, 1994.

20. Burrin, D. G., Davis, T. A., Ebner, S., Schoknecht, P. A., Fiorotto, M. L., Reeds, P. J., and McAvoy, S., Nutrient-independent and nutrient-dependent factors stimulate protein synthesis in colostrum-fed newborn pigs, *Pediatr. Res.*, 37, 593, 1995.

21. Davis, T. A., Burrin, D. G., Fiorotto, M. L., and Nguyen, H. V., Protein synthesis in skeletal muscle and jejunum is more responsive to feeding in 7- than in 26-day-old pigs, *Am. J. Physiol.*, 270, E802, 1996.

22. Davis, T. A., Fiorotto, M. L., Burrin, D. G., Pond, W. G., and Nguyen, H. V., Intrauterine growth restriction does not alter response of protein synthesis to feeding in newborn pigs, *Am. J. Physiol.*, 272, E877, 1997.

23. Schoknecht, P. A., Ebner, S., Skottner, A., Burrin, D. G., Davis, T. A., Ellis, K., and Pond, W. G., Exogenous insulin-like growth factor-I increases weight gain in intrauterine growth-retarded neonatal pigs, *Pediatr. Res.*, 42, 201, 1997.

24. McNurlan, M. A., Tomkins, A. M., and Garlick, P. J., The effect of starvation on the rate of protein synthesis in rat liver and small intestine, *Biochem. J.*, 178, 373, 1979.

25. Reeds, P. J., Haggarty, P., Wahle, K. W. J., and Fletcher, J. R., Tissue and whole body protein synthesis in immature Zucker rats and their relationship to protein deposition, *Biochem. J.*, 204, 393, 1982.

26. Garlick, P. J., Fern, M., and Preedy, V. R., The effect of insulin infusion and food intake on muscle protein synthesis in postabsorptive rat, *Biochem. J.*, 210, 669, 1983.

27. Goldspink, D. F. and Kelly, F. J., Protein turnover and growth in the whole body, liver, and kidney of the rat from fetus to senility, *Biochem. J.*, 217, 507, 1984.

28. Davis, T. A., Fiorotto, M. L., Nguyen, H. V., and Reeds, P. J., Protein turnover in skeletal muscle of suckling rats, *Am. J. Physiol.*, 257, R1141, 1989.

29. Southorn, B. G., Palmer, R. M., and Garlick, P. J., Acute effects of corticosterone on tissue protein synthesis and insulin-sensitivity in rats in vivo, *Biochem. J.*, 272, 187, 1990.

30. Burrin, D. G., Davis, T. A., Fiorotto, M. L., and Reeds, P. J., Stage of development and fasting affect protein synthetic activity in the gastrointestinal tissues of suckling rats, *J. Nutr.*, 121, 1099, 1991.

31. Tomas, F. M., Knowles, S. E., Owens, P. C., Read, L. C., Chandler, C. S., Gargosky, S. E., and Ballard, F. J., Increased weight gain, nitrogen retention and muscle protein synthesis following treatment of diabetic rats with insulin-like growth factor (IGF)-I and des(1-3)IGF-I, *Biochem. J.*, 276, 547, 1991.

32. Baillie, A. G. S. and Garlick, P. J., Attenuated responses of muscle protein synthesis to fasting and insulin in adult female rats, *Am. J. Physiol.*, 262, E1, 1991.

33. Vary, T. C. and Kimball, S. R., Regulation of hepatic protein synthesis in chronic inflammation and sepsis, *Am. J. Physiol.*, 262, C445, 1992.

34. Burrin, D. G., Davis, T. A., Fiorotto, M. L., and Reeds, P. J., Hepatic protein synthesis in suckling rats: effects of stage of development and fasting, *Pediatr. Res.*, 31, 247, 1992.

35. Davis, T. A., Fiorotto, M. L., Nguyen, H. V., and Reeds, P. J., Enhanced response of muscle protein synthesis and plasma insulin to food intake in suckled rat, *Am. J. Physiol.*, 265, R334, 1993.

36. Pomposelli, J. J., Palombo, J. D., Hamawy, K. J., Bistrian, B. R., Blackburn, G. L., and Moldawer, L. L., Comparison of different techniques for estimating rates of protein synthesis in vivo in healthy and bacteraemic rats, *Biochem. J.*, 226, 37, 1985.

37. Jahoor, F., Zhang, X., Baba, H., Sakuria, Y., and Wolfe, R. R., Comparison of constant infusion and flooding dose techniques to measure muscle protein synthesis rate in dogs, *J. Nutr.*, 122, 878, 1992.

38. Smith, K., Barua, J. M., Watt, P. W., Scrimgeour, C. M., and Rennie, M. J., Flooding with L-[1-^{13}C]leucine stimulates human muscle protein incorporation of continuously infused L-[1-^{13}C]valine, *Am. J. Physiol.*, 262, E372, 1992.

39. Rennie, M. J., Smith, K., and Watt, P. W., Measurement of human tissue protein synthesis: an optimal approach, *Am. J. Physiol.*, 266, E298, 1994.

40. Garlick, P. J., McNurlan, M. C., and Preedy, V. R., A rapid and convenient technique for measuring the rate of protein synthesis in tissues by injection of [^{3}H]phenylalanine, *Biochem. J.*, 192, 719, 1980.

41. Lobley, G. E., Harris, P. M., Skene, P. A., Brown, D. S., Milne, E., Calder, A. G., Anderson, S. E., Garlick, P. J., Nevison, I., and Connell, A., Responses in tissue protein synthesis to sub- and supra-maintenance intake in ruminant lambs: comparison of large dose and continuous infusion techniques, *Br. J. Nutr.*, 68, 373, 1992.

42. Southorn, B. G., Kelly, J. M., and McBride, B. W., Phenylalanine flooding dose procedure is effective in measuring intestinal and liver protein synthesis in sheep, *J. Nutr.*, 122, 2398, 1992.

43. Garlick, P. J., McNurlan, M. A., Essen, P., and Wernerman, J., Measurement of tissue protein synthesis rates in vivo: a critical analysis of contrasting methods, *Am. J. Physiol.*, 266, E287, 1994.

44. Elwyn, D. H., Parikh, H. C., and Shoemaker, W. C., Amino acid movements between gut, liver, and periphery in unanesthetized dogs, *Am. J. Physiol.*, 215, 1260, 1968.

45. Harris, P. M., Skene, P. A., Buchan, V., Milne, E., Calder, A. G., Anderson, S. E., Connell, A., and Lobley, G. E., Effect of food intake on hind-limb and whole body protein metabolism in young growing sheep: chronic studies based on arterio-venous techniques, *Br. J. Nutr.*, 68, 389, 1992.

46. Abumrad, N. N., Kim, S., and Molina, P. E., Regulation of gut glutamine metabolism: role of hormones and cytokines, *Proc. Nutr. Soc.*, 54, 525, 1995.

47. Pell, J. M. and Bergman, E. N., Cerebral metabolism of amino acids and glucose in fed and fasted sheep, *Am. J. Physiol.*, 244, E282, 1983.

48. Ferrell, C. L. and Reynolds, L. P., Uterine and umbilical blood flows and net nutrient uptake by fetuses uteroplacental tissues of cows gravid with either single or twin fetuses, *J. Anim. Sci.*, 70, 426, 1992.

49. Trottier, N. L., Shipley, C. F., and Easter, R. A., Plasma amino acid uptake by the mammary gland of the lactating sow, *J. Anim. Sci.*, 75, 1266, 1997.

50. Ebner, S., Schoknecht, P. A., Reeds, P. J., and Burrin, D. G., Growth and metabolism of gastrointestinal and skeletal muscle tissues in protein-malnourished neonatal pigs, *Am. J. Physiol.*, 266, R1736, 1994.

51. Ten, G. A. M., Bost, M. C. F., Suyk-Wierts, J. C. A. W., van den Bogaard, A. E. J. M., and Duetz, N. E. P., Simultaneous measurements of metabolic flux in portally-drained viscera, liver, spleen, kidney and hindquarter in the conscious pig, *Laboratory Animals*, 30, 347, 1996.

52. Eisemann, J. H., Huntington, G. B., and Catherman, D. R., Patterns of nutrient interchange and oxygen use among portal-drained viscera, liver, and hindquarters of beef steers from 235 to 525 kg body weight, *J. Anim. Sci.*, 74, 1812, 1996.

53. Pell, J. M., Calderone, E. M., and Bergman, E. N., Leucine and α-ketoisocaproate metabolism and interconversion in fed and fasted sheep, *Metabolism*, 35, 1005, 1986.

54. Oddy, H. V. and Lindsay, D. B., Determination of rates of protein synthesis, gain and degradation in intact hind-limb muscle of lambs, *Biochem. J.*, 233, 417, 1986.

55. Barrett, E. J., Revkin, J. H., Young, L. H., Zaret, B. L., Jacob, R., and Gelfand, R. A., An isotopic method for measurement of muscle protein synthesis and degradation in vivo, *Biochem. J.*, 245, 223, 1987.

56. Boisclair, Y. R., Bauman, D. E., and Bell, A. W., Nutrient utilization and protein turnover in the hindlimb of cattle treated with bovine somatotropin, *J. Nutr.*, 124, 664, 1994.

57. Lobley, G. E., Connell, A., Revell, D. K., Bequette, B. J., Brown, D. S., and Calder, A. G., Splanchnic-bed transfers of amino acids in sheep blood and plasma, as monitored through use of multiple U-^{13}C-labelled amino acid mixture, *Br. J. Nutr.*, 75, 217, 1996.

58. Bergman, E.N., Sphlanchnic and peripheral uptake of amino acids in relation to the gut, *Fed. Proc.*, 45, 2277, 1986.

59. Backwell, F. R. C., Hipolito-Reis, M., Wilson, D., Bruce, L. A., Buchan, V., and MacRae, J. C., Quantification of circulating peptides and assessment of peptide uptake across the gastrointestinal tract of sheep, *J. Anim. Sci.*, 75, 3315, 1997.

60. Leevy, C. M., Mendenhall, C. L., Lesko, W., and Howard, M. M., Estimation of hepatic blood flow with ICG, *J. Clin. Invest.*, 71, 1169, 1962.

61. Katz, M. L. and Bergman, E. N., Simultaneous measurements of hepatic and portal venous blood flow in the sheep and dog, *Am. J. Physiol.*, 216, 946, 1969.

62. Meschia, G., Cotter, J. R., Makowski, E. L., and Barron, D. H., Simultaneous measurement of uterine and umbilical blood flows and oxygen uptakes, *Q. J. Exp. Physiol.*, 52, 1, 1966.

63. Heyman, M. A., Payne, B. D., Hoffman, J. L., and Rudolph, A. M., Blood flow measurements with radionuclide-labeled particles, *Prog. Cardiovasc. Dis.*, 20, 55, 1977.

64. Oddy, H. V., Brown, B. W., and Jones, A. W., Measurement of organ blood flow using tritiated water. I. Hindlimb muscle blood flow in conscious ewes, *Aust. J. Biol. Sci.*, 34, 419, 1981.

65. Rerat, A., Jung, J., and Kande, J., Absorption kinetics of dietary hydrolysis products in conscious pigs given diets with different amounts of fish protein. 2. Individual amino acids, *Br. J. Nutr.*, 60, 105, 1988.

66. Huntington, G. B., Eisemann, J. H., and Whitt, J. M., Portal blood flow in beef steers: comparison of techniques and relation to hepatic blood flow, cardiac output and oxygen uptake, *J. Anim. Sci.*, 68, 1666, 1990.

67. Sheperd, A. P., Riedel, G. L., Kiel, J. W., Haumschild, D. J., and Maxwell, L. C., Evaluation of an infrared laser-Doppler blood flowmeter, *Am. J. Physiol.*, 252, G832, 1987.

68. Morrison, P. R., Muller, G. W., and Booth, F. W., Actin synthesis rate and mRNA level increase during early recovery of atrophied muscle, *Am. J. Physiol.*, 253, C295, 1987.

69. Dudley, M. A., Burrin, D. G., Quaroni, A., Rosenberger, J., Cook, G., Nichols, B. L., and Reeds, P. J., Lactase phlorizin hydrolase turnover *in vivo* in water-fed and colostrum-fed newborn pigs, *Biochem. J.*, 320, 735, 1996.

70. Dudley, M. A., Hachey D. L., Quaroni, A., Hutchens, W. T., Nichols, B. L., Rosenberger, J., Perkinson, S. J., Cook, G., and Reeds, P. J., *In vivo* sucrase-isomaltase and lactase-phlorizin hydrolase turnover in the fed adult rat, *J. Biol. Chem.*, 268, 13609, 1993.

71. Robins, S. P., Metabolism of rabbit skin collagen. Differences in apparent turnover rates of type-I- and type-III-collagen precursors determined by constant intravenous infusion of labelled amino acids, *Biochem. J.*, 181, 75, 1979.

72. Dudley, M. A., Burrin, D. G., Wykes, L. J., Toffolo, G., Cobelli, C., Nichols, B. L., Rosenberger, J., Jahoor, F., and Reeds, P. J., Protein kinetics determined in vivo with a single tissue sample, multiple tracer overlapping infusion: application to the lactase system, *Am. J. Physiol.*, 274, G591, 1998.

73. Balagopal, P., Nair, K. S., and Stirewalt, W. S., Isolation of myosin heavy chain from small skeletal muscle samples by preparative continuous elution gel electrophoresis: application to measurement of synthesis rate in human and animal tissue, *Anal. Biochem.*, 221, 72, 1994.

74. Samarel, A. M., Parmacek, M. S., Magid, N. M., Decker, R. S., and Lesch, M., Protein synthesis and degradation during starvation-induced cardiac atrophy in rabbits, *Circ. Res.*, 60, 933, 1987.

75. Gregory, P., Gagnon, J., Essig, D. A., Reid, S. K., Prior, G., and Zak, R., Differential regulation of actin and myosin isoenzyme synthesis in functionally overloaded skeletal muscle, *Biochem. J.*, 265, 525, 1990.

76. Dudley, M. A., Wykes, L. J., Dudley, A. W., Fiorotto, M., Burrin, D. G., Rosenberger, J., Cook, G., Jahoor, F., and Reeds, P. J., Lactase phlorizin hydrolase synthesis is decreased in protein-malnourished pigs, *J. Nutr.*, 127, 687, 1997.

77. Nicholas, G. A., Lobley, G. E., and Harris, C. I., Use of the constant infusion technique for measuring rates of protein synthesis in New Zealand White rabbits, *Br. J. Nutr.*, 38, 1, 1977.

78. Buse, M. G. and Reid, S. S., Leucine, a possible regulator of protein turnover in muscle, *J. Clin. Invest.*, 56, 1250, 1975.

79. Fulks, R. M., Li, J. B., and Goldberg, A. L., Effects of insulin, glucose, and amino acids on protein turnover in rat diaphragm, *J. Biol. Chem.*, 250, 290, 1975.

80. McNurlan, M. A., Fern, E. B., and Garlick, P. J., Failure of leucine to stimulate protein synthesis in vivo, *Biochem. J.*, 204, 831, 1982.

81. Watt, P. W., Lindsay, Y., Scrimgeour, C. M., Chien, P. A. F., Gibson, J. N. A., Taylor, D. J., and Rennie, M. J., Isolation of aminoacyl-tRNA and its labeling with stable-isotope tracers: Use in studies of human tissue protein synthesis, *Proc. Natl. Acad. Sci.*, 88, 5892, 1991.

82. Baumann, P. Q., Stirewalt, W. S., O'Rourke, B. D., Howard, D., and Nair, K. S., Precursor pools of protein synthesis: a stable isotope study in a swine model, *Am. J. Physiol.*, 267, E203, 1994.

83. Young, L. H., Stirewalt, W., McNulty, P. H., Revkin, J. H., and Barrett, E. J., Effect of insulin on rat heart and skeletal muscle phenylalanyl-tRNA labeling and protein synthesis in vivo, *Am. J. Physiol.*, 267, E337, 1994.

84. Ljungqvist, E. H., Persson, M., Ford, G. C., and Nair, K.S., Functional heterogeneity of leucine pools in human skeletal muscle, *Am. J. Physiol.*, 273, E564, 1997.

85. Davis, T. A., Fiorotto, M. L., Burrin, D. G., Wray-Cahen, D., and Nguyen, H. V., Aminoacyl-tRNA and tissue free precursor pools are equilibrated with a flooding dose of phenylalanine, *FASEB J.*, 10, A285, 1996.

86. Martin, A. F., Rabinowitz, M., Blough, R., Prior, G., and Zak, R., Measurements of half-life of rat cardiac myosin heavy chain with leucyl-tRNA used as precursor pool, *J. Biol. Chem.*, 252, 3422, 1977.

87. Schwenk, W. F., Beaufrere, B., and Haymond, M., Use of reciprocal pool specific activities to model leucine metabolism in humans, *Am. J. Physiol.*, 249, E646, 1985.

88. Vazquez, J. A., Paul, H. S., and Adibi, S. A., Relationship between plasma and tissue parameters of leucine metabolism in fed and starved rats, *Am. J. Physiol.*, 250, E615, 1986.

89. Horber, F. F., Horber-Feyder, C. M., Krayer, S., Frederick, W., and Haymond, M. W., Plasma reciprocal pool specific activity predicts that of intracellular free leucine for protein synthesis, *Am. J. Physiol.*, 250, E615, 1986.

90. Attaix, D., Aurousseau, E., Bayle, G., Rosolowska-Huszca, D., and Arnal, M., Respective influences of age and weaning on skeletal and visceral muscle protein synthesis in the lamb, *Biochem. J.*, 256, 791, 1988.

91. Robinson, M. E. and Samarel, A. M., Regional differences in in vivo myocardial protein synthesis in the neonatal rabbit heart, *J. Mol. Cell. Cardiol.*, 22, 607, 1990.

92. Karim, M., Ferguson, A. G., Wakim, B. T., and Samarel, A. M., In vivo collagen turnover during development of thyroxine-induced left ventricular hypertrophy, *Am. J. Physiol.*, 260, C316, 1991.

4 The Measurement of the Rate of Synthesis of Liver-Derived Plasma Proteins

Farook Jahoor and Peter J. Reeds

CONTENTS

4.1. INTRODUCTION

4.1.1 METABOLIC AND PHYSIOLOGIC ROLES OF PLASMA PROTEINS

The hepatic-derived plasma proteins perform a variety of functions necessary for the maintenance of physiological and metabolic homeostasis, and the increased morbidity and mortality associated with lowered plasma concentrations of these proteins underscores their physiological importance.[1] The plasma proteins can be loosely divided into two groups: proteins involved in the transport of nutrients, hormones, metabolites, and drugs; and proteins involved in host defense. In the acute-phase response to the stress of infection or injury, the plasma concentrations of many transport proteins decrease; hence, they are described as negative acute-phase proteins.[2,3] The plasma concentrations of those proteins involved in host defenses increase under the same circumstances, and members of this group are often referred to as the positive acute-phase proteins.[2,3]

The negative acute-phase proteins are a diverse group which includes albumin, the lipoproteins, transferrin, retinol binding protein, and transthyretin. Adequate quantities of these proteins are necessary for survival, because they serve a variety of functions which contribute to physiological and metabolic homeostasis through the regulation of hemodynamics and nutrient transport.[3] The positive acute-phase proteins serve equally important functions related to restoration of health when the integrity of the organism is altered by injury or infection.[2-4] These functions include: the containment and destruction of infectious agents by assisting and promoting the immune response, the repair of damaged tissues and the protection of healthy tissues, the salvaging of useful components released from damaged tissues, and the indirect alteration of substrate metabolism via the induction of cytokine synthesis.[2-4]

4.1.2 HISTORY OF KINETIC TECHNIQUES

Although the physicochemical properties of plasma proteins have been studied in great detail, there is relatively little information on the *in vivo* metabolism of most of these proteins, particularly in different pathological states. For example, although the extent to which the circulating pools of acute-phase proteins increase or decrease during injury or infection has been well established, there is very little information on the kinetic changes responsible for the alterations in their respective pool sizes. Until recently, this paucity of kinetic information reflected a lack of appropriate and convenient methods to measure liver-derived plasma protein turnover, especially in a clinical setting. The limited information available from the earliest studies was based upon the analysis of the rate of loss of injected radio-iodinated proteins.[5,6] A major problem of these studies was that the synthesis rate was not measured directly, but inferred from the catabolic rate. Furthermore, apart from the radiation hazards, a major concern with this approach was that the addition of the bulky iodine atom alters the physicochemical properties of the protein, which alter its susceptibility to proteolysis, and, ultimately, the applicability of the catabolic rate determined with the tracer to that of the natural protein.[7] With the advent of radioisotope-labeled amino acids, studies of plasma protein turnover were easily carried out, first in animals and later in humans, using a constant infusion of the tracer and the precursor product equation.[8,9] In this approach, it is necessary to measure the specific activity of the protein-bound amino acid tracer at two time points during the quasi-linear incorporation of the labeled amino acid into protein, and the steady-state specific activity of the tracer at the site of protein synthesis in the liver.[10] This method also requires that an adequate amount of the protein of interest be isolated from plasma in a pure form for radioactive counting. Apart from the fact that the radiation hazard associated with this method precluded its use in children and women of child-bearing age, its only limitation was the unavailability of suitable methods to isolate individual plasma proteins. Over the last decade, as stable isotope-labeled amino acids became widely available and mass spectrometers improved markedly in sensitivity, accuracy, and precision, radioactive tracers have been almost totally replaced by stable isotope-labeled tracers. We will focus our discussion on the use of these tracers.

4.2   CHOICE OF TRACER AND MASS SPECTROMETRY

The choice of tracer is largely dependent on the available instrumentation and the rate of turnover of the protein of interest. In the earliest studies, because only singly labeled amino acids were available and gas chromatograph-mass spectrometers (GC-MS) were unable to measure low isotope ratios accurately, the method of choice was the constant infusion of ^{15}N-labeled glycine, followed by measurement of the isotope enrichment of protein-derived amino acid nitrogen by gas isotope ratio mass spectrometry (G-IRMS).[11,12] Although the G-IRMS instruments were capable of measuring extremely low levels of isotope enrichments, they required large amounts of gas because of large inlet systems. Hence, a major drawback of this approach was the requirement of a relatively large blood sample in order to isolate an amount of the protein that would provide a sufficient quantity of nitrogen gas from the tracer amino acid for G-IRMS analysis. Secondly, a large amount of the tracer amino acid had to be isolated in a pure form for combustion, a requirement that involved laborious ion exchange chromatography. This limited the use of this approach mostly to the study of albumin and fibrinogen, proteins that are present in high concentrations in plasma. A third major drawback was the requirement for long infusions because the urinary metabolites (urea, hippuric acid) that were used to estimate the isotopic enrichment of the tracer in the hepatic precursor pool needed a long time (e.g., 36 h) to reach a plateau.[11,12]

However, a number of developments have made current analysis by GC-MS routine. Improvements in GC-MS instruments, especially in computer-aided control and data acquisition, coupled to the high sensitivity afforded by negative chemical ionization (NCI), now enable accurate measurements of low isotope ratios in very small samples.[13] These factors, plus the availability of amino acids labeled with multiple ^2H- or ^{13}C-atoms, mean that it is now possible to measure the isotopic enrichment of the protein-derived amino acid tracer by GC-MS (see Chapter 6 by Patterson). In general, the accuracy of an isotope ratio measurement improves at each incremental mass higher than the base peak, [M]. The reliable measurement of small isotopic increments superimposed on an intense ion signal is technically difficult to achieve. The use of tracers of masses beyond [M+3] yield better results, because any detectable signal is due solely to the tracer.[13] Consequently, tracers with three or more isotopic substitutions provide more accurate isotopic abundance measurements over a wider dynamic range than molecules with a single isotopic substitution. The advantage of a method that employs a multiply labeled tracer plus GC-MS analysis is that the amount of protein-derived amino acid required for analysis is very small, thereby permitting studies of the turnover of plasma proteins that are present in low concentrations.[14] The disadvantages are that multiply-labeled tracers can be expensive, and that this approach may not be suitable for proteins that turn over very slowly, such as albumin, because a longer isotope infusion is required. In the case of the slower turning over proteins, the amount of tracer incorporated into the protein may still be too low for measurement by GC-MS, making it necessary to use G-IRMS analysis. Although the latter is less desirable as an analytical approach, it is more economical because these instruments can accurately measure isotope ratios as low as 10^{-3} atom % excess. Hence, the study can be done at a significantly lower cost, because much cheaper singly labeled ^{13}C- or ^{15}N-labeled tracers can be infused at lower rates. Finally, with the advent of the gas chromatograph combustion isotope ratio mass spectrometer (GC-C-IRMS), the difficulties associated with the G-IRMS analysis are obviated. This instrument separates individual amino acids by GC and has a typical requirement of only ~20 nmol of carbon dioxide for adequate analysis.

4.3   A SIMPLE METHOD TO ISOLATE THE PROTEIN

A major deterrent to the study of plasma proteins was the unavailability of a simple and efficient method to isolate individual proteins in a pure form, and in sufficient quantity for mass spectrometric analysis of the protein-derived tracer amino acid. Until recently, isolation and purification of plasma proteins were mainly accomplished by classical physicochemical methods that used salt-solubility, density-gradient sedimentation, affinity chromatography, and solvent extraction.[15] Not only are these methods tedious, but it is difficult to obtain sufficient amounts of a preparation of sufficiently high purity for mass spectrometric analysis. Once again, this limited kinetic studies to only those proteins that were present in large concentrations, such as albumin and fibrinogen,[16] and more recently, the apolipoproteins.[17] Although individual plasma proteins can be separated by affinity chromatography, these are very laborious procedures requiring large volumes of plasma, and the presence of albumin as a contaminant is always a possibility.

This problem is of particular importance in studies of infants, in whom the volume of blood that can be safely withdrawn is limited. To overcome this problem, we have developed protein extraction procedures that require a minimal volume of plasma. The procedures use either protein-specific chemical extraction for those proteins (e.g., albumin, fibrinogen) present in high concentrations,[18,19] or a combination of immunoprecipitation and sodium dodecyl sulfate polyacrylamide gel electrophoresis (SDS-PAGE) under denaturing conditions for those proteins present in smaller quantities in plasma (e.g., transferrin, prealbumin, retinol binding protein, haptoglobin, α1-acid glycoprotein, and α1-antitrypsin).[14,20,21] By judicious use of sequential extraction with specific immune sera, sufficient quantities of each protein can be extracted from 1 mL of whole blood for accurate determination of isotopic enrichment.

The method involves immunoprecipation of a particular protein by reacting 50 to 100 mL of plasma with the specific human antibody, washing the antigen-antibody complex free of albumin and other contaminating proteins, and further purifying the protein by SDS-PAGE, which also separates the protein from its antibody.[14,20-22] The remaining plasma can then be reacted with another protein-specific antibody in order to minimize the amount of plasma needed for the isolation of several proteins. The gel bands of pure protein are then hydrolyzed, and the released amino acids purified by ion exchange chromatograph, and derivatized for GC-MS (or GC-C-IRMS) analysis. In theory, providing the appropriate antibody is available, virtually any plasma protein can be separated by sequential immunoprecipitation.

4.4   SAMPLE SIZE

The concentration of a particular protein in plasma and the amount of blood that can be safely removed from a subject are factors that determine the amount of protein that can be obtained for analysis. The isolated protein must provide a sufficient amount of the tracer amino acid to satisfy the requirements of the particular mass spectrometer that is being used. Although this may not be a problem in studies in adult subjects, it is a critical concern in studies of premature neonates, infants, severely malnourished and septic infants, and young children, in whom both the amount of blood that can be removed is limited, and the concentrations of most plasma proteins are lower. For example, a typical GC-MS can readily measure ~50 picogram of a single amino acid. We have determined that ~1 nmol of leucine must be derivatized, which means that ~2 mg protein must be obtained from plasma for adequate NCI-GC-MS analysis of leucine. In the case of retinol binding protein (RBP) with a plasma concentration of ~40 mg/mL in a healthy individual, this will require at least 50 mL of plasma. In an infected, malnourished child, however, the amount of blood required would be two-fold larger, because plasma RBP concentration in these patients is only ~20 mg/mL.[22]

On the other hand, if the isotope measurement is to be done by GC-C-IRMS, the amount of tracer amino acid, hence protein required, increases further. For example, the requirement of a typical GC-C-IRMS is ~20 nmol of carbon dioxide for adequate analysis. If the tracer is leucine, and the methyl trifluoroacetic anhydride derivative is used, then this is equivalent to 2 nmol leucine per GC injection. A good rule of thumb is that the sample should contain ~10 times this amount, necessitating the isolation of 30 mg of protein. In the case of RBP, this will require 0.75 mL of plasma or ~1.2 mL of whole blood. Thus, whereas it will require 1.2 mL of blood from a healthy child, it will require 2.4 mL from a severely malnourished child to isolate sufficient RBP for GC-C-IRMS analysis. Since a minimum of two such samples will be required to obtain the rate of incorporation of the tracer into the protein, and additional blood will be required to establish that the hepatic precursor pool is at steady state, at least 7 to 10 mL of blood will be necessary. Thus, it may not be possible to study RBP kinetics using GC-C-IRMS in a severely malnourished infant.

4.5   ISOTOPIC ENRICHMENT OF TRACER IN HEPATIC
PRECURSOR POOL

The minimum requirement for the calculation of the rate of protein synthesis with the precursor-product model is the measurement of the isotopic enrichment at two time points during the quasi-linear portion of the exponential rise in protein-bound amino acid labeling.[10] In addition, it is critical to obtain an estimate of the isotopic enrichment of the amino acid tracer at the site of protein incorporation, i.e., in the liver protein synthetic precursor pool. This is a major problem, because it is well established that a labeled amino acid taken up by the liver from the blood is substantially diluted in the hepatic free pool by amino acids released from hepatic proteolysis. The ideal solution is to measure the steady-state labeling of the appropriate amino acyl t-RNA.[23] However, this measurement is not only technically very difficult, but requires samples of liver tissue, which severely limits its practicality in human studies.

An alternative is to use an indirect measurement of the intrahepatic protein synthetic precursor pool. Much of the early literature used urinary amino acid metabolites that were known to be synthesized from the tracer amino acid in the liver.[11,12] This approach has two disadvantages. First, it requires exceedingly long tracer infusions, because the fractional rates of turnover of the body pools of the metabolites are slow. Second, there is no assurance that the isotopic enrichment of a metabolite (e.g., hippuric acid) will be the same as the amino acid (e.g., glycine) being utilized for protein synthesis. More recent studies have used a prime-constant intravenous infusion of labeled leucine, followed by measurements of the isotopic enrichment of plasma alpha keto isocaproic acid (α-KICA; the keto acid derived from leucine transamination) to estimate the intrahepatic leucine precursor pool.[9,24] It has been argued, however, that plasma α-KICA isotopic enrichment may not be an accurate marker of leucine isotopic enrichment in the hepatic protein synthetic precursor pool, because the major site of α-KICA synthesis is the peripheral tissues (especially skeletal muscle). Data from our studies in pigs and humans support this argument. Significant differences between the steady-state isotopic enrichments of circulating α-KICA and VLDL-apoB-100-bound leucine in both studies suggest that plasma α-KICA may not be an accurate marker of intrahepatic precursor pool leucine under all conditions.[18,25] For example, in a study where labeled leucine was infused intravenously in adult human subjects in both the fed and fasted states, plasma VLDL-apoB-100-bound leucine was only ~70% as enriched as α-KICA in the fed state.[25]

Garlick and co-workers have adopted a separate approach, in which a large mass of tracer amino acid is injected intravenously with the objective of equilibrating ("flooding") the intracellular pool.[26] This approach also has the technical advantage that the time required for appropriate labeling of the intracellular hepatic pool is considerably shorter than for the constant infusion method (1.5 h vs. 4 to 8 h) because the equilibration of the tracer into the hepatic free pool is rapid.[26] Unfortunately, the flooding dose method may not be suitable for studies in infants because multiple blood samples are necessary for the accurate estimation of the plasma free amino acid labeling kinetics. In addition, some questions have been raised about the validity of this approach.[23,27-29] For example, it is still not known with certainty whether, in humans, the hepatic free amino acid pool is completely equilibrated with the accessible plasma amino acid pool. Furthermore, the values for the rates of synthesis of muscle protein and of albumin obtained with the flooding dose technique are consistently higher than the values obtained by the constant infusion method,[27-29] and there is evidence that the large dose of the tracer amino acid stimulates the rate of albumin synthesis.[28] Although the absolute value obtained with the flooding dose technique may not be totally accurate, the practical advantages of the method, such as a considerably shorter experimental period, make it useful for testing the effects of a treatment in the same subject.

More recently, we[18-22,25] and others[17,30] have used the steady-state enrichment of a labeled amino acid in a rapidly turning over hepatic-synthesized plasma protein, very low density lipoprotein apolipoprotein B-100 (VLDL-apoB-100), as a marker of the intra-hepatic enrichment of the tracer. This method is convenient, because the VLDL-apoB-100-bound tracer amino acid reaches a plateau enrichment in 4 to 6 h and requires only ~0.5 mL of plasma for isolation of sufficient apoB-100 at several time points for GC-MS analysis. In a study in fasted pigs, we demonstrated that the rates of synthesis of albumin and fibrinogen were the same with three different tracers, labeled leucine, lysine, and alanine.[18] Although we did not simultaneously measure liver t-RNA enrichments in this study, we showed that for the leucine and lysine tracers, the enrichment in apoB-100 was ~62% arterial plasma lysine (or leucine) enrichment and ~75% arterial plasma α-KICA. These results are almost identical to the ratios of the enrichments of hepatic t-RNA/arterial leucine (64%) and of t-RNA/arterial α-KICA (73%) reported by Bauman et al.[31] in fasted pigs. The similarity of these findings suggests that the VLDL-apoB-100-bound tracer enrichment at plateau is the same as the hepatic t-RNA enrichments when the tracer is given by a prime-constant intravenous infusion. We have now adopted this approach in all of our human studies.

Another fortuitous outcome of one of our studies was the observation that when labeled alanine is used as the tracer, the steady-state enrichment of plasma pyruvate agrees very closely with that of apoB-bound alanine in both the fed and fasted states.[25] On the basis of that observation, we infused pigs with uniformly labeled glucose (because of the unavailability of uniformly labeled alanine) to produce uniformly labeled alanine via pyruvate. We found that both plasma alanine and pyruvate were similarly enriched as apoB-bound alanine. Hence, plasma alanine or pyruvate may be used as surrogates to accurately reflect intra-hepatic precursor pool alanine enrichment.[18] The advantage of this approach is that plasma alanine reached isotopic equilibrium in a much shorter period of time compared to the time taken by VLDL-apoB-100 leucine and lysine.[18] A disadvantage of this approach is that both uniformly labeled glucose and alanine are expensive.

4.6 ROUTE OF ADMINISTRATION OF TRACER

We[32] and others[33] have found that the degree of labeling of the hepatic precursor pool, and hence of the hepatic-derived plasma proteins, are influenced by the route of administration of the tracer amino acid. In a study in which ^{13}C-leucine and ^{2}H$_3$-leucine were simultaneously infused intravenously (IV) and intragastrically (IG) in adult human subjects, Cayol et al.[33] reported that the steady-state isotopic enrichment of plasma VLDL-apoB-100-bound leucine (used as a surrogate for the hepatic precursor pool enrichment) was one-fold more enriched when the tracer was administered IG. Similarly, more than two times as much labeled leucine was incorporated into the hepatic-derived plasma proteins albumin and fibrinogen when the tracer was infused IG, compared to when it was infused IV.[33] We have recently confirmed these findings in both animal and human studies.[32] In a study in which ^{2}H$_5$-phenylalanine (IV) and ^{13}C-phenylalanine (IG) were simultaneously infused in fed piglets, the steady-state isotopic enrichments of hepatic-free phenylalanine and plasma VLDL-apoB-100-bound phenylalanine were 43% and 75% higher with the IG tracer. Furthermore, the ratio of the isotopic enrichments of VLDL-apoB-100-bound phenylalanine to arterial plasma phenylalanine was 0.92 with the IG tracer, compared to

0.65 with the IV tracer. We found the same relationship between the steady-state isotopic enrichments of VLDL-apoB-100-bound leucine and plasma α-KICA in fed young children who were infused simultaneously with ^{13}C-leucine (IV) and [2]H[3]-leucine (IG). The ratio was 0.90 with the IG tracer, compared to 0.60 with the IV tracer (Figure 4.1). Taken together, these findings suggest that in the fed state, portal

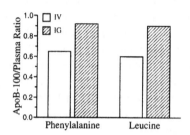

FIGURE 4.1 Ratio of steady-state tracer/tracee ratios of apoB-100-bound and arterial plasma phenylalanine in fed piglets infused simultaneously with [2]H[5]- and ^{13}C-labeled phenylalanine through the intravenous and intragastric routes, respectively;[32] and of apoB-100-bound leucine and plasma α-KICA in fed children infused simultaneously with [13]C- and [2]H[3]-labeled leucine through the intravenous and intragastric routes, respectively.

blood is the primary contributor of amino acids to the hepatic precursor pool from which plasma proteins are synthesized. Hence, to determine the rate of synthesis of hepatic-derived plasma proteins, it will be physiologically more correct and cost effective (from the standpoint of level of isotopic enrichment achieved with a given infusion rate) to infuse the tracer intragastrically.

4.7 CLINICAL SITUATION

Finally, the method employed will be dictated by the particular clinical situation. For a critically ill patient in the hospital, a shorter experiment will be more convenient. In such a situation, the flooding-dose method becomes a better option, especially if the goal is to compare one treatment to another in the same subject. In situations where the accurate absolute rate of synthesis is needed, the constant infusion method may be preferred. As discussed above, this method can be made shorter by administering a priming dose of the tracer and using the isotopic enrichment of the tracer in VLDL-apoB-100 as a surrogate for the isotopic enrichment of the tracer in the hepatic precursor pool.

4.8 PREALBUMIN AND VLDL-apoB-100 KINETICS

Because we use the steady state isotopic enrichment of VLDL-apoB-100 to estimate the isotopic enrichment of the hepatic precursor pool in all of our studies, the fractional rate of synthesis of VLDL-apoB-100 can also be obtained in any study performed to measure the rate of synthesis of a particular hepatic-derived plasma protein. This is easily done by taking frequent additional blood samples to define the rise to plateau portion of the enrichment-time curve of VLDL-apoB-100. We will illustrate this with a study designed to measure the rate of synthesis of prealbumin in adult human subjects, using $^2H_3$-leucine as the tracer.

4.8.1 TRACER INFUSION PROTOCOL

Following a 10 h overnight fast, the subjects' weights and heights were measured, and venous catheters were inserted under local anesthetic into each forearm. One catheter was used for infusion of isotope, the other for blood sampling. A sterile solution of $^2H_3$-leucine was prepared in 4.5 g/L saline, and infused continuously for 8 h at 9 $\mu mol.kg^{-1}.h^{-1}$ through the catheter in one forearm after a priming dose of 9 $\mu mol/kg$ was injected. A 4 mL blood sample was drawn before the start of the infusion, followed by additional blood samples at 1.0 h intervals for the rest of the infusion.

4.8.2 SAMPLE ANALYSES

Blood is drawn in pre-chilled tubes containing 10 μL of a solution consisting of 10% Na_2EDTA, 2% sodium azide, 1% merthiolate, and 2% soybean trypsin inhibitor, immediately centrifuged at 2000 x g for 15 min at 4°C. The plasma is removed and stored at -70°C for later analysis.

Prealbumin is isolated from plasma by immunoprecipitation with anti-human prealbumin (Behring, Somerville, NJ). Plasma (0.05 mL) is mixed with an equal volume of antihuman prealbumin (5mg/mL), and the solution made to 0.7 mL with 0.15 M NaCl containing 0.02% merthiolate. The mixture is incubated at 25°C for 2 h, and then at 4°C for 72 h. To precipitate the protein-antibody complex, the tubes are centrifuged (2000 x g) at 4°C for 20 min, and the supernatant removed.

The protein-antibody precipitates are washed three times with 0.7 mL of 0.15 M NaCl, and centrifuged. The precipitates are taken into 35 μl of sample buffer (0.187 M Tris, 0.104 M sodium docecyl sulfate, 3.26 M glycerol, 0.85 M 2-mercaptoethanol, pH 6.8) containing 0.03% (w/v) bromophenol blue. The 2-mercaptoethanol is added to the buffer just prior to use. The mixture is heated at 95°C for 5 min, then cooled and centrifuged at 3000 x g for 5 min. A standard of pure prealbumin is similarly treated. The samples are loaded into 22.5 x 16 cm slabs of 3.5% stacking and 12% resolving polyacrylamide gels. The gels are electrophoresed in 25 mM Tris buffer (pH 8.3) containing sodium dodecyl sulfate and glycine for about 5.5 h at 80 mA current. As the bromophenol blue marker reaches the edge of the plates, the gels are removed and stained with Coomassie brilliant blue R-250 in 7% acetic acid. After destaining with two changes in 7% (w/v) acetic acid, the excess acid is removed by washing the gels repeatedly with deionized water, and the protein bands corresponding to the prealbumin standard are cut out and transferred into screw-top Pyrex tubes.

VLDL-apoB-100 is separated by ultracentrifugation, followed by isopropanol precipitation. 0.5 mL of plasma is placed into a polycarbonate ultracentrifuge tube, and overlayed with 1 mL of a 0.1012 M EDTA-NaBr solution (density = 1.0063 g/mL). The solution is spun at 100,000 rpm at 20°C for 4 h in a TLA-100.3 rotor, using a Beckman TL-100 tabletop ultracentrifuge (or any other ultracentrifuge). The tube is carefully removed and placed on a rack under a light against a black background, and the upper 3 mm grayish layer is removed with a fine tip pipette into a 5 mL Pyrex tube. The volume is made up to 0.5 mL with phosphate-buffered saline (PBS), an equal volume of isopropanol is added, the mixture vortexed for 1 min, and left overnight at room temperature. The tube is centrifuged for 30 min at (5000 x g), and the supernatant carefully removed. The protein pellet is ready for hydrolysis.

Although the precipitation of VLDL-apoB-100 by isopropanol is a simple and convenient method, there is concern that if the subjects are in the fed state there will be significant contamination of the isopropanol-precipitated VLDL-apoB-100 with gut-derived VLDL-apoB-48, a protein which can also be precipitated by iso-propanol. In any fed study, however, pure apoB-100 can be immunoprecipitated from the VLDL isolate obtained by ultracentrifugation. The VLDL isolate is mixed with 100 µL of 66 mg/mL antihuman apoB-100 (Calbiochem, La Jolla, CA), and the solution made to 0.7 mL with 0.15 M NaCl containing 0.02% merthiolate. The mixture is incubated at 25°C for 1 h, and then at 4°C for 24 h. To precipitate the protein-antibody complex, the tubes are centrifuged (5000 x g) at 4°C for 20 min, and the supernatant removed. The protein-antibody precipitates are delipidated by adding 1 mL of a 4:1 hexane/isopropanol solution, the mixture vortexed, centrifuged for 15 min at (5000 x g), and the supernatant carefully removed. The precipitate is washed three times with 0.15 M NaCl, and the precipitates treated with sample buffer for SDS-PAGE as described above. The samples are loaded into 22.5 x 20 cm slabs of 3.5% stacking and 5% resolving polyacrylamide gels. The gels are electrophoresed in 25 mM Tris buffer (pH 8.3) containing sodium dodecyl sulfate and glycine for about 7.5 h at 80 mA current. The gels are stained and destained as described above, and the protein bands cut out and transferred into screw-top tubes.

The dried protein precipitates and gel bands are hydrolyzed in 6 mol/L HCl at 110°C for 12 h. The amino acids released from the protein are purified by cation exchange chromatography, and the tracer/tracee ratio of the protein-derived leucine determined by negative chemical ionization gas chromatography-mass spectrometry on a Hewlett-Packard 5988A GC-MS (Palo Alto, CA). The amino acid is converted to the n-propyl ester, heptafluorobutyramide derivative, and leucine isotope ratio is determined by monitoring ions at m/z 349 to 352, as previously described.[18] Each sample is run on the GC-MS in triplicate, and the average value used in the calculation.

4.8.3 CALCULATIONS

The fractional synthesis rate (FSR) of prealbumin is calculated with the precursor-product equation:

$$FSR(\%/d) = \frac{PEt_2 - PEt_1}{E_{pl}} \times \frac{2400}{t_8 - t_6}$$

where PEt_2 - PEt_1 is the increase in isotope ratio of prealbumin-bound leucine over the period t_8 - t_6 h of the infusion, and E_{pl} is the plateau enrichment of VLDL-apoB-100-bound leucine. In the case of VLDL-apoB-100, PEt_2 - PEt_1 is the increase in isotopic enrichment of VLDL-apoB-100-bound leucine during the time period t_2 - t_1 before a plateau is reached.

As shown in Figure 4.2, VLDL-apoB-100-bound leucine reached a plateau in

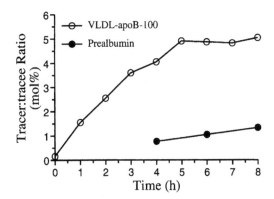

FIGURE 4.2   The tracer/tracee molar ratio of leucine incorporated into plasma VLDL-apoB-100, and into plasma prealbumin during an 8 h infusion of $^2H_3$-leucine in an adult human subject.

isotopic enrichment after 5 h of the isotope infusion, and there was a linear increase in the isotopic content of prealbumin during this period of time. Based on these isotopic enrichment time curves, it can be calculated that the FSR of VLDL-apoB-100 is 21%/h, and that of prealbumin is 68%/d.

ACKNOWLEDGMENT

This chapter is a publication of the U.S. Department of Agriculture/Agricultural Research Service, Children's Nutrition Research Center, Department of Pediatrics, Baylor College of Medicine and Texas Children's Hospital, Houston, TX. The contents of this publication do not necessarily reflect the views or policies of the U.S. Department of Agriculture, nor does mention of trade names, commercial products or organizations imply endorsement by the U.S. Government.

REFERENCES

1. McLaren, D. S., Shirajian, E., and Shadarevian, S., Short-term prognosis in protein-calorie malnutrition, *Am. J. Clin. Nutr.*, 22, 863, 1969.
2. Fleck, A., Clinical and nutritional aspects of changes in acute-phase proteins during inflammation, *Proc. Nutr. Soc.*, 48, 347, 1989.

3. Kushner, I., The phenomenon of the acute phase response, in *C-Reactive Protein and the Plasma Protein Response to Tissue Injury*, Vol. 389, I. Kushner, J.E. Volanakis, H. Gewurz, Eds., *Ann. N.Y. Acad. Sci.*, 1982, 39.

4. Schreiber, G., Synthesis, processing, and secretion of plasma proteins by the liver and other organs and their regulation, in *The Plasma Proteins*, Vol. 5, Putnam, F. W., Ed., Academic Press, New York, 1988, 293.

5. Picou, D. and Waterlow, J. C., The effect of malnutrition on the metabolism of plasma albumin, *Clin. Sci.*, 22, 459, 1962.

6. James, W. P. T. and Hay, A. M., Albumin metabolism: Effect of the nutritional state and the dietary protein intake, *J. Clin. Invest.*, 47, 1958, 1968.

7. Malaba, L., Kindberg, G. M., Norum, K.R., Berg, T., and Blomhoff, R., Receptor-mediated endocytosis of retinol-binding protein by liver parenchymal cells: interference by radioactive iodination, *Biochem. J.*, 291, 187, 1993.

8. Swick, R. W., Measurement of protein turnover in rat liver, *J. Biol. Chem.*, 231, 751, 1958.

9. De Feo, P., Horber, F. F., and Haymond, M. W., Meal stimulation of albumin synthesis: a significant contributor to whole body protein synthesis in humans, *Am. J. Physiol.*, 263, E794, 1992.

10. Waterlow, J. C., Garlick, P. J., and Millward, D. J, Measurement of the rate of incorporation of labelled amino acids into tissue proteins, in *Protein Turnover in Mammalian Tissues and in the Whole Body*, North-Holland, Amsterdam, 1978, 339.

11. Stein, T. P., Leskiw, M. J., and Wallace, H. W., Measurement of half-life of human plasma fibrinogen, *Am. J. Physiol.*, 234, E504, 1978.

12. Gersovitz, M., Munro, H. N., Udall, J., and Young, V. R., Albumin synthesis in young and elderly subjects using a new stable isotope methodology: Response to level of protein intake, *Metabolism*, 29, 1075, 1980.

13. Hachey, D. L., Stable isotopes for measurement of nutrient dynamics during pregnancy and lactation, in *Nutrient Regulation During Pregnancy, Lactation, and Infant Growth*, Vol. 24, Allen, L., King, J., and Lönnerdal, B., Eds. Plenum Press, N.Y., 1994, 265.

14. Sivakumar, B., Jahoor, F., Burrin, D. G., Frazer, M., and Reeds, P. J., Fractional synthetic rates of retinol binding protein and transthyretin measured by stable isotope technique in neonatal pigs, *J. Biol. Chem.*, 269, 26196, 1994.

15. Putnam F. W., Perspectives — past, present, and future, in *The Plasma Proteins*, Vol. 1, Putnam F. W., Ed., Academic Press, New York, 1975, 2.

16. Stein, T. P., Buzby, G. P., Gertner, M. H., Hargrove, W. C., Leskiw, M. J., and Mullen, J. L., Effect of parenteral nutrition on protein synthesis and liver fat metabolism in man, *Am. J. Physiol.*, 239, G280, 1980.

17. Lichtenstein, A. H., Cohn, J. S., Hachey, D. L., Millar, J. S., Ordovas, J. M., and Schaefer, E. J., Comparison of deuterated leucine, valine, and lysine in the measurement of human apolipoprotein A-1 and B-100 kinetics, *J. Lipid Res.*, 31, 1693, 1990.

18. Jahoor, F., Burrin, D. G., Reeds, P. J., and Frazer, M. E., Measurement of plasma protein synthesis rate in the infant pig: An investigation of alternative tracer approaches, *Am. J. Physiol.*, 267, R221, 1994.

19. Morlese, J. F., Forrester, T., Badaloo, A., Del Rosario, M., Frazer, M. E., and Jahoor, F., Albumin kinetics in edematous and non-edematous protein-energy malnourished children, *Am. J. Clin. Nutr.*, 64, 952, 1996.

20. Jahoor, F., Sivakumar, B., Del Rosario, M., and Fraser, M. E., Isolation of positive acute phase proteins for determination of fractional synthesis rates by a stable isotope tracer technique, *Anal. Biochem.*, 236, 95, 1996.

21. Morlese, J. F., Forrester, T., Del Rosario, M., Frazer, M. and Jahoor, F., Transferrin kinetics are altered in children with severe protein-energy malnutrition, *J. Nutr.*, 127, 1469, 1997.

22. Morlese, J. F., Forrester, T., Del Rosario, M., Frazer, M. E., and Jahoor, F., Repletion of the plasma pool of nutrient transport proteins occurs at different rates during the nutritional rehabilitation of severely malnourished children, *J. Nutr.*, 128(2), 214, 1998.

23. Watt, P. W., Lindsay, Y., Chien, P. A.F., Gibson, J. N. A., Taylor, D. J., and Rennie, M. J., Isolation of aminoacyl tRNA and its labelling with stable-isotope tracers: use in studies of human tissue protein synthesis, *Proc. Natl. Acad. Sci. U.S.A.*, 88, 5892, 1991.

24. Horber, F. F., Horber-Feyder, C. M., Krayer, S., Frederick, W., and Haymond, M. W., Plasma reciprocal pool specific activity predicts that of intracellular free leucine for protein synthesis, *Am. J. Physiol.*, 257, E385, 1989.

25. Reeds, P. J., Hachey, D. L., Patterson, B. W., Motil, K. J., and Klein, P. D., VLDL apolipoprotein B-100, a potential indicator of the isotopic labeling of the hepatic protein synthetic precursor pool in humans: Studies with multiple stable isotopically labeled amino acids, *J. Nutr.*, 122, 457, 1992.

26. Ballmer, P. E., McNurlan, M. A., Milne, E., Heys, S. D., Buchan, V., Calder, A. G., and Garlick, P. J., Measurement of albumin synthesis in humans: a new approach employing stable isotopes, *Am. J. Physiol.*, 259, E797, 1990.

27. Rennie, M. J., Edwards, R. H. T., Halliday, D., Matthews, D. E., Wolman, S. L., and Millward, D. J., Muscle protein synthesis measured by stable isotope techniques in man: the effects of feeding and fasting, *Clin. Sci.*, 63, 519, 1982.

28. Smith, K., Downie, S., Barua, J. M., Watt, P. W., Scrimgeour, C. M., and Rennie, M. J., Effect of flooding dose of leucine in stimulating incorporation of constantly infused valine into albumin, *Am. J. Physiol.*, 266, E640, 1994.

29. Jahoor, F., Zhang, X., Baba, H., Sakurai, Y., and Wolfe, R. R., Comparison of constant infusion and flooding dose techniques to measure muscle protein synthesis rate in dogs, *J. Nutr.*, 122, 878, 1992.

30. Venkatesan, S., Pacy, P. J., Wenham, D., and Halliday, D., Very-low-density lipo-protein-apolipoprotein B turnover studies in normal subjects: a stable isotope study, *Biochem. Soc. Trans.*, 18, 1192, 1990.

31. Bauman, P. Q., Stirewalt, W. S., O'Rouke, O., Howard, B. D., and Nair, K.S., Precursor pools of protein synthesis: a stable isotope study in a swine model, *Am. J. Physiol.*, 267, E203, 1994.

32. Stoll, B., Burrin, D. G., Henry, J., Jahoor, F., and Reeds, P. J., Phenylalanine utilization by the gut and liver measured with intravenous and intragastric tracers in pigs, *Am. J. Physiol.*, 273, G1208, 1997.

33. Cayol, M., Boirie, Y., Prugnaud, J., Gachon, P., Beaufrere, B., and Obled, C., Precursor pool for hepatic protein synthesis in humans: Effects of tracer route infusion and dietary proteins, *Am. J. Physiol.*, 270, E980, 1996.

5   Evaluation of the Adaptation to Protein Restriction in Humans

L. John Hoffer

CONTENTS

5.1   INTRODUCTION

What are the least amounts of protein or essential amino acids a normal person may consume without danger of nutritional deficiency? The answer to this question is unclear, despite more than a century of investigation and debate.[1-5] In part, this is because research in this area is hampered by methodologic and conceptual problems, and in part because our understanding of the mechanisms that control adaptation to variations in dietary protein and amino acid intake is still rudimentary. Thus, Hegsted[6] argues that all current methods for estimating the adult protein requirement are inadequate, for they lack an appropriate measure of health. Waterlow[7] notes that

0-8493-9612-3/99/$0.00+$.50
© 1999 by CRC Press LLC

even at the simple metabolic level, we still do not understand how the body maintains nitrogen balance in response to varying nitrogen intakes.

In spite of these difficulties, there is no doubt that adaptation to protein restriction remains an important topic for research. The earliest efforts to measure and interpret human whole-body protein metabolism were not so much motivated by theoretical interest as they were by an urgent desire to find practical answers to pressing problems caused by human protein malnutrition.[8] Even in well-off societies, where average protein consumption is far greater than necessary to meet nutritional needs, situations occur in which a disease process (or its treatment) restricts protein intake. How much protein restriction can be tolerated in such situations? In other situations, a disease (or its treatment) could impair the metabolic processes that govern the adaptation to protein restriction, leading to protein deficiency disease despite a protein intake reduction that would normally be well tolerated. Another reason for studying human protein restriction is its relationship to starvation. Starvation disease develops when total food intake is chronically inadequate, so it is usually the result of a combination of energy and protein deficiency. A better understanding of the separate adaptations to protein and energy deficiency will go a long way towards understanding the adaptation to protein-energy malnutrition, one of the commonest diseases of mankind.

This chapter provides a survey of the conceptual and technical issues involved in studying human adaptation to a change of protein or amino acid intake from one customary level to a different one. Although the focus is naturally on protein restriction, it is necessary to discuss a range of protein intakes; indeed, the definition of what constitutes "reduced" and "increased" protein intakes requires comment.

5.2 CONCEPTS AND DEFINITIONS

5.2.1 ADAPTATION, ACCOMMODATION, AND HABITUATION

Under most conditions, the body's total protein store is nearly constant. So, as measured over hours or days, it must catabolize amino acids and excrete their nitrogen (chiefly as urinary urea) at the same rate nitrogen is being consumed. Normal adaptation to an increase or a reduction in protein intake requires the body to detect this change, and adjust the sum of endogenous and dietary amino acid catabolism upwards or downwards to match the new rate of intake. Since humans exist in an environment in which protein intake may vary considerably from season to season, day to day, and even from meal to meal, sensitive adjustment of whole-body amino acid catabolism to a changing protein intake may be considered a part of normal homeostasis. There appears to be no practical upper limit to the rate amino acids can be catabolized by a normal human,[9] but a lower limit does exist, since amino acid oxidation is never zero, even on a protein-free diet. The protein intake below which whole-body amino acid catabolism cannot be equivalently reduced is considered to be an individual's minimum protein requirement.

This definition of the minimum protein (or amino acid) requirement turns out to be difficult to apply in practice. When a moderately protein-deficient diet is eaten, nitrogen balance predictably becomes negative, but after a certain amount of body protein has been lost, nitrogen balance typically comes back to zero and homeostasis is reestablished. Was the "deficient" protein intake really deficient?

To account for this situation, the terms *adaptation* or *normal adaptation* have been used to describe normal homeostatic adjustments to changes in protein intake *at or above* the minimum requirement, whereas metabolic changes that restore nitrogen equilibrium only after significant lean tissue loss, and hence at a physiologic cost to the organism, are termed *accommodation* or *pathologic adaptation*. *Adaptation* is thus an aspect of normal homeostasis, whereas *accommodation* implies that homeostasis has been regained only at the cost of a physiologic compromise with adverse health implications.[10,11]

This refinement brings other problems. Even adjustments in protein intake within the normal adaptive range are associated with small, but real transients in nitrogen balance. The German physiologist Voit ignored this phenomenon (even though he was the first to describe it in 1867) when he concluded that the protein requirement of normal men must be 120 g/day after finding their nitrogen balance became negative for the first few days after a reduction of their protein intake below this level. As Carpenter[1] has pointed out, Voit's subjects did not *require* 120 g of protein daily, they were merely *habituated* to it. The term "habituation" has the same meaning as completed normal adaptation, but draws attention to the harmlessness of the metabolic adjustments that accompany changes in protein intake above the requirement level.

5.2.2 ADAPTATIONS ABOVE AND BELOW THE MINIMUM REQUIREMENT

A person adapted to a deficient protein intake will respond differently to a standard protein meal than one adapted to surfeit protein. In the first situation, the prior diet has primed the body to conserve incoming dietary amino acids with high efficiency by minimizing their oxidation, both during meals and in the basal state between meals. The aim of reduced amino acid oxidation can be achieved either by reducing proteolysis, or by increasing protein synthesis from exogenous and endogenous amino acids. Either or both of these adaptations will reduce the size of the free amino acid pools under basal conditions and limit their increase in the fed state, thereby reducing "overflow" oxidation.[12] The goal of reduced amino acid oxidation can also be achieved by reducing the amounts or specific catalytic activities of key amino acid degradative enzymes.[11,13] In quantitative terms, the body's major decisions as to whether tissue amino acids will be oxidized or deposited in newly synthesized proteins occur in the fed state.[14-16] The opportunity to modulate endogenous amino acid oxidation continues throughout the periods between meals, however; indeed, it is hard to conceive of an adaptive process aimed at improving the efficiency of dietary amino acid utilization that is not measurably in effect in the basal period that precedes meal consumption. (As Waterlow explains, while all aspects of adaptation are, by definition, regulated, much of what constitutes accommodation is "automatic," for the body's protein requirement is proportional to its active protein mass. Thus, a person whose diet is moderately deficient in protein may eventually regain nitrogen equilibrium merely by losing enough body protein to reduce his or her protein requirement to the level provided in the diet.[5])

The organism adapted to surfeit protein consumption has a different, but no less important, agenda. Amino acids in excess are toxic; since they cannot be stored, all surfeit consumption must rapidly be disposed of by catabolism, and the resulting free nitrogen converted to urea and ammonia, and the sulfur to sulfate. This situation requires that dietary protein be metabolized with "zero" efficiency. As Voit observed, it is normal for a person adapted to a very high protein intake, then switched to a lower but still excessive one, to waste some of the protein in the first several meals of the new diet, exhibiting negative nitrogen balance, before coming into full adaptation. This shows that even "zero" efficiency of dietary amino acid utilization is regulated, for it successfully avoids "negative" efficiency.

5.2.3 BREAKPOINT

Of greatest practical interest to the nutritionist is the protein or amino acid intake at which the body switches from high-efficiency nutrient retention to zero-efficiency surfeit amino acid elimination, for this is the minimum requirement. The nitrogen balance curve shown in Figure 5.1 illustrates the process by which the current adult protein requirement was estimated.[17] When increasing amounts of high-quality protein are added to a protein-free diet, nitrogen balance improves steeply and steadily at low levels of intake, proof of highly efficient dietary protein retention.[18] In contrast, protein intakes at and above the requirement are associated with zero nitrogen balance. The intersection of these two functions — one a straight line with a positive slope, the other a straight line with a slope of zero — is the *breakpoint* which represents the minimum theoretical requirement.

However, the theoretical breakpoint is a mathematical discontinuity, which does not exist in biology. As Figure 5.1 illustrates, the slope of the line relating nitrogen balance to protein intake decreases as protein intakes near the requirement level.[18] Because of this, the *theoretical* requirement extrapolated from a straight line equation based on protein intakes well below the requirement (0.34 g per kg of normal adult body weight per day) turns out to be substantially less than the *actual* requirement — the protein intake at which zero nitrogen balance actually first occurs (0.6 g per kg per day). Available measurements are too imprecise to indicate the extent to which the shape of this curve (and the resulting uncertainty in defining the actual requirement) is determined by factors acting within each individual and to what extent it is determined by differences between individuals.[19] It is plausible to predict that the switch from a metabolic agenda of "high-efficiency" nutrient retention at sub-requirement protein intakes to "surfeit elimination" once the requirement has been met, is a gradual transition *for each individual*, as implied by Figure 5.1. What would this tell us about how that process is regulated? Are there two separate processes which kick in or kick out for protein intakes below and above the requirement? Or is there only a single set-point seeking process which can be mathematically modeled and predictably generate a smooth physiologic response with these characteristics?

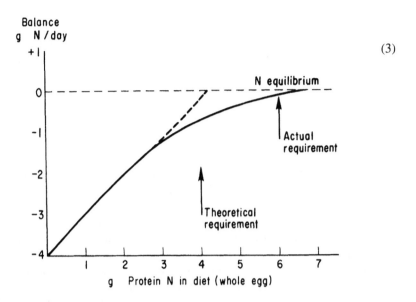

(3)

FIGURE 5.1 Nitrogen balance response to increasing amounts of high-quality protein added to a protein-free diet. (From Munro, H.N. and Crim, M.C., The proteins and amino acids, in *Modern Nutrition in Health and Disease,* Seventh Ed., Shils, M.E. and Young, V.R., Eds., Lea & Febiger, 1988. With permission.)

In tracer-based amino acid research, breakpoints have been sought in the pattern of changing plasma essential amino acid oxidation, when protein or amino acids are fed below and above the requirement level. When a test amino acid is fed below its minimum requirement, its oxidation rate is low since most of it is used for protein synthesis. Once the minimum requirement is exceeded, a surfeit is created and oxidation strongly increases at higher intakes. The level of amino acid intake at which the break from low to rapidly rising oxidation occurs is the minimum requirement.[20] A different way to locate the same breakpoint is *the indicator amino acid oxidation (IAAO) technique.*[21] This involves measuring the oxidation of an essential amino acid different from the one whose requirement is being tested. The indicator is fed at an unchanging, adequate rate, and its oxidation rate is measured at the same times that different levels of the test amino acid are fed. When adequate amounts of the test amino acid are provided, body protein synthesis occurs normally, so oxidation of the indicator should equal its constant rate of provision. At the point where the intake of the test amino acid falls below its requirement, protein synthesis becomes partially compromised for lack of the limiting amino acid. The result is an overabundance of the other amino acids, including the indicator, whose oxidation rate shoots up.[21]

5.2.4 Equivalence of Amino Acid and Nitrogen Balance

While different in method, the IAAO technique and the classical nitrogen balance approach shown in Figure 5.1 are conceptually the same. When measured in the basal state, the oxidation of any essential amino acid must be accompanied, sooner or later, by the catabolism of all the amino acids in the protein it came from. This should remain true even for fed-state essential amino acid oxidation, as long as the exogenous protein entering has an amino acid composition similar to that of the mixed body proteins that are contributing to whole-body protein turnover. In any event, it is clear that the oxidation of a given essential amino acid ought to provide information equivalent to total nitrogen excretion. Researchers have tested this by comparing nitrogen excretion and leucine oxidation (using an isotope labeled at the 1-C position). The stoichiometry is readily calculated if one assumes that mixed body proteins are 16% nitrogen and 8% leucine by weight, in which case 1 mmol leucine oxidized corresponds to 260 mg nitrogen released from catabolized amino acids.[22] Simultaneous comparison of these two measures of net protein catabolism is actually quite complicated, since leucine oxidation is an instantaneous rate measurement[23] whereas nitrogen excretion represents the result of amino acid oxidation over many hours, owing to the slow turnover of the urea pool. It might be thought that a better comparison would be obtained using leucine oxidation and tracer-determined urea appearance, but we have found this is not the case: even a nonsteady-state urea appearance model is not sensitive enough to detect rapid changes in the urea appearance rate. [24]

After adaptation to a protein-free diet, leucine oxidation and urinary nitrogen excretion both become constant over the entire 24-h period. [25] This makes it feasible to directly compare these two measures of whole-body amino acid catabolism. We found leucine oxidation on a protein-free diet was 5.2 μmol.kg^{-1}.h^{-1} (assuming plasma ketoisocaproate enrichment is 80% that of leucine).[26] If the stoichiometry is correct, this is equivalent to the concurrent elimination of 1.4 mg N.kg^{-1}.h^{-1} = 33 mg N.kg per day (The urinary nitrogen excretion we actually measured was 39 mg. kg^{-1}. day^{-1}; $P > 0.05$.)[26]

Although leucine oxidation should, under most conditions, provide the same information as the sum of urea and ammonia formation, it has the important advantage of indicating amino acid catabolism over periods as short as several minutes.[23,27] As with any balance determination,[28] leucine balance is technically demanding. The oxidation measurement must be both accurate and precise, since the balance calculated (leucine input from diet and tracer minus leucine oxidation) is usually a small difference between two much larger numbers.

5.3 WHAT IS PROTEIN RESTRICTION?

In practice, "protein restriction" refers to any reduction of protein intake below the customary level. Since customary protein intakes in well-off countries are typically at least twice the estimated minimum requirement, most protein restriction is merely an example of habituation to one surfeit intake or another. Such moderate adaptations may not require the body to evoke regulatory mechanisms aimed to maximum efficiency, and hence may not bear on the factors that determine the minimum requirement. When designing a protein turnover study, it is important to ask what metabolic state is being studied — surfeit amino acid elimination or increased metabolic efficiency? The answer may depend both on the protein intake subjects are adapted/accommodated to, and on their hormonal or metabolic state.

5.4. OBLIGATORY NITROGEN

When a normal adult is switched from a typical high-protein diet (e.g., 100 g protein per day) to one that is protein-free, there is a gradual reduction in daily urinary nitrogen excretion until, after an adaptation period of about 4 to 7 days, daily urinary nitrogen excretion stabilizes at the rate of 37 ± 7 (SD) mg per kg of adult body weight. The other sources of nitrogen loss, which do not change, are in the feces and secretions (including sweat and shed skin).[17,18,29] This "endogenous" or "obligatory" nitrogen loss is the lowest rate to which endogenous protein loss can be adaptively reduced, and hence has been deemed to represent the minimum amount of dietary protein necessary to replace it.[17,20] Rubner referred to this nitrogen loss as the "wear and tear quota," expressing the view held during the first third of this century that body proteins are static, needing replacement from the diet only after they "wear out."[30] Many experiments of this type have been conducted in order to estimate the minimum protein requirement by the "factorial" method. This method involves adding up the factors that contribute to body nitrogen loss after adaptation to a protein-free diet, and equating the sum to the dietary protein requirement.[31,32] The requirement figure that results is less than the actual protein requirement. For the same reason, the theoretical protein requirement shown in Figure 5.1 is less than the actual one — obligatory nitrogen only provides information about endogenous protein metabolism; it cannot take into account the decreasing efficiency with which dietary protein is incorporated into tissue proteins as protein intake nears the requirement level. In the past, somewhat arbitrary correction factors were used to correct the "replacement" requirement for the inefficiency of dietary protein retention;[31] ultimately, the whole approach was discarded in favor of detailed nitrogen balance studies at several levels of intake below and above the requirement level, upon which the current estimate of the minimum protein requirement is based.[17]

Nevertheless, obligatory nitrogen remains of interest. Its constancy and precision suggest that it represents a biological constant; indeed it has been considered the metaphoric equivalent of the basal metabolic rate.[33] Rather than representing the "wear out" rate of old proteins, as it was originally conceived, obligatory nitrogen actually indicates the maximum efficiency at which endogenous amino acids can be recycled. This is a measure of some interest for understanding metabolic adaptation in situations in which adaptation might be impaired. Thus, for example, we found the obligatory nitrogen excretion of persons with insulin-dependent diabetes mellitus was greater than normal, even during intensive insulin therapy.[26]

5.5 LABILE PROTEIN

Voit first pointed out the existence of a protein pool within the body whose amount was determined by the protein content of the diet, and which was mobilized during the first few days of fasting or upon changing from a higher to a lower protein intake.[30] Munro[34] characterized this "labile protein" as a general phenomenon of rapid body protein gain or loss in response to variations in protein and energy intake, or to a variety of hormonal and physiologic stimuli. When a normal adult is switched from a high-protein diet to a protein-free diet, urinary nitrogen excretion remains considerable for 4 to 6 days, before diminishing to the steady state of obligatory nitrogen loss. This represents a loss from the body of about 30 g nitrogen or 180 to 200 g of rapidly mobilizable proteins. If the former protein intake is resumed nitrogen balance becomes positive until the previous losses are made up. Defined in this way, labile protein constitutes about 3% of body protein in well-nourished rats[34] and the same or somewhat less in humans.[34,35] This is a trivial figure in terms of body nitrogen economy, but one which could be important for assessing the adaptive response to protein deficiency. Although small, the amount of labile protein is greater than the free amino acid pool, which accounts for only about 0.5 – 1.0% of the body's amino acids, and an even smaller percentage of the essential ones.[36-38] The free amino acid pool, because of its small size and rapid turnover, might be thought to play an essential role in regulating tissue protein synthesis and breakdown.[38] Since, by its nature, labile protein undergoes the most rapid exchange with the free amino acid pool, it is tempting to regard it as important in indicating (if not regulating) the oxidation of amino acids, particularly those newly entering the body from the diet.[34]

In general terms, at least, the existence of this small, rapidly turning over protein pool in the body could help explain how the efficiency of dietary protein retention improves after adaptation (or accommodation) to a reduction in protein intake. According to this view, when ample amounts of protein are being consumed the pool is large, rapidly turning over, and amino acid oxidation is high. In protein deficiency, the store is depleted but ready to be *preferentially* repleted when the nutritional environment permits, providing a mechanism for the increased efficiency of amino acid assimilation that occurs during refeeding after protein or energy starvation or during muscular hypertrophy. This process could also explain how the body unifies its response to a diversity of nutrient inputs (e.g., changes in habitual diet, meal composition, size, and frequency).[39]

5.5.1 WHAT AND WHERE IS LABILE PROTEIN?

Labile protein primarily resides in the splanchnic tissues.[33,40] This is in keeping with their rapid protein turnover, and consistent with observations that the greatest acute loss of protein in the protein-deficient rat is from the liver, with the other visceral organs making up large contributions.[29,41] In humans the splanchnic tissues preferentially take up administered amino acids, even when infused intravenously.[42,43] Is labile protein a homogeneous pool which increases or decreases in size over hours or days? If so, what is its turnover rate? If fitted to a simple exponential function, the rate of reduction in urinary nitrogen excretion that occurs after switching to a

protein-free diet indicates a fractional turnover of about 38% per day.[34,44] We calculated that normal men adapted to a 1.1 g protein/kg diet lost about 360 mg N/kg
(2.2 g protein/kg) after adaptation to a protein-free diet.[26] (Young et al.[35] reported a
smaller value, 110 mg N/kg, but this is because they subtracted obligatory nitrogen
over the 6 to 7 day adaptation period from their total.) Since the turnover rate of
a substrate is equal to the product of its pool size and fractional turnover rate,
labile protein proteolysis should contribute 2.2 g protein/kg x 38% per day =
0.836 g protein/kg per day = 35 mg protein. kg^{-1}. h^{-1} to total proteolysis in a
person habituated to a high-protein diet. Therefore, this person's rate of proteolysis
should fall by at least this much after adaptation to a protein-free diet.

Do measured protein turnover data confirm this prediction? Basal proteolysis of
our normal subjects was reduced from 108 to 88 μmol. kg^{-1}. h^{-1} after adaptation to
the protein-free diet, assuming plasma ketoisocaproate enrichment is 80% that of
leucine.[26] This represents a reduction of 20 μmol leucine. kg^{-1}. h^{-1} = 33 mg
proteolysis. kg^{-1}. h^{-1}, a value extremely close to the one calculated from cumulative
urinary nitrogen excretion and its rate of reduction in the same subjects. Urinary 3-
methylhistidine excretion did not decrease (unpublished), suggesting that the reduction in whole-body proteolysis was not due to reduced muscle proteolysis. In two
other comparable studies, Motil et al. found basal proteolysis of normal men fell
from 156 μmol. kg^{-1}. h^{-1} on a 1.5 g/kg protein diet to 106 μmol. kg^{-1}. h^{-1} after
adaptation to a virtually protein-free diet.[45] Yang et al. reported a reduction from
122 to 94 μmol. kg^{-1}. h^{-1}.[46]

As interesting as this calculation may be, it is presumptuous to think one can
use such simple reasoning to distinguish between concepts of labile protein as either
(1) a large increase or decrease in the size of a small, rapidly turning over pool; (2)
slight changes in the rate of synthesis and breakdown of a large, slowly turning over
protein pool of nearly constant mass; or, most likely (3) a combination of both. The
contributions of the different protein pools to whole-body protein turnover remain
poorly defined. Until they are clarified, the specific contribution made by labile
protein synthesis and breakdown to whole-body protein turnover will be
speculative.[47]

Two types of nitrogen balance transients have been referred to as labile protein.
The first refers to nitrogen gains and losses that occur over several days. The second
refers to the acute deposition of protein that must take place in the fed state to
balance inevitable protein losses during the fast after every meal. Plasma concentrations of the essential amino acids are only modestly perturbed during normal
protein consumption, despite the large influx of amino acids in relation to the size
of the body's free amino acid pools.[43,48] This relative stability of the free amino acid
pools could be achieved by an increase in protein synthesis (accelerating removal
of amino acids from their free pools), by a decrease in endogenous protein breakdown
(decreasing entry into the pools), or by an increase in amino acid oxidation. Fed-
state enhancement of protein synthesis and diminished protein breakdown, particularly in the splanchnic tissues, will divert amino acids from oxidation by limiting
the increase in the size of free amino acid pools. The result is a transient increase
in the body's protein content — labile protein. According to this view, the amount
of labile protein present at any moment is determined by the activity of the amino

acid-metabolizing enzymes, which are programmed in activity and amount by the preceding diet. In the interval between meals, a finer-tuned regulation continues, as some of the amino acids in the labile proteins accumulated acutely during the dietary influx are released and redistributed for the synthesis of more slowly turning over proteins.[34] Since amino acid oxidation is not negligible during this period, the body retains the ability to maintain or mobilize some body protein.

This has been documented by a study, in which fed-state and basal N, leucine, and phenylalanine balance were separately measured in the fed and basal states of men adapted to daily protein intakes ranging from low (0.36 g/kg) to medium (0.8 g/kg) to high (2 g/kg).[49,50] As protein intake increased, there was increasingly large fed-state protein deposition, precisely balanced by increasing losses in the basal state that followed each meal. This pattern of increasingly large fed-state gain suggests a simple explanation for labile protein losses upon switching from a diet high in protein to a lower but still ample protein intake. Assuming the body is primed to oxidize a large fraction of each meal's amino acids, switching to a diet that provides less protein will result in amino acid wastage until the body recognizes and adapts to the lower (but still surfeit) protein intake.[51] The reverse process will occur if the person switches to a high protein intake. If this temporary deposit is all there is to "labile protein," then it might not make much of a contribution to basal whole-body protein turnover.[50,51] The opinion[5] that labile protein is of little importance in directly *regulating* protein balance may then be correct, at least when one is describing variations of protein intake *in the surfeit range*. There are too few studies of protein metabolism at protein intakes in the deficient range to draw conclusions about a role for labile protein in determining the minimum requirement or in the process of accommodation to true protein deficiency.

Recent reports of a prompt increase in albumin synthesis in the fed state suggest it could represent a potential source of labile protein.[52-54] The extent to which the net gain in body protein represented by albumin synthesis accounts for the total of fed-state gains remains to be seen. Albumin synthesis and degradation are reduced by severe short-term protein restriction[29,55] (and this could be true of other liver secretory proteins as well), but albumin degradation is reduced, too, so it is unlikely that albumin loss can account for much of the labile nitrogen loss in this situation.

Although Munro[34] and most others equated the protein lost upon initiating a fast with the protein loss that occurs in protein deficiency, the sources of loss are probably not the same in these two situations. The heterogeneity of the different sources of rapid protein loss in different forms of starvation is illustrated by a study in which subjects underwent a total fast that was preceded either by a protein-replete or protein-deficient diet. In these healthy individuals, there was only a small blunting effect of prior protein depletion on fasting nitrogen loss.[47]

Finally, some of what might be considered labile protein on the basis of nitrogen excretion alone is not protein at all, but merely represents the redistribution of urea from total body water into the urine. Another possible source of urinary nitrogen could be glutamine, since changes in tissue glutamine concentration can make a surprisingly large contribution to short-term nitrogen balance.[56,57] It should be noted, however, that *muscle* glutamine appears not to vary significantly in the fed state;[58]

and postabsorptive *plasma* glutamine concentrations actually rise during protein restriction.[59,60]

5.6 BALANCE AND TURNOVER IN THE FED AND BASAL STATES

Waterlow and Fern[38] compared the body's free amino acid pool to a narrow pipe that joins large organs/tissues with greatly differing protein turnover rates and differing capacities to metabolize different amino acids. The fed state, in particular, is associated with a large influx of essential amino acids in relation to the size of the free amino acid pool. As explained in Chapter 2 by El-Khoury, our understanding of whole-body protein metabolism continues to derive from the original Waterlow equations relating amino acid flux to intake, whole-body proteolysis, amino acid oxidation, and protein synthesis.

Amino acid oxidation provides the most revealing information for following the adaptation to changes in protein intake. Several of the problems with accurate tracer measurement of amino acid oxidation are discussed by Waterlow,[5] and in Chapter 2 of this book. Most short-term oxidation measurements (8 h or less) indicate that the increased or decreased fed-state leucine oxidation evoked by high or low leucine intakes is carried over into the basal periods between meals,[50,51,61,62] but this is not the case in all of them.[14,63] A discussion of this issue and the role of the diurnal pattern of tracer amino acid oxidation may be found in Chapter 2.

As measured using tracers of leucine or phenylalanine, basal proteolysis appears to be little affected by changes of customary protein intake above the requirement level in most[14,50,51,63] studies, but this is not a universal finding.[45,64] Basal proteolysis is markedly reduced after adaptation to protein restriction below the minimum requirement.[26,45,46] Essential amino acid deficiency also promptly reduces whole-body protein turnover.[65] There has been much debate about the effect of the fed state on whole-body proteolysis and protein synthesis.[66,67] But as Pacy et al.[50] point out, the results of any such measurements, including ones based on sophisticated tracer models,[23,54,68-70] may depend critically on what protein level the subject is adapted to, how much protein is fed, and even how it is fed. As a general rule, any measurement can only be interpreted in light of the specific biologic hypothesis it is testing, and the subject's prior state of adaptation has to be appropriately chosen for the test.

5.6.1 FORM OF TEST MEALS

It is plausible to assume that the body regulates its affairs in a way to make details about the frequency and composition of individual meals, subsidiary to its main concern of meeting its tissue requirements for depositing or mobilizing protein. This assumption does not preclude the need for a little time to adapt to abrupt changes in meal format. The technical designs currently used in clinical research implicitly make this assumption, as, for example, when they involve lengthy, continuous-fed states in order to achieve the metabolic and isotopic steady state required by tracer models. Conventionally, humans consume food over relatively short periods of 10 to 30 minutes, two or three times daily.

In a study described earlier, Price et al.[49] observed that during surfeit protein consumption postabsorptive protein losses actually drive fed-state gains (since the negative nitrogen balance that occurs in the post-absorptive state can only be compensated by a strongly positive nitrogen balance during the subsequent meal), and these authors draw important conclusions from this observation. But it is unclear how important the phenomenon is in light of the way the subjects were fed. For technical reasons, leucine oxidation was measured during only the first 4 h of the fed state; but, as the authors acknowledged, this might not have accurately depicted leucine oxidation during the latter part of the 12 h fed period. The reason for suspecting this is clear if one imagines a fed state being extended all the way to 24 h. During such continuous feeding, nitrogen excretion must very soon rise to equal nitrogen intake. It is therefore quite likely that during the final hours of even a 12 h high-protein fed state, leucine oxidation will be greater than during the initial few hours. In fact, the authors' assumption that leucine oxidation as measured only during the first few hours of their fed period represented leucine oxidation throughout the entire 12 h led to an apparent underestimation of whole-body protein oxidation, when compared to measured urinary nitrogen loss. There is also a flaw in assuming that leucine oxidation measured during the final few hours of the basal state, as was done[49], represents leucine oxidation throughout. It is plausible to imagine that as protein intake increases, fed-state leucine oxidation increases, not just in rate, but also in its *duration* after the meal is concluded. Flatt[71] has shown that this occurs with glucose oxidation during carbohydrate overfeeding, and it is strongly suggested by some of the instantaneous leucine oxidation data of El-Khoury et al.[72]

While it may be desirable to provide more physiologic test meals, the temptation to use nonsteady-state amino acid turnover models[23] in this situation should, in my view, be resisted. Such models are elegantly used in glucose studies, but glucose is distributed where it can be measured in the extracellular space, and it enters the circulation only from the liver. Amino acids enter the circulation from all the tissues, and they are mostly distributed inside the cells; plasma measurements do not permit an accurate prediction of that distribution. Most importantly, unlike glucose, there is no way at present to validate the accuracy of any nonsteady-state amino acid turnover model. This may not be true of leucine oxidation, however. It is theoretically valid to argue[23,72] that leucine oxidation can be measured under nonsteady-state conditions, as long as the conditions are sufficiently invariant that expired labeled CO_2 appearance pertains to plasma ketoisocaproate enrichment, which should reflect the intracellular enrichment of the ketoisocaproate that was oxidized to release the expired $^{13}CO_2$.

We have developed a different approach for measuring fed-state amino acid catabolism that is not dependent on steady-state analysis, called the "oral protein tolerance test." The test is simply a short-term "metabolic" nitrogen balance study, in which urinary urea nitrogen excretion is measured over the 9 h following consumption of a test meal of precise composition, and from this body protein balance (N consumed minus urea nitrogen produced) and net protein utilization (N retained/N consumed) are calculated. The problem of the slow turnover of the body urea pool is mitigated by making an appropriate adjustment to urinary urea excretion to account for any change in whole-body urea over the same time period, as indicated by a changing plasma concentration. The test meal protocol has the advantage that it is a natural, normal-sized meal, for steady state is not required. [15N]alanine may be included in each test meal, and its recovery as [15N]urea in urine and plasma used as an index of "first pass" catabolism of the amino acids in the test meal.[15,60] It should be noted that this method considers only urinary urea excretion and any change in the urea in total body water, ignoring urea that is lost by nonurinary routes (chiefly bacterial hydrolysis in the large intestine). This can be corrected by including a tracer amount of [13C]urea in the test meal, and measuring its recovery in plasma and urine. For example, if 70% of the tracer is recovered, it is assumed that 70% of true urea production ended up in urine and body water and 30% elsewhere, and this correction is applied.[60]

5.6.2 WHICH TRACER MODEL?

As described in Chapter 2, the most widely used and validated tracer used in whole-body amino acid research is [1-13C]leucine, with measurement of plasma ketoiso-caproate enrichment as the precursor for flux and oxidation. For regional studies, phenylalanine has the advantage that it is not oxidized by muscle. The 15N end-product model is also described in Chapter 2. In my view, this model is theoretically unsatisfactory, but this does not mean it is without any merit at all.[8] The results of its use in protein restriction studies have not been particularly revealing. In one early study that used 60 h of continuous [15N]glycine administration (thus encompassing both the fed and fasting states), protein restriction to 0.4 g/kg per day substantially increased proteolysis and protein synthesis,[73] but in two subsequent studies of similar design, protein restriction neither increased or decreased proteolysis and protein synthesis.[74,75] Most current studies have, for reasons of simplicity and convenience, employed the technique of single dose [15N]glycine administration, followed by a 9 or 12 h urine collection period, in which ammonia and/or urea are used as end products.[76,77] In a fed-state study, Pacy et al.[50] observed no significant effect of dietary protein level on proteolysis and protein synthesis, whereas Pannemans et al., in a basal study,[78] found proteolysis and protein synthesis significantly lower on a 0.8 g protein/kg per day diet than on one that provided 1.25 g protein/kg per day. Basal leucine turnover was measured in the same subjects, and was unaffected by the protein level of the diet, directly contradicting the end-product model results.

We analyzed the 15N enrichment in plasma amino acids and in urea after subjects consumed a test meal that included [15N]alanine. Subjects first were studied after adaptation to a typical high-protein diet, then once again after 5 days of protein restriction.[60] Our data suggest that a person adapted to protein deficiency absorbs and distributes the 15N introduced by [15N]alanine as widely in the free amino acid pool in both situations. However, following adaptation to severe protein restriction, an important fraction of the 15N in the test meal is saved from ureagenesis by first-pass sequestration within newly synthesized splanchnic or hepatic proteins. If this is correct, the end-product model cannot be valid in this setting, for label seques-tration prior to mixing in the entire free nitrogen pool will lead the model to factitiously overestimate Q (and hence S and B).

5.7 PROLONGED PROTEIN DEFICIENCY

In a study of protein restriction to treat chronic renal failure, six months' adherence to a protein intake of only 0.4 g/kg per day caused weight loss and reduced serum transferrin, but not albumin concentrations.[79] The investigators attributed the weight loss to aversion to components of the diet. But energy supplementation did not lead to weight regain, suggesting that at least some of the weight loss was due to lean tissue loss. Thus, protein-restricted, conventionally treated diabetic patients lost muscular strength that was not accompanied by weight loss because of a concurrent increase in fat mass.[61] Also in concurrence are the results of a detailed protein-restriction study, in which elderly but healthy women were randomized to diets providing either surfeit (0.92 g/kg) or inadequate (0.45 g/kg) daily protein intakes with adequate energy.[80,81] After 9 weeks, the women fed inadequate protein sustained no weight loss, and their nitrogen balance was only slightly negative (-0.35 g N per day), indicating successful accommodation to protein restriction, but, unlike the control subjects, their body cell mass was significantly reduced and their muscle function and immune status were impaired.[80] The protein restriction had no effect on basal plasma leucine concentration, nor on *fed-state* proteolysis or protein synthesis (measured either per kg of body weight or fat-free mass), nor on urinary 3-methylhistidine excretion.[81] Serum albumin and the concentrations of the liver secretory proteins, retinol-binding protein, and transferrin remained normal.[80] Evidently, plasma concentrations of these proteins provide less insight into the adaptation to protein deficiency than would measurement of their actual synthesis, secretion, and removal rates. This study provides evidence that plasma transthyretin (prealbumin), retinol binding protein, and transferrin concentrations, often taken as indicators of the adequacy of protein nutrition, are far more sensitive to carbohydrate and total energy intake than to protein nutrition per se.[82,83] In more severe or prolonged protein deficiency, the serum albumin concentration is reduced,[84] indicating a more severe degree of compromise, despite the presence of normal fat stores.

This recent study[80,81] is a clear demonstration of accommodation. It is intriguing that the parameters one would have most relied upon — body weight, serum secretory proteins, nitrogen balance, proteolysis and protein synthesis measured by leucine kinetics, and urinary 3-methylhistidine excretion — all proved to be insensitive for detecting the true physiologic compromise that protein restriction exacted on the subjects. Instead, this was demonstrated by changed body composition and by such functional tests as muscle function and immune system responsiveness. Regrettably, *basal* proteolysis and protein synthesis, which may indicate accommodation most reliably or precisely, were not measured. More research in this area is needed.

5.8 PROTEIN RESTRICTION IN DISEASE

Research on the effects of disease on human adaptability is conceptually easier than research aimed at explaining the normal response to protein restriction: deep insight is not required, only the demonstration that the responses of the patient group of interest are the same or different from a suitable, normal control group. The difficulties lie in recruiting sufficient numbers of suitable patients for study, and in designing practical, robust test protocols to which subjects will readily give consent. For our diabetes studies, we have taken the position that our findings may help to define the role of insulin in regulating the adaptation to protein restriction; this is surely an oversimplification, since human diabetes is more than simple insulin lack. The major conclusion from these studies is that abnormal protein metabolism will be virtually unapparent and probably inconsequential in intensively and conventionally treated insulin-dependent diabetes, as long as the protein intake is well above the normal requirement level.[25] Intensively, but not conventionally treated patients may be able to adapt to protein restriction on the normal minimum requirement level.[25,61,64]

5.9   EFFECTS OF CHANGING BODY COMPOSITION

This creates difficult problems for interpreting protein metabolic data. It is common practice to present turnover or amino acid oxidation data per kg of body weight, reasonably enough since a person with a larger active protein mass has more protein turning over and a protein requirement which can be assumed to be proportional. Some studies, especially ones that involve obese or underweight subjects, correctly present data per unit of lean body mass or body cell mass; this is helpful, despite the uncertainties involved in such measurements. Strictly speaking, however, it is not valid to express metabolic results this way. The lean tissue compartment itself is inhomogeneous with respect to energy and protein metabolism,[85,86] and losses occur unequally from its various sub-compartments in the process of accommodation. This problem has been most clearly illustrated with energy expenditure measurements,[87,88] but it must be just the same for protein turnover. For example, a study of adults with chronic energy deficiency revealed their whole-body protein turnover per kg of fat-free mass to be greater than normal. This was attributed to the markedly greater loss of slowly turning over skeletal muscle than of rapidly turning over central proteins in these adapted, starving persons.[89]

5.10 CONCLUSION

There are good reasons for wishing to understand the nature of human adaptation to variations in dietary protein intake. Even if not fully understood, these effects are not trivial and need to be recognized when designing and interpreting research studies. Hormones, body composition, and dietary protein (and energy) intake are the factors which modify human protein metabolism, yet most human protein turnover studies are conducted on subjects adapted to "conventional" protein intakes, with little regard to the modulating effects of prior protein intake. In fact, there is no standard human basal or fed-state value for any parameter of protein turnover. In particular, fed-state amino acid metabolism is determined not only by the precise composition of the meal that is eaten, but also by the prior state of adaptation. Results can be expected to differ if the prior state of adaptation is for increased efficiency, rather than elimination of an excess, as in most fed-state studies published to this date. Studies conducted only above the minimum requirement level are unlikely to provide information about the protein requirement or about its regulatory mechanisms.

REFERENCES

1. Carpenter, K. J., *Protein and Energy: A Study of Changing Ideas in Nutrition*, Cambridge University Press, New York, 1994.
2. Young, V. R., Adult amino acid requirements: the case for a major revision in current recommendations, *J. Nutr.*, 124, 1517S, 1994.
3. Fuller, M. F. and Garlick, P. J., Human amino acid requirements: can the controversy be resolved? *Ann. Rev. Nutr.*, 14, 217, 1994.
4. Millward, D. J. and Pacy, P. J., Postprandial protein utilization and protein quality assessment in man, *Clin. Sci.*, 88, 597, 1995.
5. Waterlow, J. C., The requirements of adult man for indispensable amino acids, *Eur. J. Clin. Nutr.*, 50, S151, 1996.
6. Hegsted, D. M. Protein and energy: a study of changing ideas in nutrition, *Am. J. Clin. Nutr.*, 61, 163, 1995.
7. Waterlow, J. C., Where do we go from here? *J. Nutr.*, 124, 1524S, 1994.
8. Waterlow, J. C., Whole-body protein turnover in humans — past, present, and future, *Ann. Rev. Nutr.*, 15, 57, 1995.
9. Richards, P. and Brown, C. L., Urea metabolism in an azotæmic woman with normal renal function, *Lancet*, 2, 207, 1975.
10. Waterlow, J. C., What do we mean by adaptation? in *Nutritional Adaptation in Man*, Blaxter, K. and Waterlow, J. C., Eds., John Libbey, London, 1985, 1.
11. Young, V. R. and Marchini, J. S., Mechanisms and nutritional significance of metabolic responses to altered intakes of protein and amino acids, with reference to nutritional adaptation in humans, *Am. J. Clin. Nutr.*, 51, 270, 1990.
12. Krebs, H. A. Some aspects of the regulation of fuel supply in omnivorous animals, *Adv. Enz. Reg.*, 10, 397, 1972.
13. Millward, D. J. and Rivers, J. P. W., The nutritional role of indispensable amino acids and the metabolic basis for their requirements, *Eur. J. Clin. Nutr.*, 42, 367, 1988.
14. Zello, G. A., Telch, J., Clarke, R., Ball, R. O., and Pencharz, P. B., Reexamination of protein requirements in adult male humans by end-product measurements of leucine and lysine metabolism, *J. Nutr.*, 122, 1000, 1992.
15. Taveroff, A., Lapin, H., and Hoffer, L. J., Mechanism governing short-term fed-state adaptation to dietary protein restriction, *Metabolism*, 43, 320, 1993.
16. Taveroff, A. and Hoffer, L. J., Are leucine turnover measurements valid in the intravenously fed state? *Metabolism*, 43, 1338, 1993.
17. FAO/WHO/UNU Expert Consultation, *Energy and Protein Requirements. Technical Report Series No. 724*, World Health Organization, Geneva, 1985.
18. Crim, M. C. and Munro, H. N., Proteins and amino acids, in *Modern Nutrition in Health and Disease*, 8th Ed., Shils M. E., Olson J. A., and Shike M., Eds., Lea and Febiger, Philadelphia, 1994, 3.
19. Rand, W. M., Scrimshaw, N. S., and Young, V. R., Determination of protein allowances in human adults from nitrogen balance data, *Am. J. Clin. Nutr.*, 30, 1129, 1977.
20. Young, V. R., Bier, D. M., and Pellett, P. L., A theoretical basis for increasing current estimates of the amino acid requirements in adult man, with experimental support, *Am. J. Clin. Nutr.*, 50, 80, 1989.

21. Zello, G. A., Wykes, L. J., Ball, R. O., and Pencharz, P. B., Recent advances in methods of assessing dietary amino acid requirements for adult humans, *J. Nutr.*, 125, 2907, 1995.

22. Hoffer, L. J., Taveroff, A., Robitaille, L., Hamadeh, M. J., and Mamer, O. A., Effects of exogenous leucine on whole-body leucine, valine and threonine metabolism in man, *Am. J. Physiol.*, 272, E1037, 1997.

23. Boirie, Y., Gachon, P., Corny, S., Fauquant, J., Maubois, J-L., and Beaufrere, B., Acute postprandial changes in leucine metabolism as assessed with an intrinsically labeled milk protein, *Am. J. Physiol.*, 271, E1083, 1996.

24. Hamadeh, M. J. and Hoffer, L. J., Tracer methods underestimate short-term variations in urea production in humans, *Am. J. Physiol.*, 274, E547, 1998.

25. Hoffer, L. J., Adaptation to protein restriction is impaired in insulin-dependent diabetes mellitus, *J. Nutr.*, 128, 333S, 1998.

26. Lariviere, F., Kupranycz, D., Chiasson, J-L., and Hoffer, L. J., Plasma leucine kinetics and urinary nitrogen excretion in intensively-treated diabetes mellitus, *Am. J. Physiol.*, 263, E173, 1992.

27. El-Khoury, A. E., Fukagawa, N. K., Sanchez, M., Tsay, R. H., Gleason, R. E., Chapman, T. E., and Young, V. R., Validation of the tracer-balance concept with reference to leucine: 24-h intravenous tracer studies with L-[1-^{13}C]leucine and [^{15}N-^{15}N]urea, *Am. J. Clin. Nutr.*, 59, 1000, 1994.

28. Scrimshaw, N. S., Criteria for valid nitrogen balance measurements of protein requirements, *Eur. J. Clin. Nutr.*, 50, S196, 1997.

29. Waterlow, J. C., Metabolic adaptation to low intakes of energy and protein, *Ann. Rev. Nutr.*, 6, 495, 1986.

30. Lusk, G., *The Science of Nutrition,* 4th Ed., W.B. Saunders, Philadelphia, 1928.

31. Joint Food and Agriculture Organization/World Health Organization Expert Committee, *Energy and Protein Requirements. WHO Technical Report Series No. 522,* World Health Organization, Geneva, 1973.

32. Munro, H. N., Historical perspective on protein requirements: objectives for the future, in *Nutritional Adaptation in Man,* Blaxter K. and Waterlow J. C., Eds., John Libbey, London, 1985, 155.

33. Peret, J. and Jacquot, R., Nitrogen excretion on complete fasting and on a nitrogen-free diet — endogenous protein, in *Protein and Amino Acid Functions,* Bigwood E. J., Ed., Pergamon Press, Oxford, 1972, 73.

34. Munro, H. N., General aspects of the regulation of protein metabolism by diet and hormones, in *Mammalian Protein Metabolism.,* Vol.1, Munro H. N. and Allison J. B., Eds., Academic Press, New York, 1964, 381.

35. Young, V. R., Hussein, M. A., and Scrimshaw, N. S., Estimate of loss of labile body nitrogen during acute protein deprivation in young adults, *Nature*, 218, 568, 1968.

36. Munro, H. N., Free amino acid pools and their regulation, in *Mammalian Protein Metabolism.* Vol. 4., Munro H. N., Ed., Academic Press, New York, 1970, 299.

37. Bergström, J., Fürst, P., Noree, L-O., and Vinnars, E., Intracellular free amino acid concentration in human muscle tissue, *J. Appl. Physiol.*, 36, 693, 1974.

38. Waterlow, J. C. and Fern, E. B., Free amino acid pools and their regulation, in *Nitrogen Metabolism in Man.,* Waterlow J. C. and Stephen J. M. L., Eds., Applied Science Publishers, London, 1981, 1.

39. Millward, D. J., The hormonal control of protein turnover, *Clin. Nutr.*, 9, 115, 1990.

40. Millward, D. J., Human protein requirements: the physiological significance of changes in the rate of whole-body protein turnover, in *Substrate and Energy Metabolism in Man*, Garrow J. S. and Halliday D., Eds., John Libbey, London, 1985, 135.

41. McNurlan, M. A., Pain, V. M., and Garlick, P. J., Conditions that alter rates of tissue protein synthesis in vivo, *Biochem. Soc. Trans.*, 8, 283, 1980.

42. Gelfand, R. A., Glickman, M. G., Jacob, R., Sherwin, R. S., and DeFronzo, R. A., Removal of infused amino acids by splanchnic and leg tissues in humans, *Am. J. Physiol.*, 250, E407, 1986.

43. Abumrad, N. N., Williams, P., Frexes-Steed, M., Geer, R., Flakoll, P., Cersosimo, E., Brown, L. L., Melki, I., Bulus, N., Hourani, H., Hubbard, M., and Ghishan, F., Inter-organ metabolism of amino acids in vivo, *Diabetes Metab. Rev.*, 5, 213, 1989.

44. Rand, W. M., Young, V. R., and Scrimshaw, N. S., Change of urinary nitrogen excretion in response to low-protein diets in adults, *Am. J. Clin. Nutr.*, 29, 639, 1976.

45. Motil, K. J., Matthews, D. E., Bier, D. M., Burke, J. F., and Munro, H. N., Whole-body leucine and lysine metabolism: response to dietary protein intake in young men, *Am. J. Physiol.*, 240, E712, 1981.

46. Yang, R. D., Matthews, D. E., Bier, D. M., Wen, Z. M., and Young, V. R., Response of alanine metabolism in humans to manipulation of dietary protein and energy intakes, *Am. J. Physiol.*, 250, E39, 1986.

47. Lariviere, F., Wagner, D. A., Kupranycz, D., and Hoffer, L. J., Prolonged fasting as conditioned by prior protein depletion: effect on urinary nitrogen excretion and whole-body protein turnover, *Metabolism*, 39, 1270, 1990.

48. Wahren, J., Felig, P., and Hagenfeldt, L. J., Effect of protein ingestion on splanchnic and leg metabolism in normal man and in patients with diabetes mellitus, *J. Clin. Invest.*, 57, 987, 1976.

49. Price, G. M., Halliday, D., Pacy, P. J., Quevedo, R. M., and Millward, D. J., Nitrogen homeostasis in man: influence of protein intake on the amplitude of diurnal cycling of body nitrogen, *Clin. Sci.*, 86, 91, 1994.

50. Pacy, P. J., Price, G. M., Halliday, D., Quevedo, M. R., and Millward, D. J., Nitrogen homeostasis in man: the diurnal responses of protein synthesis and degradation and amino acid oxidation to diets with increasing protein intakes, *Clin. Sci.*, 86, 103, 1994.

51. Quevedo, M. R., Price, G. M., Halliday, D., Pacy, P. J., and Millward, D. J., Nitrogen homeostasis in man: diurnal changes in nitrogen excretion, leucine oxidation and whole body leucine kinetics during a reduction from a high to a moderate protein intake, *Clin. Sci.*, 86, 185, 1994.

52. De Feo, P., Horber, F. F., and Haymond, M. W., Meal stimulation of albumin synthesis: a significant contributor to whole body protein synthesis in humans, *Am. J. Physiol.*, 263, E794, 1992.

53. Hunter, K. A., Ballmer, P. E., Anderson, S. E., Broom, J., Garlick, P. J., and McNurlan, M. A., Acute stimulation of albumin synthesis rate with oral meal feeding in healthy subjects measured with [ring-^{2}H$_5$]phenylalanine, *Clin. Sci.*, 88, 235, 1995.

54. Cayol, M., Boirie, Y., Rambourdin, F., Prugnaud, J., Gachon, P., Beaufrere, B., and Obled, C., Influence of protein intake on whole body and splanchnic leucine kinetics in humans, *Am. J. Physiol.*, 272, E584, 1997.

55. Kelman, L., Saunders, S. J., Frith, L., Wicht, S., and Corrigal, A., Effects of dietary protein restriction on albumin synthesis, albumin catabolism, and the plasma aminogram, *Am. J. Clin. Nutr.*, 25, 1174, 1972.

56. Giesecke, K., Magnusson, I., Ahlberg, M., Hagenfeldt, L., and Wahren, J., Protein and amino acid metabolism during early starvation as reflected by excretion of urea and methylhistidines, *Metabolism*, 38, 1196, 1989.

57. Walser, M. Misinterpretation of nitrogen balances when glutamine stores fall or are replenished, *Am. J. Clin. Nutr.*, 53, 1337, 1991.

58. Bergström, J., Fürst, P., and Vinnars, E., Effect of a test meal, without and with protein, on muscle and plasma free amino acids, *Clin. Sci.*, 79, 331, 1990.

59. Weller, L. A., Margen, S., and Howes Calloway, D.,Variation in fasting and postprandial amino acids of men fed adequate or protein-free diets, *Am. J. Clin. Nutr.*, 22, 1577, 1969.

60. Hoffer, L. J., Taveroff, A., and Schiffrin, A., Metabolic adaptation to protein restriction in insulin-dependent diabetes mellitus, *Am. J. Physiol.*, 272, E:59, 1997.

61. Brodsky, I. G., Robbins, D. C., Hiser, E., Fuller, S. P., Fillyaw, M., and Devlin, J. T., Effects of low-protein diets on protein metabolism in insulin-dependent diabetes mellitus patients with early nephropathy, *J. Clin. Endocrinol. Metab.*, 75, 351, 1992.

62. Hoffer, L. J., Taveroff, A., and Hamadeh, M. J., Dietary protein restriction alters glucose but not protein metabolism in NIDDM, *Metabolism*, 47(9), 1145, 1998.

63. Goodship, T. H. J., Mitch, W. E., Hoerr, R. A., Wagner, D. A., Steinman, T. I., and Young, V. R., Adaptation to low-protein diets in renal failure: leucine turnover and nitrogen balance, *J. Am. Soc. Nephrol.*, 1, 66, 1990.

64. Brodsky, I. G. and Devlin, J. T., Effects of dietary protein restriction on regional amino acid metabolism in insulin-dependent diabetes mellitus, *Am. J. Physiol.*, 270, E148, 1996.

65. Marchini, J. S., Cortiella, J., Hiramatsu, T., Chapman, T. E., and Young, V. R., Requirements for indispensable amino acids in adult humans: longer-term amino acid kinetic study with support for the adequacy of the Massachusetts Institute of Technology amino acid requirement pattern, *Am. J. Clin. Nutr.*, 58, 670, 1993.

66. McNurlan, M. A. and Garlick, P. J., Influence of nutrient intake on protein turnover, *Diabetes Metab. Rev.*, 5, 165, 1989.

67. Garlick, P. J., McNurlan, M. A., and Ballmer, P. E., Influence of dietary protein intake on whole-body protein turnover in humans, *Diabetes Care*, 14, 1189, 1991.

68. Nissen, S. and Haymond, M. W., Changes in leucine kinetics during meal absorption: effects of dietary leucine availability, *Am. J. Physiol.*, 250, E695, 1986.

69. Matthews, D. E., Marano, M. A., and Campbell, R. G., Splanchnic bed utilization of leucine and phenylalanine in humans, *Am. J. Physiol.*, 264, E109, 1993.

70. Biolo, G., Tessari, P., Inchiostro, S., Bruttomesso, D., Fongher, C., Sabadin, L., Fratton, M. G., Valerio, A., and Tiengo, A., Leucine and phenylalanine kinetics during mixed meal ingestion: a multiple tracer approach, *Am. J. Physiol.*, 262, E455, 1992.

71. Flatt, J. P., Diet, lifestyle, and weight maintenance, *Am. J. Clin. Nutr.*, 62, 820, 1998.

72. El-Khoury, A. E., Fukagawa, N. K., Sanchez, M., Tsay, R. H., Gleason, R. E., Chapman, T. E., and Young, V. R., The 24-h pattern and rate of leucine oxidation, with particular reference to tracer estimates of leucine requirements in healthy adults, *Am. J. Clin. Nutr.*, 59, 1012, 1994.

73. Steffee, W. P., Goldsmith, R. S., Pencharz, P. B., Scrimshaw, N. S., and Young, V. R., Dietary protein intake and dynamic aspects of whole body nitrogen metabolism in adult humans, *Metabolism*, 25, 281, 1976.

74. Gersovitz, M., Bier, D. M., Matthews, D. E., Udall, J., Munro, H. N., and Young, V. R., Dynamic aspects of whole body glycine metabolism: influence of protein intake in young adult and elderly males, *Metabolism*, 29, 1087, 1980.

75. Meredith, C. N., Zackin, M. J., Frontera, W. R., and Evans, W. J., Dietary protein requirements and body protein metabolism in endurance-trained men, *J. Appl. Physiol.*, 66, 2850, 1989.

76. Fern, E. B., Garlick, P. J., McNurlan, A., and Waterlow, J. C., The excretion of isotope in urea and ammonia for estimating protein turnover in man with [15N]-glycine, *Clin. Sci.*, 61, 217, 1981.

77. Fern, E. B., Garlick, P. J., Sheppard, H. G., and Fern, M., The precision of measuring the rate of whole-body nitrogen flux and protein synthesis in man with a single dose of [15N]-glycine, *Human Nutr.: Clin. Nutr.*, 38C, 63, 1984.

78. Pannemans, L. E., Halliday, D., Westerterp, K. R., and Kester, A. D. M., Effect of dietary protein on bed-rest-related changes in whole-body-protein synthesis, *Am. J. Clin. Nutr.*, 61, 69, 1995.

79. Ihle, B. U., Becker, G., Whitworth, J. A., Charlwood, R. A., and Kincaid-Smith, P. S., The effect of protein restriction on the progression of renal insufficiency, *N. Engl. J. Med.*, 321, 1773, 1989.

80. Castaneda, C., Charnley, J. M., Evans, W. J., and Crim, M. C., Elderly women accommodate to a low-protein diet with losses of body cell mass, muscle function, and immune response, *Am. J. Clin. Nutr.*, 62, 30, 1995.

81. Castaneda, C., Dolnikowski, G. G., Dallal, G. E., Evans, W. J., and Crim, M. C., Protein turnover and energy metabolism of elderly women fed a low-protein diet, *Am. J. Clin. Nutr.*, 62, 40, 1995.

82. Shetty, P. S., Watrasiewicz, K. E., Jung, R. T., and James, W. P. T., Rapid-turnover transport proteins: an index of subclinical protein-energy malnutrition, *Lancet*, 2, 230, 1979.

83. Hoffer, L. J., Bistrian, B. R., Young, V. R., Blackburn, G. L., and Wannemacher, R. W., Metabolic effects of carbohydrate in low-calorie diets, *Metabolism*, 33, 820, 1984.

84. Barac-Nieto, M., Spurr, G. B., Lotero, H., and Maksud, M. G., Body composition in chronic undernutrition, *Am. J. Clin. Nutr.*, 31, 23, 1978.

85. Weinsier, R. L., Schutz, Y., and Bracco, D., Reexamination of the relationship of resting metabolic rate to fat-free mass and to the metabolically active components of fat-free mass in humans, *Am. J. Clin. Nutr.*, 55, 790, 1992.

86. Elia, M., The inter-organ flux of substrates in fed and fasted man, as indicated by arterio-venous balance studies, *Nutr. Res. Rev.*, 4, 3, 1991.

87. Ravussin, E. and Bogardus, C., Relationship of genetics, age, and physical fitness to daily energy expenditure and fuel utilization, *Am. J. Clin. Nutr.*, 49, 968, 1989.

88. Allison, D. B., Paultre, F., Goran, M. I., Poehlman, E. T., and Heymsfield, S. B., Statistical considerations regarding the use of ratios to adjust data, *Int. J. Obes.*, 19, 644, 1995.

89. Soares, M. J., Piers, L. S., Shetty, P. S., Jackson, A. A., and Waterlow, J. C., Whole body protein turnover in chronically undernourished individuals, *Clin. Sci.*, 86, 441, 1994.

6 Determination of Amino Acid Isotopic Enrichment: Methods, Difficulties, and Calculations

Bruce W. Patterson

CONTENTS

0-8493-9612-3/99/$0.00+$.50
© 1999 by CRC Press LLC

6.1　INTRODUCTION

Stable isotopically labeled amino acids are used extensively in studies of protein and amino acid metabolism at the whole-body and tissue levels. The gas chromatograph-mass spectrometer (GC-MS) is a versatile instrument to measure the isotopic enrichment of amino acids. Investigators today are faced with diverse GC-MS methods, which combine a variety of derivatives available for amino acid separation by gas chromatography (GC) with different ionization modes for mass spectrometer (MS) operation. Adding to this diversity is a variety of approaches that are used to calculate isotopic enrichments from GC-MS measurements.

This chapter provides a critical review of methods commonly used to measure amino acid and keto acid enrichment by conventional GC-MS. The reader is directed to Chapter 7 by Metges and Petzke which discusses the complementary technique of GC-C-IRMS, whereby a GC is connected to a gas isotope ratio mass spectrometer through a combustion interface.

6.2.　GC-MS METHODS

6.2.1　GAS CHROMATOGRAPHY

Amino acids are not volatile, and therefore need to be derivatized in order to be separated by GC. An extensive variety of derivatives has been used for GC analysis of amino acids.[1] Derivatives are chosen based on their ease of preparation, stability, and optimal GC performance. Most importantly, derivatives are chosen based on formation of suitable ions for MS analysis of the specific isotopically labeled position(s) in the tracer amino acid. Many derivatives require a two-step procedure: esterification of the free carboxyl group and acylation of the amino (and sometimes hydroxyl) groups. However, some reagents (especially those producing silyl derivatives) conveniently derivatize carboxyl, amino, and hydroxyl groups in a single step. A GC column and temperature parameters are chosen to provide optimal baseline separation of desired derivatized components, with minimal peak tailing. Today, most separations are performed on capillary columns, which provide excellent resolution and minimal carrier gas flow. High resolution may be required for some applications (e.g., separation of leucine and isoleucine). A fused silica capillary column with a bonded phase of 5% phenyl, 95% methyl silicone of 15- to 30-m length is generally a good choice for most amino acid applications. Alternatively, packed columns provide adequate resolution for many amino acid applications, usually with faster run times than capillary columns. The effluent from a packed column must pass through a jet separator prior to passage into the MS, with a reduction in sensitivity.

6.2.2.　MASS SPECTROMETRY

6.2.2.1　Ionization Mode

The GC effluent passes into the source of the MS, where the organic molecules become ionized. In *electron impact ionization* (EI), a molecule is hit by an energetic electron emitted by a filament, resulting in loss of an electron from the molecule to form a positively charged molecular ion $[M]^+$. The molecular ion dissipates excess energy by fragmenting into a spectrum of ions characteristic of the structure of the parent molecule. Frequently, no unfragmented molecular ions remain, and the isotopically substituted atom(s) in the parent molecule will be found in one or more fragments. This fragmentation causes a decrease in sensitivity, as the original signal carried by the molecular ions is dispersed across many fragments. This fragmentation may confer greater selectivity for an analysis in two ways. First, one fragment may produce a "cleaner" chromatogram than others. Second, fragmentation facilitates some analyses where it is necessary to differentiate the isotopic enrichment of separate portions of the parent molecule, such as the amide and amino nitrogens of glutamine.[2]

Chemical ionization (CI) is useful when fragmentation of the molecular ion is unacceptable, either because of decreased sensitivity or because it is preferable to retain the isotopically labeled position(s) in an intact molecule. In CI, a reagent gas (usually methane, but other gases can be used) is introduced into the ionization chamber at a steady rate. The reagent gas is ionized by EI, and the positively charged ions ionize the target compound through a series of reactions, typically resulting in a protonated molecular ion $[M+H]^+$. Less fragmentation of the molecular ion occurs with CI, because less excess energy is transferred to the molecular ion. A major disadvantage of CI is that greater contamination of the source occurs, such that more frequent cleanings are needed.

In *negative chemical ionization* (NCI, more appropriately termed electron capture negative ion chemical ionization), a gas such as methane is introduced into the source as in CI. This gas is used to quench the thermal energy of the electrons emitted by the filament, so they can be captured by the target molecules. Derivatives must be highly electronegative for efficient electron capture (e.g., highly fluorinated). Some fragmentation does occur with NCI, but the spectrum is typically dominated by a major fragment which retains the intact parent molecule (e.g., M-HF). A major advantage of NCI is increased sensitivity resulting from efficient ionization and reduced fragmentation. As with CI, however, the source may require more frequent cleanings.

6.2.2.2 Selected Ion Monitoring

Data for isotope ratio measurements by GC-MS is acquired by *selected ion monitoring* (SIM). Selected ions representing the unlabeled tracee and one or more labeled isotopomers are monitored for a specific fragment. Selectivity is enhanced, since nearby or co-eluting peaks may not generate the specific ions monitored for a target peak. Sensitivity (signal/noise ratio) is also enhanced, since the detector does not waste cycle time monitoring ions which are not of interest.

An instrument parameter controls the length of time (dwell time) each ion is monitored. As a general guideline, 15 to 20 data points are desired to define an ideal Gaussian-like chromatographic peak.[3] The accuracy of peak shape definition is reduced with fewer data points, whereas more data points introduce unnecessary noise (as the dwell time is too short) without a significant increase in peak shape accuracy. The optimal dwell time will depend on the width of the chromatographic peak and the number of ions that need to be monitored.

6.2.3 GC-MS METHODS

Although numerous methods have been used to measure amino acid isotopic enrichment, the most applicable methods for a wide range of amino acids fall within three major categories. Major features of the most commonly used derivatives are summarized in Table 6.1.

TABLE 6.1
Frequently Used Derivatives and Ionization Modes for Measurement of Amino Acid Isotopic Enrichment by GC-MS

Abbr.	Name	Ionization mode	Common base ion fragments*	Comments
NAP	N-acetyl n-propyl ester	CI	[M+H], [M+C$_2$H$_5$], [M+C$_3$H$_5$]	Good for most amino acids except glutamine/ asparagine
HFBPr	Heptafluorobutyryl n-propyl ester	NCI	[M-HF]	Good for most amino acids except glutamine/ asparagine
TMS	trimethylsilyl	EI	[M-CH$_3$], [M-COCH$_3$], [M-CO$_2$TMS], [M-sidechain]	Not useful for 1-^{13}C label
tBDMS	tert.- butyldimethylsilyl	EI	[M-CH$_3$], [M-C(CH$_3$)$_3$], [M-C(CH$_3$)$_3$-CO], [M-CO$_2$tBDMS], [M-sidechain]	Useful for all labels; glutamine/aspar agine measured

*The most abundant ions typically produced are underlined

6.2.3.1 N-Acetyl N-Propyl Ester

The N-acetyl n-propyl ester (NAP) derivative is used primarily in CI.[4-6] The major ion produced in CI is a protonated molecular ion [M+H]$^+$. Matthews et al.[4] used this derivative to monitor the incorporation of ^{15}N into 15 amino acids during a constant infusion of ^{15}N-leucine. The NAP derivative may be used in EI, although major fragments produced may not be useful for 1-^{13}C labeled amino acids, due to loss of the 1-C position.[7] The amide nitrogen of glutamine and asparagine is lost during the formation of NAP derivatives, as with any derivative which uses acidic alcohol (in this case, propanol) in its formation.

6.2.3.2   N-Perfluoroacyl Alkyl Esters

Many derivatives fall in this category, using various combinations of perfluorinated anhydride acylation reagents and alcohol esterification reagents. Some of these combinations include trifluoroacetyl methyl[8] or butyl[9,10] esters, pentafluoropropionyl butyl esters,[9] and heptafluorobutyryl propyl (HFBPr)[11,12] or isobutyl[13] esters. Different derivatives may be useful for specific amino acids to provide "clean" chromatographic peaks;[9] however, Berthold et al.[12] measured ^{13}C enrichment in 17 amino acids using only the HFBPr derivative. The perfluoroacyl alkyl ester derivatives are versatile for MS analysis, with applications reported using EI,[9,14] CI,[8,15] and NCI.[11-13] These derivatives are very sensitive in NCI, producing a major fragment at [M-20]$^-$ (loss of HF from the molecular ion), which retains all labeled atoms from the parent amino acid. Because of this sensitivity, the HFBPr derivative in NCI is useful to measure the enrichment of amino acids isolated from single purified proteins when only 10 to 50 μg of material is available for analysis,[11,16] or when very low enrichment of a highly substituted tracer (e.g., [2]H$_3$-leucine) is measured.[17] As with the NAP derivative, the amide nitrogen of glutamine and asparagine is lost during the derivatization process.

6.2.3.3   Silyl Derivatives

The trimethylsilyl (TMS) derivative is convenient for quantitative GC analysis of amino acids since amino, carboxyl, and hydroxyl groups are derivatized in a single step, although TMS derivatives are readily susceptible to hydrolysis.[1] Unfortunately, TMS has limited use for GC-MS analysis of tracer-labeled amino acids. Fragmentation in EI produces a major fragment at [M-117]$^+$ (M-CO$_2$TMS),[18] rendering this useless for amino acids labeled in the 1-C position. Other characteristic ions of TMS EI fragmentation (see Table 6.1) are present at low abundance, and have variable yield for different amino acids, and are not generally useful for GC-MS analysis. The TMS derivative has been useful in studies with deuterated and ^{15}N amino acids.[4,19] The use of silyl derivatives in CI is not generally recommended, due to rapid contamination of the MS source.

   In contrast, the *tert.*-butyldimethylsilyl (tBDMS) derivative is an excellent choice for general amino acid GC-MS analysis in EI. This derivative differs from TMS by the replacement of one methyl group with a tertiary butyl group; however, this derivative is much more stable to hydrolysis compared to TMS, and generates an EI fragmentation pattern that is very suitable for GC-MS analysis of amino acid tracers.[20] In particular, the characteristic [M-57] fragment (M-*tert.* butyl) is generally produced in large abundance for most amino acids and retains all labeled atoms from the parent molecule. Other fragments are also frequently produced in sufficient abundance to be useful for tracer amino acid GC-MS, notably the [M-159] fragment

(M-CO$_2$tBDMS, loss of 1-C label). The tBDMS derivative has been used to measure ^{15}N incorporation into 18 amino acids plus urea in a single GC-MS analysis.[2,21]

6.2.3.4   Glutamine/Glutamate and Arginine

The derivatives discussed above are useful for most general-purpose amino acid GC-MS analyses. However, certain amino acids require special consideration. Glutamine is converted to glutamate during derivatization procedures using acidic alcohol conditions, thereby negating the enrichment of both amino acids (the same problem occurs with asparagine/aspartate). One way to circumvent this problem is to separate glutamine and glutamate by ion exchange chromatography prior to derivatization,[6] although this precludes the measurement of amide ^{15}N glutamine enrichment. It is more convenient to use the tBDMS derivative which derivatizes glutamine (and asparagine) without loss of the amide nitrogen.[2] Furthermore, the EI fragmentation of tBDMS glutamine allows the ^{15}N enrichment of the amide and amino nitrogens to be resolved.[2,21] Arginine frequently decomposes during derivatization,[2] or undergoes fragmentation such that the enrichment of the guanidino nitrogens cannot be measured. The trifluoroacetyl methyl ester in NCI has been used to study interconversion of arginine, citrulline, and ornithine.[22]

6.2.3.5   Measuring Very Low Enrichments with GC-MS

Measurements of very low amino acid enrichment (e.g., muscle protein synthesis) traditionally require the use of ^{13}C tracers, combustion of the amino acid to CO$_2$, and the use of a gas isotope ratio mass spectrometer. However, very low enrichments (tracer:tracee ratios down to 0.002%) can be measured by conventional GC-MS. The approach requires a highly substituted tracer such as ring-^{2}H$_5$-phenylalanine,[23,24] ring-^{13}C$_6$-phenylalanine,[17] or ^{2}H$_3$-leucine,[17] and reducing the dynamic range of the ion abundance ratio measurement by using a lower abundance ion such as [m+2] to represent the unlabeled tracee, rather than the highly abundant [m+0] base ion. Phenylalanine has been analyzed as HFB[23] and tBDMS[24] derivatives in EI; phenylalanine was enzymatically converted to phenylethylamine prior to derivatization to obtain "clean" GC-MS chromatographic peaks in these reports. However, we have observed clean chromatography of phenylalanine using a conventional HFBPr derivative in EI.[17]

The approach requires a sensitive GC-MS analysis that is able to measure the natural abundance of the [m+x] substituted tracer. These measurements may be facilitated by NCI,[17] although EI may be used[17,23,24] if the analysis is sufficiently sensitive. See Patterson et al.[17] for a detailed discussion of analytical issues pertaining to this approach.

6.2.3.6   Keto Acids

A review of GC-MS methods for tracer amino acids would be incomplete without inclusion of methods for keto acids, which are frequently used as markers for intracellular amino acid precursor pool enrichment. Keto acids are typically isolated from plasma by anion exchange chromatography, and frequently analyzed as TMS[5,25] or tBDMS[26] derivatives following conversion to quinoxalinols. The TMS derivatives typically employ CI, whereas EI is used with the tBDMS derivative. Formation of quinoxalinols is tedious, and requires use of o-phenylenediamine-based reagents that are sensitive to oxygen and carcinogenic. Direct formation of a tBDMS derivative without prior conversion to quinoxalinols has been reported.[27] Hachey et al.[28] reported a convenient method to derivatize keto acids directly in plasma *in situ* by formation of pentafluorobenzyl (PFB) esters, followed by solvent extraction. The keto acid PFB esters produced intense $[M-181]^-$ ions in NCI representing loss of $CH_2C_6F_5$ from the molecular ion, as is characteristic of PFB derivatives.

6.2.3.7 Recent Advances

All methods discussed above for amino acid GC-MS analysis require isolation of amino acids (from plasma, protein, etc.), typically by ion exchange chromatography, followed by a drying step. Recent reports have demonstrated that amino acids can be derivatized directly within an aqueous milieu using chloroformate reagents. Ethyl chloroformate used with a water/ethanol/pyridine mixture produced N(O)-ethoxy-carbonyl ethyl esters suitable for EI;[29] for leucine and phenylalanine, the major fragments produced in EI lost the 1-C position, however, as with TMS amino acids in EI. Substitution of ethyl chloroformate with pentafluorobenzyl (PFB) chloro-formate produced N-pentafluorobenzyl-oxycarbonyl ethyl esters[30] suitable for NCI, with intense $[M-181]^-$ ions that retain all of the parent amino acid labels. A combination of methyl chloroformate followed by pentafluorobenzyl bromide produced N-methylformated PFB esters of amino acids and PFB esters of keto acids,[31] which were simultaneously extracted and analyzed by NCI. These methods reportedly work directly on whole blood or plasma *in situ*, and thus may eliminate the tedious procedures conventionally used to recover amino acids. Additional studies are needed to test the general utility of these methods for multiple amino acids.

6.3 PROBLEMS ASSOCIATED WITH AMINO ACID GC-MS ANALYSIS

6.3.1 SAMPLE PROCESSING ARTIFACTS

Amino acids are conventionally isolated from plasma, tissue pools, or protein hydrolysates by cation exchange chromatography.[32] Amino acid contamination of ion exchange resins has been reported;[33,34] such contamination may be reduced by preconditioning the resin before use with ultrapure acid/base solutions. Contamination can be monitored by including "blanks" during processing. Contamination may not be a problem if a sufficient quantity of amino acids is being isolated, e.g., from plasma or muscle protein hydrolysate. However, contamination was a significant problem when amino acids were recovered from 10 to 50 μg of plasma proteins isolated by polyacrylamide gel electrophoresis.[11] With stringent quality controls, contamination of less than 5% was documented by the inclusion of blanks in the processing. Based on the selectivity of the derivative, ionization mode, and SIM, it may not be necessary to use an ion exchange resin to purify amino acids from hydrolyzed polyacrylamide gels.[34]

Loss of label during sample processing can occur, especially with deuterated tracers. Hydrogen/deuterium (H/D) exchange can occur under certain conditions. For example, deuterium was lost from ring-^{2}H$_5$-phenylalanine during 24-h hydrolysis at 110°C in 10 N and 6 N HCl, but not in 4 N HCl.[14] Deuterium was not lost from 5,5,5-^{2}H$_3$-leucine under the same conditions. Exchange of isotopic label should always be considered when working with deuterated tracers; such exchange can occur within metabolic pathways *in vivo*, during sample isolation, and derivatization. Absence of exchange should be verified using labeled standards. Exchange of ^{13}C and ^{15}N labels is less likely to occur.

6.3.2 GAS CHROMATOGRAPHY ARTIFACTS

Artifacts associated with GC are usually easy to identify and eliminate. Peak overloading results in distorted peaks that may not integrate properly. Furthermore, overloaded peaks may obscure other components underlying the chromatographic peak. Overloading can be eliminated by reducing the amount of sample injected. The absence of interfering components can be verified by varying the GC temperature ramp conditions. Once the absence of extraneous components in biological samples is verified with a slow temperature ramp, the ramp rate can be increased for faster run times and improved sensitivity (provided resolution from nearby chromatographic peaks is maintained). The absence of co-eluting contaminants should be verified with a full scan acquisition in addition to SIM; a co-eluting component may interfere with the MS analysis, although the component may not be visible during SIM acquisition.

6.3.3 MASS SPECTROMETRY ARTIFACTS

6.3.3.1 Instrument Tuning

Instrument tuning parameters that affect the spectral peak shape, peak width (spectral resolution), and mass axis calibration will affect measured ion abundance ratios for a given analysis. These tuning parameters are difficult, if not impossible, to control in a precise manner. The measured ion abundance ratios for a given application may thus be variable from one tuning condition to another. Furthermore, tuning conditions may drift over time, especially as the source becomes dirty (which affects the electromagnetic fields). Some instruments are equipped with an "autotune" feature to set tuning to a nominal condition. However, this may not be adequate for reproducible ion abundance ratio measurements.[35] Manual adjustment of tuning parameters to reproducible spectral resolution and mass axis calibration conditions may be preferred over autotune for precise ion abundance ratios.

6.3.3.2 Isotope Effects in MS Fragmentation

The strength of a molecular bond differs for isotopes of the atoms involved. The relative yield of fragment ions can thus be affected by the presence of isotopically substituted positions within the parent molecule. The measured ion abundance ratio of isotopically labeled fragments reflects the relative yield of that structural fragment from the labeled and unlabelled molecules.

TABLE 6.2

Example of Isotope Effects in the EI Fragmentation of tBDMS-Alanine

	Ions monitored			
	[M-159], *m/z* 158 [M-CO$_2$tBDMS]	[M-85], *m/z* 232 [M-tButyl-CO]	[M-57], *m/z* 260 [M-tButyl]	[M-15], *m/z* 302 [M-methyl]
Tracer:tracee molar ratios:				
1-^{13}C-alanine	No label	No label	0.942	0.916
^{15}N-alanine	1.061	0.975	1.040	1.051
^{2}H$_4$-alanine	1.074	0.934	1.430	1.306

An example of isotope effects for the tBDMS derivative of alanine is shown in Table 6.2. Solutions of unlabelled alanine and three labeled tracers (1-^{13}C-, ^{15}N-, and ^{2}H$_4$-alanine) were prepared and mixed to approximate 1:1 mol ratios of labeled:unlabeled alanine. Aliquots were derivatized (tBDMS) and analyzed on a Hewlett Packard 5989 GC-MS system in EI.[2] The isotopic enrichment for each label was monitored in four fragments which retained the labels. Tracer:tracee ratios (TTR) were measured as R-R$_0$, where R and R$_0$ represent the measured ion abundance ratios for the mixture and unlabeled alanine, respectively (Section 6.4.2). The TTRs for two fragments that retained the 1-^{13}C label were similar, 0.916 and 0.942. The ^{15}N sample had a TTR between 0.975 and 1.061 for the four fragments. In the absence of an isotope effect, the TTR for a given tracer should be identical in all fragments (the value may differ from the expected TTR of 1.0 if the composition of the labeled:unlabeled mixture was inaccurate). The ^{13}C and ^{15}N tracers thus exhibited little fragmentation effect, since various fragments had similar enrichments. However, deuterated alanine exhibited a profound isotope effect: the range of TTR was 0.934 to 1.430 for the four fragments. The [M-57] ion is particularly useful for GC-MS analysis of amino acids as it represents loss of *tert.*-butyl with retention of the intact alanine molecule. However, this fragment had the largest isotope effect for the deuterated tracer, indicating that the measured ion abundance ratio did not equal the true tracer:tracee molar ratio. Isotope effects should decrease in the order: ^{2}H > ^{13}C > ^{15}N, as the influence of the nucleus on the properties of shell electrons decreases. Isotope effects will affect the accuracy of isotopic enrichment measurements from measured ion abundance ratios, unless accounted for in the analysis (Section 6.4.3).

6.3.3.3 Concentration Effects and Non-Linearities

Many GC-MS applications exhibit some degree of concentration dependency, as the measured ion abundance ratio varies with the amount of sample analyzed.[35] The degree of this effect is variable for different applications, instruments, and ionization modes. Many processes contribute to such concentration-dependent non-linearities, including detector non-linearity and scatter due to ion-molecule collisions or charge repulsions. Some molecules are particularly prone to undergo self-CI in EI as the molecular ion is protonated to form $[M+H]^+$ ions in a concentration-dependent manner.[36] Extensive self-CI of the molecular ion has been observed for HFBPr amino acids in EI (B.W. Patterson, personal observation). In NCI, concentration dependency may result from saturation of the source electrons if too much material is introduced into the source.

The presence of concentration effects should be tested for each application on each instrument. Ion abundance ratios should be measured for various quantities of sample to establish a valid working range where measured ratios are reasonably independent of peak areas. Alternately, concentration dependency may be incorporated into the analysis to determine isotopic enrichment from measured ion abundance ratios[35] (Section 6.4.3.2). Non-linearities may be reduced by increasing the sensitivity of the analysis to obtain suitable ion intensities with less material analyzed. Many factors that affect sensitivity are features of instrument design beyond the operator's control. However, sensitivity can be increased by elimination of atmospheric leaks (higher pressure in the MS reduces sensitivity), manipulation of tuning parameters, regular source cleanings, and replacement of aged detectors. Furthermore, applications can be chosen with sensitivity issues in mind, as sensitivity typically increases in the order EI < CI < NCI.

6.3.4   DEUTERATED AMINO ACID TRACERS

Deuterated tracers are frequently used in studies of protein and amino acid metabolism. One reason for their popularity stems from economical issues: deuterated tracers typically cost less than ^{13}C and ^{15}N tracers. Furthermore, a broad array of highly substituted deuterated tracers are available for applications requiring measurement of very low enrichment, such as using $^2H_3$-leucine or ring-$^2H_5$-phenylalanine for muscle protein synthesis[17] (Section 6.2.3.5). Nevertheless, more artifacts are encountered with deuterated compared to ^{13}C and ^{15}N tracers, which require special attention.

Deuterated tracers may be less isotopically pure than ^{13}C. For example, 1-^{13}C-leucine may be 99 atom % ^{13}C, whereas 5,5,5-$^2H_3$-leucine may be 98 atom % ^2H. With three isotopically labeled positions each having a 2% chance of *not* being labeled with ^2H, there is a 6% chance that at least one position is not labeled; 6% of the tracers will be labeled as m+2 rather than m+3. This may affect calculations of isotopic enrichment unless corrections are applied (Section 6.4.2).

Deuterated tracers tend to have more processing and GC-MS artifacts. Hydrogen/deuterium exchange can occur during sample processing (especially during hydrolysis of isotopically labeled proteins) leading to loss of label (Section 6.3.1). Deuterated tracers are more likely to exhibit isotope effects during fragmentation inside the ionization source such that the measured ion abundance ratios do not equate to true tracer:tracee molar ratios (Section 6.3.3.2). Capillary GC columns tend to fractionate deuterated and native components, such that they do not exactly co-elute, which affects the accuracy of ion abundance ratios.[37] Finally, concentration-dependent artifacts (Section 6.3.3.3) are more pronounced and instrument response factors more variable for deuterated than ^{13}C and ^{15}N tracers, due to this lack of co-elution.[35] For example, ring-$^2H_5$-phenylalanine was partially resolved from the native unlabeled component and exhibited concentration-dependent ion abundance ratios in EI on a VG 12-250 GC-MS system (VG Biotech, Altrincham, U.K.).[23] In contrast, ring-$^{13}C_6$-phenylalanine exactly co-eluted with the native unlabeled component, and did not exhibit concentration-dependent ion abundance ratios in EI on the same type of instrument.[17]

Finally, one of the first principles of tracer methodology is that the tracer is metabolically indistinguishable from the native tracee. This principle may be violated for deuterated tracers.[38] At isotopic steady state during a constant infusion of 1-^{13}C-phenylalanine, the ratio of enrichments in plasma and urine (P:U ratio) was 1.06 ± 0.05. During an infusion of ring-$^2H_5$-phenylalanine, the P:U ratio was 0.60 ± 0.10, demonstrating an isotope effect on amino acid transport systems.[38] Additional studies are needed to evaluate potential *in vivo* isotope effects with deuterated tracers.

6.4 CALCULATIONS OF ISOTOPIC ENRICHMENT

6.4.1 GENERAL CONSIDERATIONS

Many expressions and terms have been used as measures of isotopic enrichment. Some terms, such as atom % excess (APE) or delta (δ) are more appropriately used with IRMS applications. The mol % excess (MPE) from GC-MS measurements is analogous to APE, and measures the relative proportion of labeled molecules in a population. These terms express relative enrichment, and are not directly applicable to the formalism of metabolic kinetics initially developed with radiotracers using specific activity (SA), e.g., dpm/mol. The preferred measure of stable isotopic enrichment is the tracer:tracee ratio (TTR), which is analogous to radiotracer SA as it relates the absolute quantity of tracer to the absolute quantity of tracee.[32,39]

Various approaches to determine the TTR from GC-MS measured ion abundance ratios are described below. Space precludes a detailed presentation of the various formulations and correction factors that are used. However, it will become evident that many commonly used approaches do not take into account all of the artifacts discussed in Section 6.3, which can affect measured ion abundance ratios.

6.4.2 APPROACHES BASED ON LINEAR COMBINATION OF SPECTRA

One approach to determine the TTR (or the ratio of labeled:unlabeled molecules) is based on a linear combination of spectra.[40] The complete ion spectrum for the chosen fragment is measured by SIM for the pure tracee and tracer molecules. The fractional distribution of ions within each spectrum is normalized to sum to unity. The normalized ion spectrum for a mixture of tracee and tracer is then a linear combination of these normalized spectra. The fractional contribution of the tracer and tracee spectra to the combined spectrum can be determined by least squares analysis. This approach has the practical advantage that the tracer and tracee ion distribution spectra are actually measured rather than based on theoretical calculations, since the measured ion spectrum may not equate to the true isotopomer spectrum due to artifacts (Section 6.3.3). Furthermore, this approach can be readily extended to include multiple tracers (e.g., if one tracer is used *in vivo* and a second tracer is added for isotope dilution quantitative analysis). One practical disadvantage of this approach is that the GC-MS detector spends time measuring ions that do not make a significant contribution to the total ion distribution spectrum. Precision and/or accuracy may be reduced, because the detector dwell time on each ion has to be short so that more ions can be monitored. It may be difficult to obtain the desired 15 to 20 time points across the chromatographic peak[3] when the SIM acquisition has to monitor too many ions (Section 6.2.2.2).

To avoid these problems of monitoring the complete ion spectrum, another approach uses a reduced form that only monitors the major tracer ion of interest with the unlabeled (m+0) ion.[32] For an (m+x) labeled tracer, the TTR is determined as:

$$TTR = R - R_0 \qquad\qquad (1)$$

where R and R_0 represent the measured (m+x)/(m+0) ion abundance ratio for the sample and natural abundance material, respectively. This formula assumes the tracer is 100 mol % isotopically labeled; a correction term is necessary if the tracer is not isotopically pure. This approach does not measure the ion distribution spectrum of the pure tracer. The theoretical isotopomer distribution of an (m+x) labeled tracer molecule is not simply identical to the natural abundance isotopomer distribution with an offset of x mass units; rather, the distribution is "skewed" because the presence of a labeled atom in a specific position removes the possibility that it is present at natural abundance. The theoretical "skewed" distribution can be calculated, and a correction applied to the TTR calculation.[32]

Additional complications are introduced when the sample includes two or more tracers. Wolfe[32] illustrates corrections for a mixture of singly (^{13}C) and doubly (^{15}N-^{13}C) labeled leucine. Due to spectral overlap, the singly labeled (m+1) leucine will increase the measured (m+2) abundance, even when no (m+2) tracer is present. This overlap must be taken into consideration and subtracted from the measured (m+2) abundance to determine the residual abundance due to the (m+2) tracer. These corrections may appear complicated but are actually straightforward.[32] It may be more practical to use the total ion distribution approach with linear combination of spectrum than the reduced form when multiple tracers are present.

Cobelli et al.[39] have introduced another formulation to determine TTR from measured ion abundance ratios. Their formulation explicitly uses the measured ion abundance ratio of an infusate solution, which corrects for the case when the infused tracer is not isotopically pure. This formulation has not been extended to the case of multiple tracers.

These approaches to calculate TTR from measured ion abundance ratios are mathematically sound, based on a theoretical framework of tracer and tracee isotopomer distributions. Unfortunately, the ion abundance ratios or profiles measured by GC-MS do not always equate to the true isotopomer abundance ratios or profiles.

Many factors, such as tuning parameters (Section 6.3.3.1), isotope effects in fragmentation (Section 6.3.3.2), and concentration effects (Section 6.3.3.3) can alter the measured ion abundance ratios or distribution profiles. The measured ion abundance ratios frequently do come reasonably close to true isotopomer abundance ratios for many GC-MS methods. However, this cannot be assumed *a priori*, and must be validated for each application.

6.4.3   STANDARD CURVES

6.4.3.1   General Approach

Because measured ion abundance ratios do not necessarily equate to true tracer:tracee isotopomer ratios (Section 6.3.3), instrument response should be calibrated using a standard curve. Standards of tracee and tracer are prepared and mixed in accurately known proportions, to produce standards of known TTR that span the range of enrichments of interest. (Care should be taken to ensure that the tracer and tracee components are chemically pure and dry before use.) The measured ion abundance ratio, R, for these standards is regressed against the known TTR. Standard curves are usually linear up to reasonable enrichments (typically TTR < 0.20), but may be curvilinear at higher enrichments or due to instrument artifacts. Slopes of linear standard curves are frequently close to unity, although significant deviations from unity exist for many applications for the reasons discussed throughout Section 6.3. The slope of the standard curve may drift considerably as tuning conditions and the cleanliness of the source change;[35] calibration standards should therefore be included with each series of samples being analyzed.

The conventional standard curve approach corrects for many artifacts such as variable instrument response, "skewed" isotopomer distribution profiles, and isotope fragmentation effects. The approach is more cumbersome when two or more tracers are present, as spectral overlap (Section 6.4.2) causes crossover interference between tracers. Vogt et al.[41] have reported an approach that is applicable to multiple tracers, which combines a complete measured isotopomer distribution with a standard curve.

6.4.3.2   Incorporating Concentration Dependency

Although a standard curve corrects for many GC-MS artifacts, it cannot account for concentration dependency of measured ion abundance ratios (Section 6.3.3.3). Such problems can be reduced by adjusting the concentrations, so that the standards and biological samples generate approximately equivalent peak areas, although this is not always practical. We recently reported an approach that incorporates concentration dependencies into a standard curve analysis.[35] An example of this approach for an (m+2) labeled tracer is illustrated in Figure 6.1.

Various quantities of each isotopic enrichment standard of known TTR are analyzed to cover a range of peak areas that spans those obtained for the biological samples analyzed. The analysis proceeds in two stages. The observed tracer (m+2) peak areas are first correlated against the observed tracee (m+0) peak areas. These "area vs. area" plots are described by second-order regressions which do not pass exactly through the origin. The second-order coefficients account for non-linearities

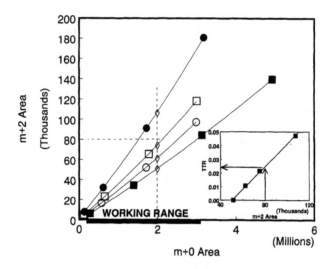

FIGURE 6.1   General procedure for incorporating concentration effects into a standard curve for a (m+2) labeled tracer. Each isotopic enrichment standard is analyzed over a range of peak areas. The measured tracer peak areas are correlated against the measured tracee peak areas using second-order regressions. The TTR of a given sample is determined from a linear regression of TTR against the tracer peak areas, which each enrichment standard would have generated for the tracee (m+0) peak area observed for that sample (inset). (From Patterson, B.W., Zhao, G., and Klein, S., Improved accuracy and precision of gas chromatography/mass spectrometry measurement for metabolic tracers, *Metabolism*, 47(6), 706, 1998. With permission.)

which result in concentration-dependent ion abundance ratios with larger peak areas, whereas non-zero intercepts account for ion abundance ratio irregularities that are observed for small peak areas. These second-order regressions are then used to construct a linear standard curve of TTR vs. tracer (m+2) peak areas, based on the tracer (m+2) peak areas that each TTR standard would have produced for the same tracee (m+0) peak area obtained for a given sample (inset, Figure 6.1).

This approach can be applied to any application where a standard curve can be used; illustrations for HFBPr-1-^{13}C-leucine, tBDMS-^{15}N$_2$-urea, and ^{2}H$_2$-palmitate methyl ester have been presented.[35] Although this approach is more cumbersome than a conventional standard curve, it improves the accuracy and precision for applications where concentration dependencies significantly affect measured ion abundance ratios.

6.5   CONCLUSIONS

Many methods are available to measure enrichment of amino acids by GC-MS. Most methods work well for most amino acids, although certain amino acids require special consideration. Some derivative/ionization mode combinations do not work well for certain labeled tracers, particularly 1-^{13}C amino acids in EI. Many artifacts may affect measured ion abundance ratios with implications for certain approaches used to calculate isotopic enrichment. With attention to details to minimize these artifacts and incorporate them into a framework to determine isotopic enrichment, GC-MS analysis of amino acids is accurate, precise, and reliable.

REFERENCES

1. Husek, P. and Macek, K., Gas chromatography of amino acids, *J.Chromatogr.*, 113, 139, 1975.
2. Patterson, B. W., Carraro, F., and Wolfe, R. R., Measurement of ^{15}N enrichment in multiple amino acids and urea in a single analysis by gas chromatography/mass spectrometry, *Biol. Mass Spectrom.*, 22, 518, 1993.
3. Matthews, D. E. and Hayes, J. M., Systematic errors in gas chromatography-mass spectrometry isotope ratio measurements, *Anal. Chem.*, 48, 1375, 1976.
4. Matthews, D. E., Ben-Galim, E., and Bier, D. M., Determination of stable isotopic enrichment in individual plasma amino acids by chemical ionization-mass spectrometry, *Anal. Chem.*, 51, 80, 1979.
5. Matthews, D. E., Schwarz, H. P., Yang, R. D., Motil, K. J., Young, V. R., and Bier, D. M., Relationship of plasma leucine and α-ketoisocaproate during a L-[1-^{13}C]leucine infusion in man: a method for measuring human intracellular leucine tracer enrichment, *Metabolism*, 31, 1105, 1982.
6. Darmaun, D., Manary, M. J., and Matthews, D. E., A method for measuring both glutamine and glutamate levels and stable isotopic enrichments, *Anal. Biochem.*, 147, 92, 1985.
7. Darmaun, D., Froguel, P., Rongier, M., and Robert, J. J., Amino acid exchange between plasma and erythrocytes *in vivo* in humans, *J. Appl. Physiol.*, 67, 2383, 1989.
8. Shanbhogue, R. L. K., Bistrian, B. R., Lakshman, K., Crosby, L., Swenson, S., Wagner, D., Jenkins, R. L., and Blackburn, G. L., Whole body leucine, phenylalanine, and tyrosine kinetics in end-stage liver disease before and after hepatic transplantation, *Metabolism*, 36, 1047, 1987.
9. Nissim, I. and Lapidot, A., Plasma amino acid turnover rates and pools in rabbits: in vivo studies using stable isotopes, *Am. J. Physiol.*, 237, E418, 1979.
10. Leimer, K. R., Rice, R. H., and Gehrke, C. W., Complete mass spectra of N-trifluoro-acetyl-n-butyl esters of amino acids, *J. Chromatogr.*, 141, 121, 1977.
11. Patterson, B. W., Hachey, D. L., Cook, G. L., Amann, J. M., and Klein, P. D., Incorporation of a stable isotopically labeled amino acid into multiple human apolipoproteins, *J. Lipid Res.*, 32, 1063, 1991.
12. Berthold, H. K., Hachey, D. L., Reeds, P. J., Thomas, O. P., Hoeksema, S., and Klein, P. D., Uniformly ^{13}C-labeled algal protein used to determine amino acid essentiality *in vivo*, *Proc. Natl. Acad. Sci. U.S.A.*, 88, 8091, 1991.
13. Ford, G. C., Cheng, K. N., and Halliday, D., Analysis of (1-^{13}C)leucine and (^{13}C)KIC in plasma by capillary gas chromatograph/mass spectrometry in protein turnover studies, *Biomed. Mass Spectrom.*, 12, 432, 1985.
14. Maugeais, C., Ouguerram, K., Maugeais, P., Simoneau, C., Gardette, J., Magot, T., and Krempf, M., Comparison of [5,5,5-[2]H$_3$]leucine and [ring-[2]H$_5$]phenylalanine tracers for the measurement of human apolipoprotein B100 kinetics, *J. Mass Spectrometry*, 30, 478, 1995.

15. Robinson, J. R., Starratt, A. N., and Schlahetka, E. E., Estimation of nitrogen-15 levels in derivatized amino acids using gas chromatography quadrupole mass spectrometry with chemical ionization and selected ion monitoring, *Biomed. Mass Spectrom.*, 5, 648, 1978.

16. Jahoor, F., Sivakumar, B., Del Rosario, M., and Frazer, E. M., Isolation of acute-phase proteins from plasma for determination of fractional synthesis rates by a stable isotope tracer technique, *Anal. Biochem.*, 236, 95, 1996.

17. Patterson, B. W., Zhang, X-J., Chen, Y., Klein, S., and Wolfe, R. R., Measurement of very low stable isotope enrichments by gas chromatography/mass spectrometry: application to measurement of muscle protein synthesis, *Metabolism*, 46, 943, 1997.

18. Leimer, K. R., Rice, R. H., and Gehrke, C. W., Complete mass spectra of the pertrimethylsilylated amino acids, *J. Chromatogr.*, 141, 355, 1977.

19. Haymond, M. W., Howard, C. P., Miles, J. M., and Gerich, J. E., Determination of leucine flux in vivo by gas chromatography-mass spectrometry utilizing stable isotopes for trace and internal standard, *J. Chromatogr.*, 183, 403, 1980.

20. Mawhinney, T. P., Robinett, R. S. R., Atalay, A., and Madson, M. A., Analysis of amino acids as their *tert.*-butyldimethylsilyl derivatives by gas-liquid chromatography and mass spectrometry, *J. Chromatogr.*, 358, 231, 1986.

21. Patterson, B. W., Carraro, F., Klein, S., and Wolfe, R. R., Quantification of incorporation of [^{15}N]ammonia into plasma amino acids and urea, *Am. J. Physiol.*, 269, E508, 1995.

22. Yu, Y-M., Ryan, C. M., Burke, J. F., Tompkins, R. G., and Young, V. R., Relations among arginine, citrulline, ornithine, and leucine kinetics in adult burn patients, *Am. J. Clin. Nutr.*, 62, 960, 1995.

23. Calder, A. G., Anderson, S. E., Grant, I., McNurlan, M. A., and Garlick, P. J., The determination of low d_5-phenylalanine enrichment (0.002-0.09 atom percent excess), after conversion to phenylethylamine, in relation to protein turnover studies by gas chromatography/electron ionization mass spectrometry, *Rapid Comm. Mass Spectrom.*, 6, 421, 1995.

24. Slater, C., Preston, T., McMillan, D. C., Falconer, J. S., and Fearon, K. C. H., GC-MS analysis of [^{2}H$_5$]phenylalanine at very low enrichment: Measurement of protein synthesis in health and disease, *J. Mass Spectrometry*, 30, 1325, 1995.

25. Rocchiccioli, F., Leroux, J. P., and Cartier, P., Quantitative gas chromatography-chemical ionization mass spectrometry of 2-ketoglutarate from urine as its O-trimethylsilyl-quinoxalinol derivative, *J. Chromatogr.*, 226, 325, 1981.

26. Langenbeck, U., Luthe, H., and Schaper, G., Keto acids in tissues and biological fluids: O-*t*-butyldimethylsilyl quinoxalinols as derivatives for sensitive gas chromatographic/mass spectrometric determination, *Biomed. Mass Spectrom.*, 12, 507, 1985.

27. Schwenk, W. F., Berg, P. J., Beaufrere, B., Miles, J. M., and Haymond, M. W., Use of *t*-butyldimethylsilylation in the gas chromatographic/mass spectrometric analysis of physiologic compounds found in plasma using electron-impact ionization, *Anal. Biochem.*, 141, 101, 1984.

28. Hachey, D. L., Patterson, B. W., Reeds, P. J., and Elsas, L. J., Isotopic determination of organic keto acid pentafluorobenzyl esters in biological fluids by negative chemical ionization gas chromatography/mass spectrometry, *Anal. Chem.*, 63, 919, 1991.

29. Pietzsch, J., Nitzsche, S., Wiedemann, B., Julius, U., Leonhardt, W., and Hanefeld, M., Stable isotope ratio analysis of amino acids: The use of N(O)-ethoxycarbonyl ethyl ester derivatives and gas chromatography mass spectrometry, *J. Mass Spectrometry*, S129, 1995.

30. Simpson, J. T., Torok, D. S., Girard, J. E., and Markey, S. P., Analysis of amino acids in biological fluids by pentafluorobenzyl chloroformate derivatization and detection by electron capture negative ionization mass spectrometry, *Anal. Biochem.*, 233, 58, 1996.

31. Kulik, W., Vantoledoeppinga, L., Kok, R. M., Guerand, W. S., and Lafeber, H. N., Simultaneous determination of concentrations and stable isotope enrichments of alpha-ketoisocaproic acid, leucine, phenylalanine and tyrosine in blood plasma by gas chromatography negative ion mass spectrometry, *J. Mass Spectrometry*, 30, 1260, 1995.

32. Wolfe, R. R., *Radioactive and Stable Isotope Tracers in Biomedicine: Principles and Practice of Kinetic Analysis*, Wiley-Liss, New York, 1992.

33. Cayol, M., Capitan, P., Prugnaud, J., Genest, M., Beaufrere, B., and Obled, C., Cation-exchange resins release amino acids: consequences for tracer studies, *Anal. Biochem.*, 227, 392, 1995.

34. Welty, F. K., Lichtenstein, A. H., Barrett, P. H. R., Dolnikowski, G. G., Ordovas, J. M., and Schaefer, E. J., Production of apolipoprotein B-67 in apolipoprotein B-67/B-100 heterozygotes: technical problems associated with leucine contamination in stable isotope studies, *J. Lipid Res.*, 38, 1535, 1997.

35. Patterson, B. W., Zhao, G., and Klein, S., Improved accuracy and precision of gas chromatography/mass specrometry measurements for metabolic tracers, *Metabolism*, 47(6), 706, 1998.

36. Patterson, B. W. and Wolfe, R. R., Concentration dependence of methyl palmitate isotope ratios by electron impact ionization gas chromatography/mass spectrometry, *Biol. Mass Spectrom.*, 22, 481, 1993.

37. Thomas, L. C. and Weichmann, W., Quantitative measurements via co-elution and dual-isotope detection by gas chromatography-mass spectrometry, *J. Chromatogr.*, 587, 255, 1991.

38. Zello, G. A., Marai, L., Tung, A. S., Ball, R. O., and Pencharz, P. B., Plasma and urine enrichments following infusion of L-[1-^{13}C] phenylalanine and L-[ring-^{2}H$_5$] phenylalanine in humans: evidence for an isotope effect in renal tubular reabsorption, *Metabolism*, 43, 487, 1994.

39. Cobelli, C., Toffolo, G., and Foster, D. M., Tracer-to-tracee ratio for analysis of stable isotope tracer data: link with radioactive kinetic formalism, *Am. J. Physiol.*, 262, E968, 1992.

40. Brauman, J. I., Least squares analysis and simplification of multi-isotope mass spectra, *Anal. Chem.*, 38, 607, 1966.

41. Vogt, J. A., Chapman, T. E., Wagner, D. A., Young, V. R., and Burke, J. F., Determination of the isotope enrichment of one or a mixture of two stable labelled tracers of the same compound using the complete isotopomer distribution of an ion fragment; theory and application to in vivo human tracer studies, *Biol. Mass Spectrom.*, 22, 600, 1993.

7 The Use of GC-C-IRMS for the Analysis of Stable Isotope Enrichment in Nitrogenous Compounds

Cornelia C. Metges and Klaus J. Petzke

CONTENTS

7.1   INTRODUCTION

The relative natural abundance of the main heavy stable isotopes in bioelements (^2H, ^{13}C, ^{15}N, ^{18}O) is generally considered as fixed. However, it varies in subtle limits ($\pm$ 10^{-4} - 10^{-2} atom %; AP), due to various isotope fractionation processes in nature. The specialized instrument dedicated to measure such small differences precisely is a gas isotope ratio mass spectrometer (GIRMS), which requires the introduction of the sample as pure gas.

GIRMS is used in numerous laboratories to measure the $^{13}CO_2$ enrichment in expired air samples. However, GIRMS has not been extensively used to measure enrichment of metabolites in biological fluids and tissues until relatively recently. This was, in part, due to the necessary large sample amounts (0.5 to 5 µmol) and laborious sample preparation, such as purification of the substance of interest by

0-8493-9612-3/99/$0.00+$.50
© 1999 by CRC Press LLC

preparative chromatography, off-line combustion to yield CO_2, or degradation by a Kjedahl procedure and the subsequent oxidation of NH_3 by hypobromite to yield N_2.

A new era began when a gas chromatograph (GC), modeled after the tremendously successful gas chromatography-mass spectrometry (GC-MS), was coupled online via a combustion interface to a GIRMS. The subsequent instrument, which became commercially available about a decade ago, is now commonly known under the abbreviations GC-C-IRMS (gas chromatography-combustion-isotope ratio mass spectrometer) or irm-GC-MS (isotope ratio monitoring-GC-MS). This technology combines the resolution capabilities of a GC with the accuracy and precision of a GIRMS. The development of the instrument has been reviewed recently.[1]

Unlike a conventional GC-MS (see Chapter 6 by Patterson), a GC-C-IRMS is capable of detecting differences in stable isotope enrichments below 0.01 atom% excess (APE) and covers a range of enrichments between 0.0001 to 1 APE. However, at present, measurements on a routine basis are only possible for ^{13}C and ^{15}N, although basic work to measure ^{2}H/^{1}H ratios by GC-C-IRMS is in progress.[2,3] Since the early 1990s a considerable increase in the application of this technique to metabolic research occured with an emphasis on fatty acid research; analysis of urea, cholesterol, and lactate have also been reported.[4-11] In those studies, chemically enriched tracers have been used; however, naturally stable isotope enriched substances, based on corn, also allow researchers to trace the fate of amino acids, dietary glucose, and fatty acids.[7,12,13]

The number of studies dealing with protein and amino acid metabolism in humans or animals has been increasing tremendously in the last few years. For ^{13}C analysis, mainly [^{13}C]leucine has been used as tracer.[14-18] Because of a number of difficulties, few measurements of ^{15}N enrichments in amino acids have been published so far.[19] In addition to the pioneering work of Merritt and Hayes, and a recent study by Macko et al. in which amino acid standard mixtures were analyzed, studies have investigated the incorporation of ^{15}N into protein and free amino acids of plants, animals, and human subjects.[20-28]

In this chapter, we present a brief overview of the reasons for the variations of mean natural abundances of stable isotopes. We outline instrumentation and principal methodology for the measurement of ^{13}C and ^{15}N enrichments in amino acids. After a discussion of the factors influencing precision and accuracy, we give examples of applications relevant to the investigation of amino acid and protein metabolism in order to illustrate the utility and sensitivity of this technique. Pros and cons in comparison to GC-MS are discussed. We end this chapter with an outlook on future developments of GC-C-IRMS.

7.2   MATERIAL AND METHODS

7.2.1   Stable Isotope Natural Abundances

7.2.1.1   Variations of [13]C- and [15]N Natural Abundances

The different number and symmetry of the neutrons within the nuclei of the (stable=non-radioactive) isotopes of an element (e.g., carbon ^{12}C, ^{13}C; oxygen ^{16}O,

^{17}O, ^{18}O) determine their mass polarization and nuclear spin. These in turn affect mass, polarity, and binding energies within and between the molecules. Any organic substance consists of a natural mixture of isotopomer molecules with different molecular weights, such as carbon dioxide which occurs as the isotopomeric species $^{12}C^{16}O^{16}O$, $^{13}C^{16}O^{16}O$, $^{12}C^{16}O^{17}O$, $^{13}C^{16}O^{17}O$, $^{12}C^{17}O^{17}O$, or $^{12}C^{16}O^{18}O$ having molecular weights between 44 and 46 g/mole. The isotopomers have slightly different physical properties, and show differences in the velocities of chemical or biochemical reactions. This varied behavior causes phenomena called thermodynamic, kinetic, or nuclear spin isotope effects.[29] Isotope effects are implied in natural processes and cause small but perceptible separations of isotopomers with different molecular weights. As a classical example, for carbon, two different primary reactions of the photosynthetic CO_2 fixation occur, proceeding with different kinetic isotope effects resulting in the so-called C_3- and C_4-plants, differing in the carbon isotope ratio by $\sim 10^{-2}$ AP.[30] Within animal and plant tissues, a characteristic difference in the isotopic signature exists between carbohydrates and lipids, a consequence of carbon isotope fractionation in lipogenesis.[31] Due to various metabolic branching points, isotope effects are connected to the biosynthetic pathways in the animal and plant kingdom, resulting in distinct differences in the carbon and nitrogen-stable isotope natural abundances of free and protein-bound amino acids in animals and humans.[12,26,32-35]

In contrast, a substance which is usually referred to as a "stable isotope tracer" is a molecule in which one or more atoms in the structure are replaced with stable isotopes by chemical means (e.g., a ^{12}C is replaced by a ^{13}C). This replacement can result in an enrichment of up to 99.9 atom % ^{13}C in a certain molecular position (e.g., the carboxyl position). The mean carbon enrichment of this tracer can then be calculated by addition of the contributions of unenriched carbons of natural mean ^{13}C abundance ($\sim$ AP) and the artificially enriched carboxyl carbon (i.e., for leucine $(5 \times 0.16 \times 1.1) + (1 \times 0.16 \times 99.9) = 17.57$ AP).

7.2.1.2 Delta Notation

Due to the small differences in natural isotopic composition between molecules, a special notation – the δ – is used. This designates the isotopic abundance as a permill (‰) deviation from an international standard:[36]

$$\delta\ (‰) = [(R_{sample}/R_{standard}) - 1] \times 10^3 \qquad (1)$$

The mean natural abundance for carbon (^{13}C) and nitrogen (^{15}N) is 1.108 and 0.3663 AP, respectively.[30] The abundance of the international standard for carbon, the PDB (Pee Dee Belemnite carbonate), is 1.111 AP and the respective isotope ratio (R_{PDB} $^{13}C/^{12}C$) is 0.0112372. The international nitrogen standard is atmospheric N_2 (AIR) with a $^{15}N/^{14}N$ isotopic ratio $R_{AIR} = 0.0036765$. The δ notation can be converted to AP and vice versa by the following equations:

$$AP_{sample} = [\ (1\ /\ (\ (\delta_{sample}\ /\ 1000 + 1) \times R_{standard}\ ) + 1)^{-1}\ ] \times 10^2 \qquad (2)$$

$$\delta_{sample} = [\ (1\ /\ (100\ /\ AP_{sample} - 1)\ /\ R_{standard}\ ) - 1] \times 10^3 \qquad (3)$$

APE is calculated by subtraction of the baseline abundance AP, or mean natural abundance. For example, 0.1 APE ^{15}N or ^{13}C corresponds to 274.3 ‰ δ ^{15}N and 90.9 ‰ δ ^{13}C, respectively, based on the mean abundance of the respective international standards.

7.2.2 INSTRUMENTATION

GIRMS has two prominent features. The first is that the sample is a gas (CO_2, N_2, or H_2), and the second is that the difference between isotope ratios of a sample compared to a reference gas is measured rather than absolute isotope ratios. Due to the comparably low molecular weights of the measured gases, the upper mass limit is usually approximately m/z 70 (see below). All of these features determine the high precision of 10^{-5} to 10^{-4} APE achieved by GIRMS. Figure 7.1 depicts a

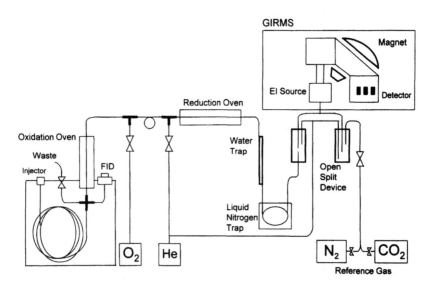

FIGURE 7.1   Schematic representation of a gas chromatography-combustion-isotope ratio mass spectrometry system (see Section 7.2.2 in text).

schematic representation of a GC-C-IRMS. The mass spectrometer comprises an ion source where the sample gas is ionized by electron impact; an analyzer section where the ions are separated; and a detector where separated groups of ions are detected. Under high vacuum (~ 4 x 10^{-6} mbar), a heated filament in the ion source (EI) emits electrons which collide with the sample gas molecules, thereby removing an electron which results in a positively charged molecular ion (e.g., CO_2^+, N_2^+). In the analyzer, a magnetic field is generated to sort the ions according to their mass to charge (m/z) ratios. For CO_2 and N_2, the m/z ratios are 44 ($^{12}C^{16}O^{16}O$), 45 ($^{13}C^{16}O^{16}O$ or $^{12}C^{16}O^{17}O$), 46 ($^{13}C^{16}O^{17}O$ or $^{12}C^{17}O^{17}O$ or $^{12}C^{16}O^{18}O$), and 28 ($^{14}N^{14}N$), 29 ($^{14}N^{15}N$), 30 ($^{15}N^{15}N$), respectively. The charged molecular ions move in a circular path, the radius of which is proportional to the particle's mass. The detector where the separated ions are collected consists of a triple Faraday cup* arrangement, allowing simultaneous detection of all three isotopomers of the measured gas (CO_2 or N_2). Due to the difference in natural abundances of masses, cups differ in response (e.g., 3 x 10^{-8} Ω, 3 x 10^{-10} Ω and 3 x 10^{-11} Ω resistors for m/z 44, 45, and 46, respectively). As the ions hit the metal Faraday cups, they discharge and generate a measurable ion current (one charge per ion). The numbers of ions at respective m/z ratios are expressed as ratios (45/44 or 29/28) and are converted into $^{13}C/^{12}C$ and $^{15}N/^{14}N$ isotope ratios, delta (δ) units or APE, respectively (see Section 7.2.1.2).

Due to the special features of the GIRMS, it is clear that a substance in the GC effluent cannot be introduced directly into the ion source. Upon separation of amino acid derivatives on a capillary column, the effluent is split into two or three parts (Figure 7.1). One part (> 90%) is directed toward the oxidation oven, and one other part leaves through a waste line connected to a time-programmable helium backflush vent valve which directs the solvent peak effluent outward. The third (optional) branch of the splitter can be mounted to another detector (e.g., flame ionization detector, FID; mass selective detector, MSD) to simultaneously monitor compound signals.

The oxidation oven comprises an alumina tube, filled with various combinations of either nichrome and copper oxide wires or copper oxide, nickel oxide, and platinum wires, kept between 800 to 1100°C, according to the type of oven used.[12,19-21,24] Eluting compounds are oxidized to CO_2, H_2O, N_2 and NO_x. A reduction furnace filled with elemental copper at 600°C reduces NO_x and scavenges a surplus of oxygen. Water is removed by a water-permeable membrane or by a liquid nitrogen or cold trap.[21,24,37] In the nitrogen mode, carbon dioxide is trapped at -196°C (liquid nitrogen trap). When carbon isotope composition is measured, the reduction furnace is not necessary; also, the liquid nitrogen trap can be replaced by another device for water removal, usually a cold trap at -100°C or a water-permeable membrane.[12,24] An open-split device allows pressure adjustment of the sample gas before it enters the GIRMS. Between the oxidation oven and the reduction oven, O_2 and He can be directed opposite the normal carrier gas stream to reoxidize the copper and nickel in the oxidation oven (Figure 7.1). A He inlet valve serves to backflush the solvent peak and undesired components of the GC effluent, when the waste valve at the gas chromatograph is opened, thereby preventing early exhaustion of the oxidation oven.

Calibration of sample N_2 or CO_2 is accomplished by addition of a N_2 or CO_2 standard gas pulse to the gas stream, from a steel bottle via a second open-split device. Sample peaks are measured in reference to a laboratory standard gas, which in turn is calibrated against the international standards (see Section 7.2.1). Typically, standard gas pulses are set before and after the sample peaks of interest, and periodically at appropriate time points inbetween sample peaks to allow correction for drifts in instrument performance.

Amino acid separation is performed using several stationary phases (Ultra 1, Ultra 2, Hewlett Packard, San Fernando, CA; DB-5, DB-1701, DB-1301, J&W Scientific Inc., Folson, CA; Chirasil-Val, Alltech Associates Inc., Deerfield, IL),

---

* Device to count charged particles, named after the physicist M. Faraday (1791-1867).

usually on column lengths of 50 m. In general, columns with a low column bleed should be selected in order to extend the life of the oxidation furnace. For $^{15}N/^{14}N$ analysis, column phases containing nitrogen may be used with caution. An inner column diameter of 0.25 or 0.32 mm and a film thickness of 0.25 or 0.52 μm was used.[12,20-22,24,38] Depending upon the instrument model and derivative used, injection quantities between 1 to 2 nmol to 10 to 20 nmol per amino acid, in 0.5 to 7.5 μl injection volume, have been reported as usually injected in the splitless mode.[21,23-25] Figure 7.2 shows a typical amino acid chromatogram as a nitrogen gas peak profile (m/z 28 chromatogram) of plasma free and fecal microbial protein amino acids.

7.2.3 SAMPLE PREPARATION AND DERIVATIZATION PROCEDURES

Proteins and amino acids are isolated by standard chromatographic, electrophoretic, or precipitation methods. For information on protein purification methods, we refer to the relevant literature.[e.g.,39,40]

To isolate amino acids from proteins, a hydrolysis procedure is performed.[e.g.,12,24] After appropriate cleanup by filters or resins, free amino acids are evaporated to dryness for derivatization. Isolation of free amino acids from plasma by cation exchange chromatography has been described with or without prior deproteinization.[12,26] Briefly, 0.5 to 1 mL plasma or serum is acidified with HCl, and an internal standard (e.g., α-aminoadipic acid, norleucine, or tranexamic acid) is added. The mixture is applied to a cation exchange column (Dowex AG 50W-X8; BioRad, Melville, NY), and amino acids are eluted by ammonium hydroxide plus distilled H_2O. Upon evaporation to dryness by a nitrogen stream, the amino acids are derivatized.

To allow separation of amino acids by gas chromatography, volatility has to be enhanced by chemical derivatization. This is achieved by conversion of ionizable molecular groups to nonionizable derivatives (e.g., carboxyl groups to esters; replacing hydrogen-bound to heteroatoms by alkyl, acyl, or silyl). Widespread use has found the tertiary butyl dimethylsilyl (t-BDMS) derivative for a wide range of amino acids in GC-MS analysis, because it is prepared by an easy one-step heating procedure, allowing differentiation between glutamic acid and glutamine, as well as between aspartic acid and asparagine.[41,42] The t-BDMS derivative has been used also for GC-C-IRMS, but there are several reasons why it is not an ideal candidate for GC-C-IRMS.[22,23] Because of the large molecular size of the derivative (i.e., one mole t-BDMS has a molecular weight of 115) a possible overloading of the GC capillary column may occur in the attempt to generate m/z 28 signals large enough for integration. Note that, for most amino acids, two moles of amino acid are required to generate one mole N_2 gas. Hence, the use of t-BDMS may lead to impaired peak shape, and an early exhaustion or a temporary overload of the oxidation catalyst.[23,37] Simultaneously, a large bulk of CO_2 is produced, which needs to be removed by the liquid nitrogen trap. This may cause it to clog, or introduce CO_2 into the ion source. The latter leads to the formation of CO^+ fragments (m/z 28, 29) which interfere with the measurement of $^{15}N/^{14}N$ ratios. Also, t-BDMS amino acid derivatives are not suitable for $^{13}C/^{12}C$ analysis because a large number of additional carbons is added (6 carbons per one mole of t-BDMS). For example, an alanine t-BDMS derivative

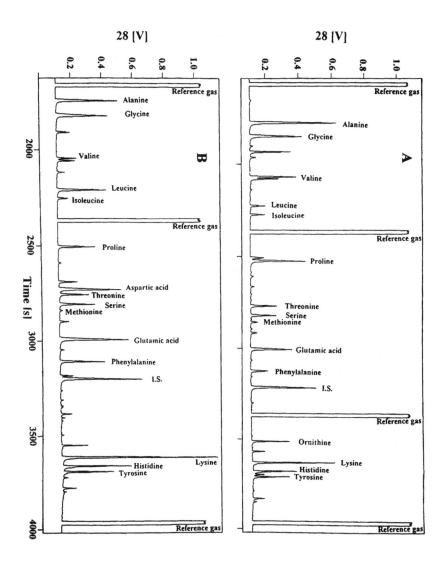

FIGURE 7.2 GC-C-IRMS chromatogram of m/z 28 (nitrogen). Panel A: N-pivaloyl-n-propyl esters of human free plasma amino acids. Panel B: N-pivaloyl-n-propyl esters of human fecal microbial protein amino acids. (Column: HP Ultra 2, 50 m, 0.32 mm internal diameter, 0.52 μm film; Injection volume: 0.5 μl; Internal standard: α-amino adipic acid, approx. 1 nmol per injection).

would contain only 3 indigenous carbons out of a total of 15 carbons; therefore, it makes it more difficult to detect small differences in the amino acid carbon isotope composition. However, if uniformly ^{13}C-labeled tracers are used, this may be of lesser importance. As suggested above, the t-BDMS derivative is the derivative of choice when it comes to the chromatographic separation of glutamine and glutamate, as well as asparagine and aspartate. For investigations of human nitrogen metabolism, measurement of the above amino acids in plasma is of special interest. However, we anticipate that only glutamine occurs in plasma at a sufficient concentration to generate an appropriate signal for ^{15}N/^{14}N analysis. Finally, the relative instability of t-BDMS during storage has to be accounted for.

A different approach is the preparation of trifluoroacetyl (TFA) esters which have been used for ^{13}C as well as ^{15}N analysis.[21,38] In contrast to t-BDMS derivatives, the additional contribution of carbon from the derivatization agent is comparably small. Per each OH and NH group, respectively, two moles of carbon are introduced and this adds up, e.g., for alanine, to a total of five moles of carbon due to propylation. However, an isotopic fractionation occurs during the derivatization process, preventing the direct calculation of the original amino acid carbon composition from mass balance equations.[43] An individual correction has to be applied for each amino acid, in order to derive δ^{13}C values of underivatized amino acid carbon.[38,43] Since no nitrogen is introduced into the derivative via derivatization agents, measured δ^{15}N values do not need to be corrected in this way. Excellent agreement has been found between δ^{15}N values of single underivatized amino acids with their derivatized counterparts measured by GC-C-IRMS, indicating absence of isotopic fractionation.[21,22]

TFA is the derivative of choice for analysis of arginine.[44] A peculiarity of its use, however, is a relatively fast deterioration of the oxidation catalyst due to generation of metal fluorides, which impair reoxidation of the copper and destroy the catalytic activity of platinum. In consequence, the oxidation furnace would need to be replaced more often (Gehre, M., personal communication). The same might be expected with the use of N-heptafluorobutyryl esters adding even more fluoride moieties.[15] However, this was not confirmed in one study (Ford, G. C. and Nair, S., personal communication) and it may be due to the fact that only leucine was monitored and not the full amino acid profile.

N-acetyl-n-propyl (NAP) esters have been used for ^{13}C amino acid analysis because of their small contribution to additional carbon and good long-term stability.[12,14,18] Merritt and Hayes, as described in the first full-length paper on ^{15}N analysis of standard amino acids, used NAP esters.[20] Apart from leucine, this derivative works well for a range of selected amino acids.[12,24] However, due to the complex nature of amino acid mixtures occurring in physiological samples, which makes analysis of isotopic composition of samples more difficult, one has to search for a specific derivative allowing good gas chromatographic separation of the target amino acid(s). For ^{15}N/^{14}N analysis on a HP Ultra 2 column, NAP esters of threonine and serine did not achieve complete separation. The same was true for aspartic acid and methionine, and lysine and histidine.[26] We therefore applied N-pivaloyl-i-propyl esters (NPP), and resolution of lysine and threonine proved to be satisfactory.[24,26] In contrast to t-BDMS, with NPP and NAP it is not possible to distinguish glutamine from glutamate, as well as asparagine from aspartic acid. Compared to NAP derivatives, NPP derivatives generate a slightly noisier background signal. However, when compared to t-BDMS derivatives, there is no problem in placing calibration gas pulses.

We conclude from the above that there is no multi-purpose derivative for the carbon and nitrogen isotopic analysis of all amino acids, but one has to select the derivative according to the specific intended purpose.

7.3 COMPARISON TO GC-MS AND PREREQUISITES FOR PRECISION AND ACCURACY

The intra-assay precision reached at natural abundance and up to approximately 0.1 APE is 0.3 ‰ $\delta^{13}C$ for carbon and 0.5 ‰ $\delta^{15}N$ for nitrogen (0.0001 to 0.0005 AP).[21,24,38,45] When approaching higher levels of enrichment (e.g., 0.8 APE) or measuring very low signals, precision may decrease.[24,43] However, compared to precision obtained by GC-MS, GC-C-IRMS analysis of low abundances of ^{15}N or ^{13}C in tracer studies is still useful for detecting enriched metabolites when precision is 0.01 AP or even less, as also pointed out by Goodman and Brenna.[45] Several authors have reported the good linear response of GC-C-IRMS over a large range of enrichments, starting from natural abundance up to 1 APE.[18,24]

Overlapping peaks result in biased isotope ratios. Therefore, excellent gas chromatographic separation is a primary issue for GC-C-IRMS.[46] This is particularly challenging in complex samples of physiological origin. Due to the presence of at least 20 different amino acids in a wide range of concentrations (e.g., Figure 7.2) well-resolved peaks are more difficult to achieve. Unlike GC-MS, where a particular fragment peak can be picked up unequivocally by monitoring a characteristic single ion even when peaks are overlapping, conventional GC-C-IRMS software usually does not provide means for correction of overlap.[46] Therefore it is imperative, for both carbon and nitrogen measurements, that the peaks of the target amino acids are pure and baseline-separated; this is because all nitrogen or carbon dioxide gas in the defined integration window, irrespective of its origin, does contribute to the recorded δ-value. Instrumental memory effects are a known phenomenon in mass spectrometry, and are caused by contamination from previous samples. Although not yet addressed for GC-C-IRMS measurements, it will have to be taken into consideration. According to our observations, nitrogen $\delta^{15}N$ values for amino acids in samples where enrichments are higher than 1500‰ (0.54 APE ^{15}N) will need to be interpreted with caution.

A characteristic feature and advantage of GC-C-IRMS, compared to GC-MS, is that enrichment of several amino acids can be measured in one chromatographic run without additional time-consuming measurements of standards. For example, depending upon the derivative used in a 60-min run, enrichments of about 10 to 15 amino acids can be obtained. However, as mentioned previously, the inevitable complexity of physiological samples may cause difficulties due to large differences of peak intensities. As a solution, it has been proposed to use curve-fitting algorithms instead of conventional summation methods for integration of noisy data, thereby improving precision for minor components.[45,46]

An important aspect for precise and accurate measurements is the quality of the maintenance routine. In our experience, and especially for nitrogen, the system has to be checked daily for absence of leaks. This is done by monitoring argon (m/z

40), and samples are run only when the argon signal is below 20 mV (collector resistance: 3×10^{-10} Ω). Stringent checks are performed also for water (m/z 18; upper limit 150 mV) and NO (m/z 30; upper limit 20 mV). The latter can be a marker for incomplete combustion or the condition of the ovens. Typically, but according to the type of derivative, number of runs, and concentration of samples, the oxidation catalyst is reoxidized every third to fourth day for 10 min. After subsequent purging of the system with He for about 60 min, sample measurement can be started. However, other investigators prefer to reoxidize the catalyst prior to each sample for a few seconds (Demmelmair, H., personal communication). As part of the daily routine, we run a quality control standard amino acid mixture, and perform series of standard gas analysis (SD $\leq \pm 0.06$ ‰ δ). The condition of the oxidation furnace affects the precision and accuracy of the measurements; consequently, the appropriate time for furnace replacement is a much-discussed question. For this, important parameters to consider are the continuous monitoring of a quality control sample, the impairment of the peak shape, and the m/z 30 signal (useful for $^{15}N/^{14}N$ analysis).

In contrast to GC-MS, no information can be obtained on stable isotope enrichments at some specific intramolecular positions, since the GIRMS requires that the whole molecule is converted to pure CO_2, N_2, and H_2. Because a GC-MS is recording mass differences, stable isotope enrichments can be measured simultaneously for all relevant elements in the molecule. This is not the case with GC-C-IRMS, because the conventional instrument set-up is dedicated to one element only (carbon or nitrogen).

7.4   SELECTED APPLICATIONS

To calculate protein synthesis rates, isotopic enrichments of the tracer amino acid usually have to be measured both in the precursor pool and in the tissue or protein of interest. The enrichment of the labeled amino acid in protein is generally low, which makes it an ideal candidate for IRMS. However, conventional IRMS techniques require a rather time-consuming sample preparation and a relatively large amount of protein.[15,47] Using GC-C-IRMS offers the possibility of reducing the necessary sample size to a few mg. Fractional muscle and tumor protein synthesis, as well as apolipoprotein metabolism, have been studied using GC-C-IRMS, based on a [^{13}C] leucine intravenous (i.v.) continuous infusion or an i.v. bolus.[14-18] Also, ^{13}C incorporation from acetate into plasma free glutamine was measured.[48]

[1-^{13}C, ^{15}N] leucine and [1-^{13}C, ^{15}N] alanine were used to demonstrate the feasibility of GC-C-IRMS analysis for studies of albumin synthesis.[25] To address questions related to collagen synthesis in humans, [^{13}C]- and [^{15}N]proline have been used.[25] The same authors also indicated the possibility of measuring RNA turnover by an intravenous infusion of [^{15}N]orotate.[25]

We measured ^{15}N enrichments of various plasma free and body protein amino acids from human and animal samples, particularly the enrichment of lysine; this amino acid is not transaminated in mammalian tissues.[24,28] The appearance of ^{15}N-labeled lysine in body proteins and amino acids upon oral administration of anorganic ^{15}N does indicate its microbial origin (and intestinal absorption) from the gut microflora. A method to trace incorporation of ^{13}C into plasma urea was recently reported. This would offer possibilities to study in vivo kinetics of urea and ureagenesis.[9]

Due to its capability of detecting very small enrichments with high precision, the application of GC-C-IRMS allows the decrease in the needed dose of stable isotope tracer. This would prevent a possible artificial increase in metabolite pool sizes, and it also decreases tracer cost.[8,10] For example, plasma amino acid turnover measurements in humans are usually performed using a singly carbon-labeled tracer, and infusion rates between 1 and 5 $\mu mol \cdot kg^{-1} \cdot h^{-1}$, depending on the pool size of the amino acid considered and the physiological state. These rates could be decreased at least by a factor of 10.

7.5 CONCLUSION AND OUTLOOK

In this chapter, we have outlined general features of GC-C-IRMS analysis for carbon and nitrogen, and have shown the feasibility and utility of this sensitive, high-precision methodology for studies of protein and amino acid kinetics. It provides the means for a dramatic expansion of opportunities to investigate metabolic issues which can be addressed using stable isotope tracer techniques. However, the future holds new, exciting opportunities which may eventually become commercially available.

The simultaneous analysis of ^{13}C and ^{15}N in a single GC-C-IRMS run should be relatively easy to achieve, since the combustion interface does generate both N_2 and CO_2, and the isotopic measurement could be performed simultaneously by two IRMS: one dedicated to ^{13}C, and the other to ^{15}N measurement. Techniques for on-line reduction of organic compounds to hydrogen gas for hydrogen isotopic analysis have already been developed.[2,3] Another new approach is the pyrolysis of organic material and subsequent separation of fragments by gas chromatography, which allows intramolecular high-precision position-specific carbon isotope analysis.[49] The pyrolysis approach is also useful for the on-line determination of ^{18}O in organic matter.[19,50]

We hope that researchers in the area of metabolism will take full advantage of the attractive analytical possibilities offered by GC-C-IRMS, and that scientists who are new in this field may obtain information on the pitfalls and their solutions.

ACKNOWLEDGMENT

We express our gratitude to P. Albrecht, D. Ulbricht, and E. Küchler for their commitment and their skilled analytical assistance.

REFERENCES

1. Brand, W. A., High precision isotope ratio monitoring techniques in mass spectrometry, *J. Mass Spectrom.*, 31, 225, 1996.

2. Tobias, H. J. and Brenna, J. T., High-precision D/H measurement from organic mixtures by gas chromatography continuous-flow isotope ratio mass spectrometry using a palladium filter, *Anal. Chem.*, 68, 3002, 1996.

3. Tobias, H. J. and Brenna, J. T., On-line pyrolysis as a limitless reduction source for high-precision isotopic analysis of organic-derived hydrogen, *Anal. Chem.*, 69, 3148, 1997.

4. Metges, C. C., Kempe, K., and Wolfram, G., Enrichment of selected serum fatty acids after a small oral dosage of (1-^{13}C)- and (8-^{13}C)triolein in human volunteers analysed by gas chromatography/combustion isotope ratio mass spectrometry, *Biol. Mass. Spectrom.*, 23, 295, 1994.

5. Carnielli, V. P., Sulkers, E. J., Moretti, C., Wattimena, J. L. D., van Goudoever, J. B., Degenhart, H. J., Zacchello, F., and Sauer, P. J. J., Conversion of octanoic acid into long-chain saturated fatty acids in premature infants fed a formula containing medium-chain triglycerides, *Metabolism*, 43, 1287, 1994.

6. Binnert, C., Laville, M. Pachiaudi, C., Rigalleau, V., and Beylot, M., Use of gas chromatography/isotope ratio mass spectrometry to study triglyceride metabolism in humans, *Lipids*, 30, 869, 1995.

7. Demmelmair, H., von Schenck, U., Behrendt, E., Sauerwald, T., and Koletzko, B., Estimation of arachidonic acid synthesis in full term neonates using natural variation of ^{13}C content, *J. Pediatr. Gastroenterol. Nutri.*, 21, 31, 1995.

8. Guo, Z., Nielsen, S., Burguera, B., and Jensen, M. D., Free fatty acid turnover measured using ultralow doses of [U-^{13}C] palmitate, *J. Lipid Res.*, 38, 1888, 1997.

9. Beylot, M., David, F., Khalfallah, Y., Normand, S., Large, V., and Brunengraber, H., Determination of (^{13}C)urea enrichment by gas chromatography/mass spectrometry and gas chromatography/isotope ratio mass spectrometry, *Biol. Mass Spectrom.*, 23, 510, 1994.

10. Guo, Z. K., Luke, A. H., Lee, W. P., and Schoeller, D., Compound specific carbon isotope ratio determination of enriched cholesterol, *Anal. Chem.*, 65, 1954, 1993.

11. Tetens, V., Kristensen, N. B., and Calder, A. G., Measurement of ^{13}C enrichment of plasma lactate by gas chromatography/isotope ratio mass spectrometry, *Anal. Chem.*, 67, 858, 1995.

12. Demmelmair, H. and Schmidt, H-L., Precise δ^{13}C-determination in the range of natural abundance on amino acids from protein hydrolysates by gas chromatography-isotope ratio mass spectrometry, *Isotopes Environ. Health Stud.*, 29, 237, 1993.

13. Rambal, C., Pachiaudi, C., Normand, S., Riou, J-P., Louisot, P., and Martin, A., Effects of specific dietary sugars on the incorporation of ^{13}C label from dietary glucose into neutral sugars of rat intestine and serum glycoproteins, *Br. J. Nutr.*, 73, 443, 1995.

14. Yarasheski, K. E., Smith, K., Rennie, M. J., and Bier, D. M., Measurement of muscle protein fractional synthetic rate by capillary gas chromatography/combustion isotope ratio mass spectrometry, *Biol. Mass Spectrom.*, 21, 486, 1992.

15. Balagopal, P., Ford, G. C., Ebenstein, D. B., Nadeau, D. A., and Nair, K. S., Mass spectrometric methods for determination of [^{13}C] leucine enrichment in human muscle protein, *Anal. Biochem.*, 239, 77, 1996.

16. Demant, T., Packard, C. J., Demmelmair, H., Stewart, P., Bedynek, A., Bedford, D., Seidel, D., and Shepherd, J., Sensitive methods to study human apolipoprotein B metabolism using stable isotope-labeled amino acids, *Am. J. Physiol.*, 270 (Endocrinol. Metab. 33), E1022, 1996.

17. Hartl, W. H., Demmelmair, H., Jauch, K-W., Schmidt, H-L., Koletzko, B., and Schildberg, F. W., Determination of protein synthesis in human rectal cancer in situ by continuous [1-^{13}C]leucine infusion, *Am. J. Physiol.*, 272 (Endocrinol. Metab. 35), E796, 1997.

18. Pont, F., Duvillard, L., Maugeais, C., Athias, A., Persegol, L., Gambert, P., and Verges, B., Isotope ratio mass spectrometry, compared with conventional mass spectrometry in kinetic studies at low and high enrichment levels: applications to lipoprotein kinetics, *Anal. Biochem.*, 248, 277, 1997.

19. Brand, W. A., Tegtmeyer, A. R., and Hilkert, A., Compound-specific isotope analysis: extending toward $^{15}N/^{14}N$ and $^{18}O/^{16}O$, *Org. Geochem.*, 21, 585, 1994.

20. Merritt, D. A. and Hayes, J. M., Nitrogen isotopic analyses by isotope-ratio-monitoring gas chromatography/mass spectrometry, *Am. Soc. Mass Spectrom.*, 5, 387, 1994.

21. Macko, S. A., Uhle, M. E., Engel, M. H., and Andrusevich, V., Stable nitrogen isotope analysis of amino acid enantiomers by gas chromatography/combustion/isotope ratio mass spectrometry, *Anal. Chem.*, 69, 926, 1997.

22. Hofmann, D., Jung, K., Segschneider, H-J., Gehre, M., and Schüürmann, G., $^{15}N/^{14}N$ analysis of amino acids with GC-C-IRMS-methodological investigation and ecotoxicological applications, *Isotopes Environ. Health Stud.*, 31, 367, 1995.

23. Segschneider, H-J., Hofmann, D., Schmidt, G., and Russow, R., Incorporation of $^{15}NO_2$ nitrogen into individual amino acids by sunflowers using GC-C-IRMS, *Isotopes Environ. Health Stud.*, 31, 315, 1995.

24. Metges, C. C., Petzke, K. J., and Hennig, U., Gas chromatography/combustion/isotope ratio mass spectrometric comparison of N-acetyl- and N-pivaloyl amino acid esters to measure ^{15}N isotopic abundances in physiological samples: a pilot study on amino acid synthesis in the upper gastro-intestinal tract of minipigs, *J. Mass Spectrom.*, 31, 367, 1996.

25. Rennie, M. J., Meier-Augenstein, W., Watt, P. W., Patel, A., Begley, I.S., and Scrimgeour, C. M., Use of continuous-flow combustion MS in studies of human metabolism, *Biochem. Soc. Trans.*, 24, 927, 1996.

26. Metges, C. C. and Petzke, K. J., Measurement of $^{15}N/^{14}N$ isotopic composition in individual plasma free amino acids of human adults at natural abundance by gas chromatography-combustion isotope ratio mass spectrometry, *Anal. Biochem.*, 247, 158, 1997.

27. Petzke, K. J., Korkushko, O. V., Semesko, T. M., and Metges, C. C., N-isotopic composition in human plasma protein amino acids at natural abundance level and after a single [$^{15}N_2$] urea administration measured by GC-C-IRMS, *Isotopes Environ. Health Stud.*, 33, 267, 1997.

28. Metges, C. C., El-Khoury, A. E., Petzke, K. J., Bedri, S., Fuller, M. F., and Young, V. R., The quantitative contribution of microbial lysine to lysine flux in healthy male subjects, *FASEB J*, 11, A149, 1997.

29. Galimov, E. M., *The biological fractionation of isotopes*, Academic Press, Orlando, 1985.

30. Schmidt, H-L. and Metges, C., Variations of the natural isotope abundance in diet — causes of artifacts or the base of new possibilities in stable isotope tracer work? in *Proc. 7th Congr. ESPEN*, Munich, Dietze, Grünert, Kleinberger, and Wolfram, Eds., Karger, Basel, 1986, 156.

31. DeNiro, M. J. and Epstein, S., Mechanism of carbon isotope fractionation associated with lipid synthesis, *Science*, 197, 261, 1977.

32. Abelson, P. H. and Hoering, T.C., Carbon isotope fractionation in formation of amino acids by photosynthetic organisms, *Proc. Natl. Acad. Sci. U.S.A.*, 47, 623, 1961.

33. Macko, S. A., Fogel, M. L., Engel, M. H., and Hare, P. E., Kinetic fractionation of stable nitrogen isotopes during amino acid transamination, *Geochimica et Cosmochimica Acta*, 50, 2143, 1986.

34. Hare, P. E., Fogel, M. L., Stafford, T. W., Mitchell, A. D., and Hoering, T. C., The isotopic composition of carbon and nitrogen in individual amino acids isolated from modern and fossil proteins, *J. Archaeol. Sci.*, 18, 277, 1991.

35. Gaebler, O. H., Vitti, T. G., and Vukmirovich, R., Isotope effects in metabolism of ^{14}N and ^{15}N from unlabeled dietary proteins, *Can. J. Biochem.*, 44, 1249, 1966.

36. Craig, H., Isotope standards for carbon and oxygen and correction factors for mass-spectrometric analysis of carbon dioxide, *Geochimica et Cosmochimica Acta*, 12, 133, 1957.

37. Meier-Augenstein, W., The chromatographic side of isotope ratio mass spectrometry – pitfalls and answers, *LC-GC*, 15, 244, 1997.

38. Silfer, J. A., Engel, M. H., Macko, S. A., and Jumeau, E. J., Stable carbon isotope analysis of amino acid enantiomers by conventional isotope ratio mass spectrometry and combined gas chromatography/isotope ratio mass spectrometry, *Anal. Chem.*, 63, 370, 1991.

39. Jakoby, W. B., Ed., Enzyme purification and related techniques, *Methods in Enzymology*, Vol. 104 Part C, Academic Press Inc., Orlando, 1984.

40. Harris, E. L. V. and Angal, S., Eds., *Protein purification methods - a practical approach*, Practical Approach Series, Rickwood, D. and Hames, B.D., Series Eds., IRL Press at Oxford University Press, Oxford, 1989.

41. Schwenk, W. F., Berg, P. J., Beaufrere, B., Miles, J. M., and Haymond, M. W., Use of t-butyldimethylsilylation in the gas chromatographic/mass spectrometric analysis of physiological compounds found in plasma using electron-impact ionization, *Anal. Biochem.*, 141, 101, 1984.

42. Fortier, G., Tenaschuk, D., and MacKenzie, S. L., Capillary gas chromatography micro-assay for pyroglutamic, glutamic and aspartic acids, and glutamine and asparagine, *J. Chrom.*, 361, 253, 1986.

43. Rieley, G., Derivatization of organic compounds prior to gas chromatographic-combustion-isotope ratio mass spectrometry analysis: identification of isotope fractionation processes, *Analyst*, 119, 915, 1994.

44. Yu, Y-M., Burke, J. F., Tompkins, R. G., Martin, R., and Young, V. R., Quantitative aspects of interorgan relationships among arginine and citrulline metabolism, *Am. J. Physiol.*, 271 (Endocrinol. Metab. 34), E1098, 1996.

45. Goodman, K. J. and Brenna, J. T., High-precision gas chromatography-combustion isotope ratio mass spectrometry at low signal levels, *J. Chromat. A.*, 689, 63–68, 1995.

46. Goodman, K. J. and Brenna, J. T., Curve fitting for restoration of accuracy for overlapping peaks in gas chromatography/combustion isotope ratio mass spectrometry, *Anal. Chem.*, 66, 1294, 1994.

47. Heys, S. D., McNurlan, M. A., Park, K. G. M., Milne, E., and Garlick, P. J., Baseline measurements for stable isotope studies: an alternative to biopsy, *Biomed. Environ. Mass Spectrom.*, 19, 176, 1990.

48. Menand, C., Pouteau, E., Marchini, S., Maugere, P., Krempf, M., and Darmaun, D., Determination of low ^{13}C-glutamine enrichments using gas chromatography-combustion-isotope ratio-mass spectrometry, *J. Mass Spectrom.*, 32, 1094, 1997.

49. Corso, N. T. and Brenna, J. T., High-precision position-specific isotope analysis, *Proc. Natl. Acad. Sci. U.S.A.*, 94, 1049, 1997.

50. Koziet, J., Isotope ratio mass spectrometric method for the on-line determination of oxygen-18 in organic matter, *J. Mass Spectrom.*, 32, 103, 1997.

8 Use of Isotope Dilution Methods to Investigate Glutamine Metabolism *in vivo* in Humans

Dominique Darmaun and
Christine Bobin-Dubigeon

CONTENTS

8.1 WHY STUDY GLUTAMINE METABOLISM?

Glutamine (Figure 8.1) represents merely 5% of bound amino acids in body protein.[1,2] Since mammals have the ability to synthesize glutamine, it is not an essential amino acid by conventional criteria. Glutamine has, however, gained a peculiar status among amino acids, and is now believed to play a prominent role at the crossroads of protein and energy metabolism.

First, glutamine is the most abundant free amino acid in the body. Indeed, the concentration of glutamine exceeds that of all other amino acids in human plasma

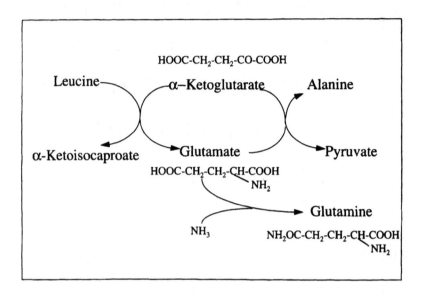

FIGURE 8.1 Role of leucine as a N donor for glutamine and alanine synthesis. During transamination, leucine's N is transferred to α-ketoglutarate, forming glutamate; the latter can either (a) donate its N to pyruvate, yielding alanine, or (b) accept a second N, forming glutamine.

(600 μmol/L), and inside cells: glutamine alone represents two-thirds of the intracellular free amino acid pool in skeletal muscle.[1,3]

Assuming 1) a muscle mass of ≈28 kg in a healthy 70-kg adult (i.e., 40% of body weight); 2) an intracellular glutamine concentration of 19.5 mmol per kg of intracellular water; and 3) an intracellular water content of 77% in muscle, intracellular glutamine content can be estimated at ≈420 mmol (6000 μmol/kg body wt), or > 60 grams for muscle alone. Since other tissues such as liver contain high concentrations of glutamine as well, it can be estimated that whole-body free glutamine is ≈80 g in a 70-kg adult, a mass somewhat similar to that of liver glycogen (120 g). In addition to its use as a building block for protein synthesis, a number of important physiological functions have been attributed to glutamine.[1] Both animal and human studies have revealed its role as a major nitrogen (N) shuttle between organs,[1,4,5,6] and a major source of N for ureagenesis.[7]

Glutamine also serves as an "ammonia trap," protecting the body against hyperammonemia; and, as the main precursor of urinary ammonia, it plays a critical role in the maintenance of acid base balance.[8] Its N is used for the synthesis of purines and pyrimidines, which are in high demand in tissues with high rates of DNA synthesis and cell replication.[9]

From a teleological standpoint, it makes sense for rapidly dividing cells to use glutamine both as an N donor for nucleic acid synthesis, and, through conversion of its carbon skeleton to CO_2 in the Krebs cycle, as a major source of energy; accordingly, glutamine is essential for mammalian cells in culture,[9] as well as the preferred fuel for cells of both the immune system[10] and intestinal lining.[1,11] More recently, glutamine was shown to be a major source of carbon for gluconeogenesis as well.[12-14] Moreover, during the last two decades, evidence has accumulated to suggest that glutamine should be considered a conditionally essential amino acid.[1,6]

Indeed, although glutamine is abundant and can be synthesized *de novo*, a rapid drop in muscle free glutamine pool is observed in severe, life-threatening conditions associated with protein wasting.[1] In the 1980s, animal studies revealed a striking correlation between the size of the intracellular glutamine pool and rates of muscle protein synthesis in rats submitted to dietary restriction or endotoxin injection.[1,6,15] Improvement in nitrogen balance was observed upon replenishment of muscle glutamine pool with intravenous glutamine supplementation in several clinical studies.[16,17] This putative protein anabolic effect may involve stimulation of protein synthesis, as nonoxidative leucine disposal, an index of whole-body protein synthesis, was enhanced by enteral glutamine infusion in healthy postabsorptive adults.[18]

8.2 DIFFICULTIES INTRINSIC TO THE INVESTIGATION OF GLUTAMINE METABOLISM WITH ISOTOPE DILUTION METHODS

Investigation of glutamine metabolism has long relied solely on the enzymatic assay of glutamine concentrations. The measurement of arterio-venous concentration gradients across organ beds conducted in the 1970s produced a wealth of information about the "geography" of glutamine metabolism,[6,19] i.e., identified sites of release and uptake.

In healthy humans, skeletal muscle was reported to be the main source of endogenous glutamine in the postabsorptive state, while splanchnic bed (gut and liver) and, to a lesser extent, kidney, were its main sites of utilization. Yet measurement of arteriovenous gradients only provides the net balance of a substrate across a tissue, and some organs (e.g., liver) may both utilize and produce glutamine at the same time. Also, arteriovenous concentration differences are often close to the limit of analytical accuracy and precision of the assay; calculation of organ glutamine balance requires the technically difficult determination of organ blood flows. Moreover, concentrations alone provide little insight into the kinetics of glutamine production, oxidation, or utilization. The latter parameters can only be approached using tracer methods.

Glutamine's chemical structure explains why tracer dilution methods which had been developed to assess amino acid kinetics since the mid-1960s[4] had not been applied to glutamine until the mid-1980s. First, there is no radioactive isotope of N (except for ^{13}N, which has too short a half-life to be conveniently used). Radioactive, ^{14}C- or ^{3}H-labeled glutamine can only be used on the condition that glutamine be well separated from glutamate and α-ketoglutarate, since all three substrates (Figure. 8.1) share the same carbon skeleton. In addition, glutamine's amide nitrogen is labile; glutamine therefore degrades spontaneously *in vitro*, producing either ammonia and glutamate, or cyclizing to pyroglutamate when heated. Degradation of glutamine to glutamate can be a significant drawback, since despite their closely related structure, glutamine and glutamate have markedly different metabolic behaviors *in vivo* (see below); thus, it is of importance to distinguish glutamate from glutamine.

In fact, early work using ^{15}N-glutamine took advantage of the lability of its amide-N. Using [5-^{15}N]glutamine as a tracer, Golden et al. determined the ^{15}N-enrichment of plasma glutamine in the [15]NH$_3$ arising from glutamine hydrolysis.[8] We adopted a different approach, and separated plasma glutamine from glutamate on disposable anion exchange columns under alkaline conditions, so that a "pure" glutamine fraction could be isolated from plasma.[20] The latter fraction could then be derivatized as glutamate (e.g., to N-acetyl, n-propyl-glutamate or NAP-glutamate) during subsequent sample preparation. Indeed, the usual derivatization procedures to produce NAP- or N-heptafluorobutyryl, n-propyl (HFBP) esters, quantitatively degrade glutamine to glutamate, because heating with either strong acid (HBr or HCl) or "aggressive" reagents (acetylchloride) is used in the alkylation reaction. Stable isotope enrichment is subsequently easily determined in the stable glutamate derivative originating from the "pure" glutamine fraction, using selected ion monitoring chemical ionization (CI) or electron impact ionization (EI) gas chromatography-mass spectrometry (GC-MS). The method has been applied to various forms of ^{15}N, ^{2}H, and ^{13}C-labeled glutamine.

The same anion-exchange separation scheme, followed by 1) subsequent enzymatic conversion of glutamate, and 2) analysis as a stable derivative of α-ketoglutarate by high-performance liquid chromatography (HPLC), allowed us to use radioactive [3]H- and ^{14}C-labeled glutamine as tracers.[21] Other research groups have performed pre-column derivatization, followed by direct HPLC separation of ^{14}C-glutamine from glutamate in plasma.[22]

When stable isotope tracers are used, conventional GC-MS has, however, relatively poor sensitivity: it cannot reliably determine enrichments below 0.3 mol% excess (MPE), so relatively large amounts of expensive glutamine tracers are required. In this regard, the use of gas chromatography-combustion-isotope ratio mass spectrometry (GC-C-IRMS) may be of interest. The same sample extraction, glutamine separation, derivatization to NAP-glutamate, and GC separation are used as with the above GC-MS method. When a GC-C-IRMS method is chosen, the NAP-glutamate isolated on GC is combusted in an online (940°C) furnace, and the CO$_2$ evolving from the combustion is subsequently analyzed for its [13]CO$_2$/[12]CO$_2$ isotope ratio, using an online isotope ratio mass spectrometer (IRMS). The latter method allows for determination of ^{13}C-enrichments as low as 0.02 MPE.[19,23]

Other research workers have set up methods to measure glutamine low ^{15}N-enrichments: a similar scheme of GC-C-IRMS is used, except that an online reduction furnace placed after the combustion furnace converts all the N in the molecule to gaseous N$_2$.[24] Instead of an initial separation of glutamine from glutamate in plasma, other groups have proposed the use of milder derivatization schemes[25] (using lower temperatures, and less aggressive derivatization reagents, avoiding HCl or HBr). These milder derivatization schemes preserve glutamine intact (at least in part), and allow the formation of different derivatives for glutamine and glutamate, which consequently have different retention times upon GC analysis.[25]

8.3 ASSESSMENT OF GLUTAMINE INTERORGAN FLUXES USING ISOTOPE DILUTION METHODS IN HUMANS

Over the last decade, tracer methods have allowed quantitation of the rates of glutamine interorgan transport in systemic circulation, and provided further insight into its sources of production and utilization in health, as well as the modulation of glutamine metabolism by nutrition, hormones, and disease.

8.3.1 GLUTAMINE INTERORGAN TRANSPORT RATES

The appearance rate (Ra) of glutamine into plasma (determined under steady-state conditions through infusion of labeled glutamine) consistently exceeds that of all other amino acids measured to date (Figure 8.2). It ranges between 280 and

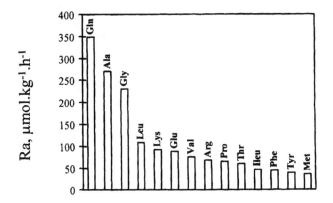

FIGURE 8.2   Rates of appearance of selected amino acids in healthy postabsorptive adults (adapted from Reference 5 and personal data).

400 $\mu mol.kg^{-1}.h^{-1}$ in healthy adults depending upon the tracer used: ^2H- and ^3H-labeled tracers yielded the highest values, followed by ^{13}C-labeled, amino-^{15}N-, and amide-^{15}N-labeled glutamine.[5,4,26] Glutamine Ra therefore is ≈80 g/d in a 70-kg adult, a flux equivalent to a third to half the rate of glucose turnover under similar conditions. No priming dose was needed to achieve isotopic steady state in plasma within 3 h of tracer infusion. Fitting the rise of plasma glutamine enrichment to plateau during an *unprimed* infusion allowed for determination of the size of glutamine tracer-miscible pool: the latter was consistently found to be ≈200 $\mu mol/kg$ of body weight in healthy adults,[5] and ≈300 $\mu mol/kg$ in healthy prepubertal children.[27,28] Assuming a plasma volume of 45 ml/kg body weight, plasma glutamine can account for only ≈20 to 30 $\mu mol/kg$; glutamine tracer-miscible pool therefore is ≈10-fold larger than plasma glutamine pool, suggesting that the labeled glutamine infused does penetrate body compartments other than plasma. The size of the tracer-miscible glutamine pool, however, represents only a small (≈5%) fraction of whole-body

glutamine content, estimated at ≈6000 μmol/kg (see above). This suggests that there is some degree of compartmentation of glutamine metabolism between the intra- and extracellular milieus. Indeed, steady-state intracellular glutamine enrichment in red blood cells was only 20% of plasma enrichment;[5] intracellular glutamine enrichment reached only 9 and 21% of plasma enrichment after 2 and 11 h of tracer infusion, respectively, in the free amino acid pool in skeletal muscle biopsy samples.[24] Compartmentation between extra- and intracellular milieus is, in fact, common to several nonessential amino acids,[29] and dramatically greater in the case of glutamate. Upon infusion of ^{15}N-glutamate, intracellular ^{15}N-glutamate remained negligible in red blood cells; even though all glutamine in the body is synthesized from glutamate, the appearance of ^{15}N-glutamine into plasma upon infusion of ^{15}N-glutamate remained extremely low.[5] Taken together, these data suggest that a very small fraction of the labeled glutamate infused into plasma entered the intracellular milieu.

Because 1) the tracer-miscible pool for glutamine tracers is much smaller than the estimated body glutamine content, and 2) equilibration of labeled glutamine across muscle cell membrane is far from complete regardless of the duration of infusion, plasma glutamine Ra should be considered an *index of glutamine interorgan transport rather than a measure of "whole-body glutamine production rate,"* a parameter that must be larger by several orders of magnitude, but is not accessible with current isotopic approaches.

In spite of these uncertainties, plasma glutamine kinetics can be reliably assessed even in the non-steady state, using a single pool model.[26]

8.3.2   SOURCES AND FATE OF PLASMA GLUTAMINE IN THE FASTING AND FED STATES

8.3.2.1   Sources of endogenous glutamine

Because glutamine is a nonessential amino acid, two sources contribute to its endogenous production: release from protein breakdown, and glutamine *de novo* synthesis. Assuming protein breakdown releases each amino acid in proportion to its abundance in body protein, the release of glutamine from protein breakdown (B,gln), can be estimated by: B,gln = k x B,leu, where B,leu is the release of the *essential* amino acid leucine from protein breakdown (synonymous with leucine Ra in the postabsorptive state), and k the ratio of glutamine to leucine content of body protein. Body protein contains 8 g of leucine per 100 g. While the glutamine + glutamate content (13.9 g/100 g) of mixed body protein is known, the contribution of glutamine per se to that total remains to be defined. Estimates of the abundance of glutamine residues in body protein range from 2% (based on the abundance of the glutamine-coding sequences in the actin gene)[1] to 13.9% for the total (glutamine + glutamate) in whole-body protein. This is because, upon acid hydrolysis of protein *in vitro*, all glutamine residues are degraded to glutamate; hence, protein composition tables only list (glutamine + glutamate).

In early studies, we assumed that glutamine residues contributed 13.9 g/100 g protein;[25,30] however, because protein glutamate content must be > 0, this results in an overestimation of glutamine release from proteolysis. More recently, calculations were performed assuming that glutamine contributed half of the total, i.e., 7 g/100 g.[31] Finally, based on recent studies using a novel analytical tool for estimating glutamine content,[2] Fürst et al. proposed that mixed body protein contains 4.5 g of glutamine per 100 g (Fürst, P., personal communication); this is consistent with the mean glutamine content calculated when averaging the gene-code frequency in a dozen proteins.[1] Depending on the estimated glutamine content of body protein, the relative contribution of glutamine *de novo* synthesis to overall glutamine Ra ranges from ≈ 60% to ≈ 85% in healthy adults.[30]

Based on ^{15}N appearing in plasma glutamine upon infusion of ^{15}N-leucine, 9% of glutamine α-amino N arises from leucine (Figure 8.1) in postabsorptive humans. This transfer accounts for 21% of overall leucine N flux, suggesting that branched-chain amino acids (BCAA) contribute similar amounts of N to glutamine and alanine.[32] The prominent role of skeletal muscle in glutamine synthesis is suggested by: 1) the fact that BCAA, which are predominantly utilized in skeletal muscle, are a major source for glutamine *de novo* synthesis; and 2) the reduction in glutamine Ra (expressed per kg of body weight) observed in children with Duchenne muscular dystrophy,[33] a disease associated with a dramatic reduction in muscle mass.

8.3.2.2   Sites of glutamine utilization

In the postabsorptive state, the rate of disappearance (Rd) of plasma glutamine (synonymous with Ra under steady-state conditions) was found as 20 to 30% lower in adults[34] or children[35] who had a very short residual small bowel after intestinal resection. Because this low Ra was measured long after surgery, and in the absence of significant malnutrition or nutritional supplementation, the data suggest that the decline in glutamine utilization was due to the reduction in the mass of small bowel per se; or, *a contrario*, that an intact small bowel would "consume" > 20% of plasma glutamine Rd.

The role of the splanchnic bed (both gut and liver) in glutamine utilization is further enhanced in the "fed" state. When exogenous glutamine is supplied through the enteral route, it is quantitatively absorbed in the proximal jejunum.[36] Simultaneous infusion of ^{3}H-glutamine via the intravenous route, along with the enteral infusion of ^{13}C-glutamine, showed that 53 to 74% of the glutamine administered via enteral route is extracted by the splanchnic bed, depending upon whether trace or nutritionally significant doses are given.[31,37] Extensive splanchnic uptake of enteral glutamine is already functional by the tenth day of life in very low birth weight premature infants.[38] The splanchnic bed most likely is a major site of glutamine oxidation: when tracer amounts of glutamine were administered intravenously, 32 to 51% (depending upon the type of tracer used) of the dose was oxidized to CO_2; with enteral administration, the oxidized fraction rose to 69% of the dose.[31]

8.4 USE OF TRACER DILUTION METHODS TO EXPLORE THE REGULATION OF GLUTAMINE METABOLISM *IN VIVO* IN HUMANS

8.4.1 DOES GLUTAMINE REGULATE ITS OWN PRODUCTION?

Glutamine may exert a negative feedback on its own rate of synthesis *in vivo*. Endogenous glutamine *de novo* synthesis declines when dietary protein intake is increased,[39] or when plasma glutamine concentration is raised via enteral glutamine delivery.[31] A decline in plasma glutamine level may not, however, enhance glutamine synthesis rate, since 1) during a 42-h fast, lower estimated rates of *de novo* synthesis were observed along with slightly lower glutamine levels,[13] and 2) a decline in plasma glutamine, induced by "trapping" plasma glutamine by the drug phenyl-butyrate, failed to enhance rates of glutamine *de novo* synthesis.[40]

8.4.2 GLUTAMINE AND GLUCONEOGENESIS

Although alanine has long been thought of as the main glucogenic amino acid, recent studies using ^{14}C-glutamine showed that the contribution of glutamine carbon to glucose equals that of alanine.[12] Labeled carbon from glutamine can, however, end up in glucose via two different routes: true conversion of glutamine to glucose (as glutamine enters the Krebs cycle as α-ketoglutarate), or, alternatively, through simple "fixation" of labeled CO_2 since 1) glutamine is extensively oxidized[31] to CO_2, and 2) fixation of CO_2 occurs in the gluconeogenic pathway during the conversion of pyruvate to oxaloacetate. Using [1-^{14}C]leucine as a probe for this "CO_2 fixation" route, we observed that 96% of the carbon transfer from [3,4-[13]C_2]glutamine to glucose occurred through "true" conversion. Overall, glutamine carbon contributes 5 to 8%[12,13] of glucose production in postabsorptive adults; its contribution rises to 16% after a 42-h fast.[13] Glutamine may not only be a substrate for gluconeogenesis, but a regulator of this pathway as well.[14] Conversely, glucose infusion enhances the relative contribution of glucose to glutamine *de novo* synthesis, without enhancing the overall rate of glutamine synthesis (Hankard, R., et al., unpublished results).

The effect of insulin deficiency on glutamine kinetics was investigated by infusing [15]N- and ^{13}C-glutamine in Type 1, insulin-dependent diabetic (IDDM) patients in whom blood sugar was "clamped" either at near normoglycemia or around 250 mg/dl: even though proteolysis (measured using leucine kinetics) was significantly increased under hyperglycemic conditions, glutamine Ra remained unaltered, whether measured with ^{15}N-glutamine[41] or ^{13}C-glutamine (Hankard, R., et al., unpublished results), and the contribution of glutamine carbon to gluconeogenesis was unchanged. Similarly, glutamine Ra measured using infusion of ^{14}C-glutamine, was found to be unaltered in patients with Type 2, non-insulin-dependent diabetes mellitus (NIDDM), compared to healthy volunteers;[42] yet the conversion of glutamine to glucose and alanine was increased nearly two-fold, while glutamine oxidation was reduced.[42]

8.4.3   GLUTAMINE IN STRESS AND GROWTH

Because life-threatening diseases induce dramatic changes in muscle glutamine pool, attention has focused on the potential role of the "stress hormones" catecholamines and cortisol, in mediating the increased glutamine efflux from muscle. Infusion of epinephrine in healthy volunteers, at doses designed to mimic the elevations in catecholamines observed in stress, only elicited a modest ≈7% rise in glutamine Ra.[43] In contrast, cortisol infusion resulting in two-fold elevations in plasma cortisol was associated with a dramatic, sustained 40 to 60% rise in glutamine *de novo* synthetic rate in healthy volunteers.[5] Similar elevations in glutamine Ra were observed in severely burned patients.[44] Taken together, the data suggest that cortisol may mediate most of the stress-induced changes in glutamine synthesis *in vivo*. Even though starvation-induced undernutrition has long been shown to be associated with a decline in energy expenditure and protein turnover, this may not hold true when malnutrition is due to gastrointestinal disease. Indeed, when leucine and glutamine fluxes were measured in malnourished patients with non-neoplastic gastrointestinal disease, a dramatic ≈28% elevation in glutamine Ra was observed, while leucine Ra was increased by ≈15%,[45] compared with matched controls. Similarly, an ≈47% elevation of glutamine Ra was observed in children with sickle cell anemia, a chronic anemia associated with hypermetabolism, compared to healthy age-matched control children.[28]

Acceleration of glutamine turnover is not, however, synonymous with protein wasting; this may reflect a state of accelerated growth as well, since 1) an ≈32% increase in glutamine Ra was observed in response to treatment with the anabolic hormone testosterone in prepubertal boys,[27] and 2) glutamine Ra expressed per unit of body weight clearly correlates with growth rates, as it continuously declines throughout growth and development (Figure 8.3).

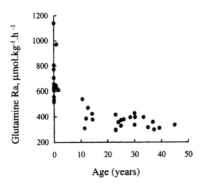

FIGURE 8.3   Glutamine Ra measured in healthy human subjects of various ages. (Data compiled from References 5, 28, 31, 34, and 35.)

REFERENCES

1. Lacey, J. M. and Wilmore, D. W., Is glutamine a conditionally essential amino acid? *Nutr. Rev.*, 48, 297, 1990.
2. Kuhn, K. S., Stehle, P., and Fürst, P., Glutamine content of protein and peptide-based enteral products, *J.P.E.N.*, 20, 292, 1996.
3. Bergström, J., Fürst, P., and Noree, L. O., Intracellular free amino acid concentration in human muscle tissue, *J. Appl. Physiol.*, 36, 693, 1974.
4. Bier, D. M., Intrinsically difficult problems: the kinetics of body proteins and amino acids in man, *Diab./Metab. Rev.*, 5, 111, 1989.
5. Darmaun, D., Matthews, D. E., and Bier, D. M. Glutamine and glutamate kinetics in humans, *Am. J. Physiol.*, 251, E117, 1986.
6. Young, V. R. and El-Khoury, A. E., The notion of the nutritional essentiality of amino acids, revisited, with a note on the indispensable amino acid requirements in adults, in *Amino Acid Metabolism and Therapy in Health and Nutritional Disease*, Cynober, L. A. Ed., CRC Press, Boca Raton, FL, 191, 1995.
7. Häussinger, D., Glutamine metabolism in the liver: overview and current concepts, *Metabolism*, 38, Suppl. 1, 14, 1989.
8. Golden, M. H. N., Jahoor, F., and Jackson, A. A., Glutamine production rate and its contribution to urinary ammonia in normal man, *Clin. Sci.*, 62, 299, 1982.
9. Engström, W. and Zetterberg, A., The relationship between purines, pyrimidines, and glutamine for fibroblast cell proliferation, *J. Cell. Physiol.*, 120, 233, 1984.
10. Calder, P. C., Glutamine and the immune system. *Clin. Nutr.*, 13, 2, 1994.
11. Souba, W. W., Glutamine: a key substrate for the splanchnic bed, *Annu. Rev. Nutr.*, 11, 285, 1991.
12. Nurjhan, N., Bucci, A., Perriello, G., Stumvoll, M., Dailey, G., Bier, D., Toft, I., Jenssen, T., and Gerich, J., Glutamine: a major gluconeogenic precursor and vehicle for interorgan carbon transport in man, *J. Clin. Invest.*, 95, 272, 1995.
13. Hankard, R. G., Haymond, M. W., and Darmaun, D., Role of glutamine as a glucose precursor in fasting humans, *Diabetes*, 46, 1535, 1997.
14. Perriello, G., Nurjhan, N., Stumvoll, M., Bucci, A., Welle, S., Dailey, G., Bier, D. M., Toft, I., Jenssen, T. G., and Gerich, J. E., Regulation of gluconeogenesis by glutamine in normal postabsorptive humans, *Am. J. Physiol.*, 272, E437, 1997.
15. Jepson, M., Bates, P., Broadbent, P., Pell, J., and Millward, D., Relationship between glutamine concentration and protein synthesis in rat skeletal muscle, *Am. J. Physiol.*, 255, E166, 1988.
16. Stehle, P., Zander, J., Mertes, N., Alhers, S., Puchstein, C., Lawin, O., and Fürst, P., Effect of parenteral glutamine dipeptide supplements on muscle glutamine loss and nitrogen balance after major surgery. *Lancet*, i:231, 1989.
17. Ziegler, T. R., Young, L. S., Benfell, K., Scheltinga, M., Hortos, K., Bye, R., Morrow, F. D., Jacobs, D. O., Smith, R. J., Antin, J. H., and Wilmore, D. W., Clinical and metabolic efficacy of glutamine-supplemented parenteral nutrition after bone-marrow transplantation, *Ann. Intern. Med.*, 116, 821, 1992.
18. Hankard, R. G., Haymond, M. W., and Darmaun, D., Effect of glutamine on leucine metabolism in humans, *Am. J. Physiol.*, 271, E748, 1996.
19. Abumrad, N. N., Darmaun, D., and Cynober L. A., Approaches to studying amino acid metabolism: from quantitative assays to flux assessment using stables isotopes, in *Amino Acid Metabolism and Therapy in Health and Nutritional Disease*, Cynober, L. A., Ed., CRC Press, Boca Raton, FL, 15, 1995.

20. Darmaun, D., Manary, M. J., and Matthews, D. E., A method for measuring both glutamine and glutamate levels and stable isotope enrichments, *Anal. Biochem.*, 147, 97, 1985.

21. Darmaun, D., D'Amore, D., and Haymond, M. W., Determination of glutamine and α-ketoglutarate concentration and specific activity in plasma using high-performance liquid chromatography, *J. Chromatogr.*, 620, 33, 1993.

22. Jenssen, T., Nurjhan, N., Perriello, G., Bucci, A., Toft, I., and Gerich, J., Determination of [^{14}C]glutamine specific activity in plasma, *J. Liq. Chromatogr.*, 17, 1337, 1994.

23. Menand, C., Pouteau, E., Marchini, J. S., Maugère, P., Krempf, M., and Darmaun, D., Determination of low ^{13}C-glutamine enrichments using gas chromatography-combustion-isotope ratio mass spectrometry, *J. Mass Spectrom.*, 32, 1094, 1997.

24. Van Acker, B. A. C., Matthews, D. E., Haisch, M., Wagenmakers, A. J. M., Hulsewé, K. W. E., Deutz, N. E. P., Soeters, P. B., and Von Meyenfeldt, M. F., Whole body appearance of glutamine calculated *via* the plasma dilution of glutamine tracers: what does it mean?, *Clin. Nutr.*, 16 (Suppl. 2), 20 (Abst.), 1997.

25. Reeds, P. J., Burrin, D. G., Stoll, B., Jahoor, F., Wykes, L., Henry, J., and Frazer, M. E., Enteral glutamate is the preferred source for mucosal glutathione synthesis in fed piglets, *Am. J. Physiol.*, 273, E408, 1997.

26. Kreider, M. E., Stumvoll, M., Meyer, C., Overkamp, D., Welle, S., and Gerich, J. Steady-state and non-steady-state measurements of plasma glutamine turnover in humans, *Am. J. Physiol.*, 273, E621, 1997.

27. Mauras, N., Haymond, M. W., Darmaun, D., Vieira, N. E., Abrams, S. A., and Yergey, A. L., Calcium and protein kinetics in prepubertal boys: positive effects of testosterone, *J. Clin. Invest.*, 93, 1014, 1994.

28. Salman, E. K., Haymond, M. W., Bayne, E., Sager, B. K., Wiisanen, A., Pitel, P., and Darmaun, D., Protein and energy metabolism in prepubertal children with sickle cell anemia, *Pediatr. Res.*, 40, 34, 1996.

29. Darmaun, D., Froguel, P., Rongier, M., and Robert, J. J., Amino acid exchange between plasma and erythrocytes *in vivo* in humans, *J. Appl. Physiol.*, 67, 2383, 1989.

30. Darmaun, D., Matthews, D. E., and Bier, D. M., Physiological hypercortisolemia increases proteolysis, glutamine, and alanine production, *Am. J. Physiol.*, 255, E366, 1988.

31. Hankard, R. G., Darmaun, D., Sager, B. K., D'Amore, D., Parsons, W. R., and Haymond, M. W., Response of glutamine metabolism to exogenous glutamine in humans, *Am. J. Physiol.*, 269, E663, 1995.

32. Darmaun, D. and Déchelotte, P., Role of leucine as precursor of glutamine-amino nitrogen *in vivo* in human, *Am. J. Physiol.*, 260, E326, 1991.

33. Hankard, R. G., Hammond, D., Haymond, M. W., and Darmaun, D., Glutamine metabolism in children with Duchenne muscular dystrophy, manuscript in preparation.

34. Darmaun, D., Messing, B., Just, B., Rongier, M., and Desjeux, J. F., Glutamine metabolism after small intestinal resection in humans, *Metabolism*, 40, 42, 1991.

35. Hankard, R. G., Goulet, O., Ricour, C., Rongier, M., Colomb, V., and Darmaun, D., Glutamine metabolism in children with short-bowel syndrome: a stable isotope study, *Pediatr. Res.*, 36, 202, 1994.

36. Déchelotte, P., Darmaun, D., Rongier, M., Hecketsweiler, B., Rigal, O., and Desjeux, J. F., Absorption and metabolic effects of enterally administered glutamine in humans, *Am. J. Physiol.*, 260, G677, 1991.

37. Matthews, D. E., Morano, M. A., and Campbell, R. G., Splanchnic bed utilization of glutamine and glutamic acid in humans, *Am. J. Physiol.*, 264, E848, 1993.

38. Darmaun, D., Roig, J. C., Auestad, N., Sager, B. K., and Neu, J. Glutamine metabolism in very low birth weight infants, *Pediatr. Res.*, 41, 391, 1997.
39. Matthews, D. and Campbell, G., The effect of dietary protein intake on glutamine and glutamate nitrogen metabolism in humans, *Am. J. Clin. Nutr.*, 55, 963, 1992.
40. Darmaun, D., Welch, S., Rini, A., Sager, B. K., Altomare, A., and Haymond, M. W., Phenylbutyrate-induced glutamine depletion in humans: effect on leucine metabolism, *Am. J. Physiol.*, 274, in press.
41. Darmaun, D., Rongier, M., Koziet, J., and Robert, J. J., Glutamine nitrogen kinetics in insulin-dependent diabetic humans, *Am. J. Physiol.*, 261, E713, 1991.
42. Stumvoll, M., Perriello, G., Nurjhan, N., Bucci, A., Welle, S., Jansson, P. A., Dailey, G., Bier, D., Jenssen, T., and Gerich, J., Glutamine and alanine metabolism in NIDDM, *Diabetes*, 45, 863, 1996.
43. Matthews, D. E., Pesola, G., and Campbell, R. G., Effect of epinephrine on amino acid and energy metabolism in humans, *Am. J. Physiol.*, 258, E948, 1990.
44. Gore, D. C. and Jahoor, F., Glutamine kinetics in burn patients, *Arch. Surg.*, 129, 1318, 1994.
45. Carbonnel, F., Messing, B., Darmaun, D., Rimbert, A., Rongier, M., Rigal, O., Kozeit, J., Thuillier, F., and Desjeux, J. F., Energy and protein metabolism in malnutrition due to nonneoplastic gastrointestinal diseases, *Metabolism*, 44, 1110, 1995.

9 The Application of Muscle Biopsy in the Study of Amino Acid and Protein Metabolism

Peter Fürst and Katharina S. Kuhn

CONTENTS

9.1 INTRODUCTION

Muscle tissue is by far the most abundant cellular tissue in the body, and is relatively uniform as to cellular composition. Profound biochemical changes in muscle are known to accompany electrolyte disorders, circulatory disturbances, nutritional deficiencies, and physical exercise. In addition, morphological changes occur in some muscle disorders and in generalized diseases. Biochemical and morphological

0-8493-9612-3/99/$0.00+$.50
© 1999 by CRC Press LLC

studies of muscle tissue in man, under various physiological and pathological conditions, have proved to be of great value in clinical research and diagnosis of various diseases.

More extensive studies of normal and pathological muscle metabolism require a simple method for muscle sampling. Percutaneous needle biopsy was introduced by Duchenne as early as 1868[1] for the investigation of patients with muscular dystrophy. The method seems, however, to have been little used during the following 90 years until 1957, when Reiffel and Stone[2] suggested that the percutaneous needle biopsy be used for the study of muscle electrolytes in man by neutron activation analysis. In 1960, a percutaneous muscle biopsy technique using a new biopsy needle[3,4] was developed by Bergström. This method of sampling with the Bergström needle is rapid and only slightly traumatic, and can therefore be repeated several times in the same individual.

The new biopsy technique was originally used for studies of intracellular water and electrolyte metabolism in muscle tissue.[3] It was, however, soon apparent that this method could also be used for the study of other tissue constituents. The advent of a repeatable technique for sampling human muscle, together with advances in histochemical techniques for studying structure and microanalytic methods for studying muscle chemistry, has been accompanied by a notable development in quantitative electromyography and measurements of muscle performance in isometric and isokinetic contractions, as well as during whole-body exercise.[5-7] This convergence of disciplines has yielded a unique opportunity to obtain a comprehensive view of the interplay between structure, function and biochemistry in normal and diseased human muscle.[7]

Today, needle biopsy plays an essential part in the clinical investigation of patients presenting a wide range of muscle symptoms, as well as those with obvious muscle disorders. Improvements in technique have allowed larger samples to be obtained, and developments in analytical methods have greatly extended the usefulness of the technique in the investigation of muscle cell structure and metabolism. One of the most fascinating implications of the percutaneous needle biopsy technique relates to investigations dealing with amino acid and protein metabolism. Needle biopsy specimens have been used for studies of intracellular muscle free amino acids, measurement of protein-bound glutamine, and assessment of protein synthesis and breakdown (turnover). This chapter describes the technique of needle biopsy of muscle, and reviews the various methods employed to study amino acid and protein metabolism with the help of muscle biopsy.

9.2 THE NEEDLE

The Bergström needle, introduced in 1960, consists of a sharp-tipped, hollow meter needle with a small opening ("window") near the tip.[3,4] A cylinder with a sharp edge fits tightly into the needle (Figure 9.1). An improved needle enables the selection of the collecting tip according to the individual conditions, and prompt cutting with a spring mechanism.[8] The University College Hospital (UCH) Muscle Biopsy Needle (4.5 mm outside diameter) is another modification of the Bergström needle, allowing single-handed control and reasonable sample sizes.[9] The UCH needle has been

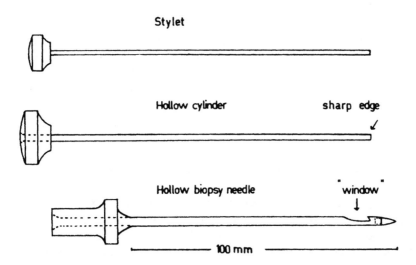

FIGURE 9.1   The Bergström biopsy needle.(Adapted from Reference 11, with kind permission from S. Karger AG, Basel, Switzerland.)

subsequently equipped with a facility of suction. The suction draws a larger portion of muscle into the lumen of the needle before it is guillotined.[7]

Fine narrow-bore needles, such as "Trucut" or modified Franklin Silverman needles, may yield small samples that are suitable for electron-microscopy but not suitable for studies of amino acid or protein metabolism.[7]

For obtaining samples from infants in whom muscle thickness is small, the current design could be modified to bring the window of the needle closer to the needle tip; at present, it may be necessary to insert the needle tip completely through the muscle bulk, to bring the window and cutting mechanisms into apposition with the muscle. Occasionally, a "stop" on the needle shaft is used when muscle is to be sampled at a standard depth, or excessively deep insertion is to be avoided.[7]

All needles should be regularly inspected for damage, and the cutting edge kept sharp.

9.3   THE CHOICE OF MUSCLES

The lateral part of the quadriceps femoris is the favored biopsy site for three reasons: it is free of major vessels and nerves, therefore the procedure is relatively safe; it is involved in most muscular disorders; and it is the major extensor of the knee joint, thus particularly suitable for studies in which structure or chemistry are to be related to function. Deltoid, supraspinatus, biceps and triceps brachii, gastrocnemius, soleus, tibialis anterior, and sacrospinal muscle have also been satisfactorily sampled. In principle, all muscles where there is no danger of damaging nerves or vessels can be used. Excessively wasted muscles are difficult to biopsy; for further information, see References 3, 7, and 10.

9.4 SAMPLING

After cleaning the skin, the needle is inserted through a small incision made in locally anaesthetized skin into the muscle, and one or more pieces of tissue bulging into the "window" are punched out with the sharp cylinder.[4] To reduce intramuscular bruising, firm pressure is applied to the site for 10 min after specimens have been obtained. The skin incision is then closed with sterile adhesive tape and covered with a protective dressing. The small scar becomes virtually invisible over time.[7] This is a "no touch" technique which can be carried out in the ward, clinic, or laboratory, used in patients ranging in age from 4 weeks to 85 years. There are particular difficulties in sampling from patients with extremely wasted muscles or with considerable fibrosis. In these cases, the suction technique has been very valuable in providing good samples.[4,9]

Only slight discomfort is experienced by most subjects, with more severe pain during the procedure or severe aching during the following days occurring only rarely. The pain experienced during biopsy is greater if the fascia lata is caught in the needle, or if a nerve is touched or damaged. On a few occasions, intramuscular haematomas have been seen but were resorbed spontaneously; only in one case out of more than 8,000 biopsies was surgical intervention required to stop arterial bleeding.[11] Other reported rare complications are infection and denervation of a small sector of vastus lateralis.[4,7,10] Muscle function is usually little impaired immediately after the biopsy, since some subjects have been able to continue competing in a 85-km cross-country ski race (Vasaloppet, Sweden) after several such biopsies.[12]

With the Bergström biopsy needle (4.5 mm), about 20 to 100 mg of muscle can be obtained.[3,4] Using the UCH technique together with suction, specimens of 70 to 140 mg are easily obtained (the largest sample obtained weighed 250 mg).[7,10] These specimens are perfectly suitable for assessment of protein turnover and amino acid and inorganic elemental analyses.

9.5 SAMPLE HANDLING

When fresh muscle is needed, the samples are dissected free from blood and visible connective tissue. They are then immediately weighed repeatedly on a sensitive electrobalance (a Cahn electrobalance, Cahn Instruments, Cettitos, CA; sensitivity of 1 μg is recommended), and the weight curve is extrapolated to zero time to compensate for water evaporation. Methods for weighing, water determination, and fat extraction of muscle samples before electrolyte analysis have been described earlier.[3,7,13,14] Wet tissue can be used for determination of enzyme activities and free amino acid concentrations (see Section 9.7.3).

Alternatively, samples can be freeze-dried after wet-weight has been established. The freeze-dried samples are weighed, fat extracted in petroleum for 60 min, dried at room temperature and reweighed.[15] This sample is referred to as dry fat-free solids (DFFS). The sample is then powdered, and the powder obtained is divided into two portions; about 2 mg for the analysis of electrolytes (required for calculation of water distribution), and about 3 mg for the determination of DNA, alkali-soluble protein (ASP) and amino acids (see Sections 9.7.2 and 9.7.3, respectively). The electrolyte sample is dried at 80°C for 30 min, and extracted with nitric acid (1 mol/l; 100 µl/mg of muscle powder) for measurement of chloride and other electrolytes of choice.

9.6 REFERENCE BASES

Amino acids and other variables derived from protein metabolism are usually referred to a series of reference bases: wet weight (WW), dry solids (DS), dry fat-free solids (DFFS), DNA, and ASP. Muscle free amino acid concentration is preferentially expressed per litre intracellular water (ICW). The use of WW might be satisfactory for normal muscle, but since no identification or removal of contaminants is possible, errors may occur when samples are taken from muscles of abnormal composition.[13] The fat content of muscle varies unpredictably, an increase in muscle fat being a non-specific finding in various groups of severely ill and/or malnourished patients.[16] Ageing and female gender are also factors associated with increased muscle fat stores.[15] Considerable variations in total water content and extracellular fluid volume are observed in diseases which involve disturbances in water and electrolyte homeostasis.[17] By using DFFS as the reference basis for intracellular muscle amino acids, the influence of variation in fat and water contents can be minimized. It is important to point out that DFFS represent not only muscle cell solids but also connective tissue solids, which may be increased in the muscle of patients with degenerative diseases and malnutrition.[15]

9.6.1 ALKALI-SOLUBLE PROTEIN

To solve the problem of increased connective tissue solids, ASP representing the non-collagen or cell protein can be introduced as a basis of reference for cell mass.[18] In normal muscle, ASP constitutes about 70% of the total DFFS, being only slightly reduced (by a mean of 2.5%) with ageing. In such a muscle sample, extracellular water is higher and potassium is lower in relation to DFFS, suggesting a minor increase in connective tissue content.[14] However, the difference in extracellular water content (and in sodium and chloride) between old and young subjects is less marked than in reports from earlier studies where similar analytical methods were used.[19] A reason for this may be that the method of dissecting the muscle specimen after freeze-drying is more efficient for removing increased amounts of connective tissue, conceivably present in the muscle of aged individuals, than the dissection of wet muscle used in earlier studies.[14] Since the skeletal musculature comprises the largest protein store in the body, the determination of muscle ASP per "cell unit" represented by the DNA content should provide the best quantitative information for evaluating the protein status of an individual.

In relation to the DNA content, ASP might be decreased with ageing and in females, compared to males, indicating lower amounts of contractile protein per cell unit. These findings are consistent with earlier observations showing a decrease of Type II fibres in the elderly[20] and smaller cross-sectional areas (fast-twitch fibres) in females.[21,22]

9.6.2 Creatine

Total creatine (TCr), the sum of phosphorylcreatine (PCr) and free creatine (Cr), has been proposed as an internal standard.[13] In early reports, it has been claimed that muscle creatine is very resistant to changes. Only after prolonged protein starvation, decreases are seen in the total Cr content in muscle.[23] Rapid exhaustion of the energy stores, as in muscular exercise[11,24] and acute illness,[25] does not deplete the total creatine store in muscle. Nevertheless, variations in the total creatine content in different muscle groups of the rat and guinea pig have been recently described, showing that muscle with predominantly fast-twitch (FT) fibres had a higher total creatine content than muscle with a high content of slow-twitch (ST) fibres.[26] The same tendency was observed in human skeletal muscle with a significantly higher creatine content in the vastus lateralis muscle which had 60% FT fibres as compared with the soleus muscle's 33% FT fibres.[26] In the same muscle (vastus lateralis), no difference in fibre-type distribution between the males and females was observed.[21,27] Therefore, special caution should be paid to the total creatine standard in conditions where there may be changes in fibre-type proportions. Total creatine is certainly a useful guide for interpreting muscle amino acid and metabolite levels when there is the possibility of sample contamination. It is especially useful for normalising data obtained from the same subject in whom several biopsies are done over a period of minutes or hours.[13,15]

9.6.3 Calculation of Muscle Water Distribution

The use of intracellular water as a basis of reference requires calculation of the share of intra- and extracellular water in the muscle sample. Intracellular water as reference minimizes the influence of variations in extracellular space on the assessment of the muscle free intracellular amino acid content. Also, it enables the calculation of the intra- to extracellular concentration gradients. The determination of extra- and intracellular water was based on the chloride method (see References 11, and 28 through 40).

The Resting Membrane Potential (RMP) is a sensitive index of metabolic derangement, low RMP being consistently found in chronically and acutely ill patients. Evidently, accurate measurements of RMP might be of great interest for understanding the underlying pathophysiology in various conditions associated with intracellular abnormalities, depletion, nitrogen catabolism, and muscle fatigue.[36]

9.7 ANALYTICAL METHODS

Multiple analyses can be performed on portions from a single muscle specimen obtained by the percutaneous muscle biopsy technique. Representative values of muscle composition in healthy and selected pathological conditions are given in Table 9.1.

9.7.1 Total Creatine and Chloride

Creatine and chloride are extracted with nitric acid (1 mol/l; 100 µl/mg of muscle powder or 5 mg of wet muscle), ultrasonicated for 15 min, left overnight, and

TABLE 9.1
Muscle Composition in Healthy and Selected Pathological Conditions (Mean ± SD)

Condition	n			Refererence
Alkali-Soluble Protein Nitrogen (ASPN), (g/100 g DFFS)				
Healthy adults	36	12.7 ± 1.7		3
	52	11.4 ± 2.3		15
Healthy children	30	12.2 ± 0.3		56
Uremic children				
Non dialysed	7	8.4 ± 0.4		56
Hemodialysis				
treated	9	8.6 ± 0.8		56
Cancer	10	9.4 ± 1.0		57
Total Creatine (μmol/g DW)				
Healthy adults	81	124 ± 11		58
	14	124 ± 16		13
Patients	19	135 ± 16		13
No apparent changes in pathological conditions				
DNA (mg/g DFFS)				
Healthy adults	51	1.83 ± 0.21		15
	19	2.00 ± 0.25		Unpub. data from own lab.
	14	1.64 ± 0.26		Unpub. data from own lab.
Protein-bound glutamine (mg/100 mg ASP)				
Healthy adults	14	4.4 ± 0.6		59
Water (ml/100 g DFFS)				
Healthy adults	85	H_2O_m	336 ± 13.8	16
		H_2O_i	289 ± 13.8	
		H_2O_e	47 ± 12.9	
Trauma	21	H_2O_m	353 ± 23.4	60
		H_2O_i	283 ± 16.5	
		H_2O_e	66 ± 17.8	
Sepsis	17	H_2O_m	366 ± 25.2	16
		H_2O_i	278 ± 33.0	
		H_2O_e	88 ± 37.9	
Chloride (mmol/100 g DFFS)				
Healthy adults	85	Cl_m	6.6 ± 1.4	16
Trauma	21	Cl_m	9.1 ± 2.4	60
Sepsis	17	Cl_m	12.1 ± 5.8	16

m; total   i;intracellular   e;extracellular

thereafter mixed in a vortex mixer and centrifuged (4,500 rpm, 15 min, 4°C). For creatine determination, the supernatant (2 x 25 µl) is boiled with 100 µl of HNO_3 (1 mol/l) for 40 min in a water-bath. In the boiling acid, all the free and phosporylated creatine is transformed into creatinine. After cooling and centrifugation (4,500 rpm, 10 min, 4°C), alkaline picric acid is added (0.75 ml of 11.5 mmol/l picric acid and 100 µl containing 1.55 mol/l NaOH and 60 mmol/l Na_2HPO_4), and the absorbance is determined at 513 nm with a suitable spectrophotometer. The colour development is stable after 1 h. Chloride content is assessed against standard solutions of NaCl in the nitric acid supernatant (2 x 25 µl) with electrometric titration against $AgNO_3$ using a Radiometer titrator.[15]

9.7.2   ALKALI-SOLUBLE PROTEIN AND DNA

Three milligrams of the freeze-dried powder or 15 mg of wet muscle is placed in a pre-weighed glass tube and precipitated (in case of wet muscle, homogenized and precipitated) with 0.5 ml of perchloric acid (PCA; 0.2 mol/l) in an ice-bath for 10 min, centrifuged (4,000 rpm, 5 min, 4°C), and the precipitate is washed twice with 0.5 ml of PCA (0.2 mol/l). The supernatants are discarded, and the washed precipitate is dissolved in 1 ml of KOH (0.3 mol/l) by incubation for 1 h at 37°C. The tube is re-weighed to obtain the true dilution volume. Portions of the solution (2 x 20 µl) are used for protein determination.[41]

DNA is precipitated with 1 ml of PCA (1.2 mol/l), and left in an ice-bath for 30 min. The precipitate is washed twice with PCA (0.2 mol/l, 0.5 ml each time), hydrolysed by adding 0.25 ml of PCA (1 mol/l) and incubated for 1 h at 70°C. The tube is weighed again to obtain a dilution volume for DNA. DNA is estimated by the diphenylamine reaction.[42] Calf thymus DNA is suitable as standard. The extraction procedure has been described by Munro and Fleck[43] as a modification of the technique used by Schmidt and Tannhauser.[44]

9.7.3   MUSCLE FREE AMINO ACIDS

When amino acid analysis is included, sulphosalicyclic acid (SSA) instead of PCA is used for the extraction procedure. Three milligrams of the freeze-dried powder is extracted with 0.35 ml of 4% (w/v) SSA in an ice-bath for 1 h, and the supernatant is used for amino acid analyses. The precipitate is treated as described above for ASP and DNA analyses.

In case wet muscle tissue is analysed, about 10 to 15 mg WW is rapidly weighed on a top-loading electrobalance, and homogenized manually in a Potter-Elvehjem homogenizer. The protein is directly precipitated with 1 ml ice-cold 4% sulfosalicylic acid. The precipitated sample is stored for 50 min at +4°C, and thereafter centrifuged (3,500 rpm, 15 min, 4°C). The supernatant material is decanted and collected. The precipitate is washed 2 times with 0.5 ml 4% sulfosalicylic acid and centrifuged each time for 10 min. The supernatants are pooled and the pH is adjusted to 2.2 by addition of 0.1 ml LiOH (2.5 mol/l). The collected "pH corrected-supernatants" are used for free amino acid determination.

Muscle free amino acids can be analysed by means of ion exchange chromatography, or using specially adapted reverse phase-high performance liquid chromatography (RP-HPLC).

9.7.3.1 Ion Exchange Chromatography

The free amino acid concentrations can be determined on a suitable automated amino acid analyzer using a one-column lithium-buffer system. High ammonia concentrations in the sample (buffer solution) may disturb the baseline reaching. This can be eliminated by introducing an extra column (Hi-Rez, type DC4, Pierce, Rockford, IL) between buffer outlets and column inlet.[33]

Ion exchange chromatography is usually performed according to the principle described by Kedenburg,[45] by using two lithium buffers with two pH (2.8 to 4.1) and temperature (39° to 60°C) changes. The original method can be "scaled down" to yield an analysis time of 90 min instead of 480 min. In our laboratory, the coefficient of variation in the determination of muscle free amino acids, calculated from duplicate samples, obtained by separate biopsies and analysed independently, revealed the highest value for cysteine (9.1%) and the lowest value for taurine (2.8%). The variation includes both a sampling error due to the heterogeneity of the muscle tissue and the combined analytical errors.[11,33]

9.7.3.2 High Performance Liquid Chromatography (HPLC)

As outlined under 9.7.3.1, the classical procedure involves separation of amino acids by ion-exchange chromatography, followed by derivatization with ninhydrin.[45,46] This method, however, suffers from the disadvantage of low mobile phase flow rate, thereby limiting the rate of sample analyses. A further drawback is the relatively poor sensitivity. Sensitive detection methods are highly desirable, considering the progress made in research on amino acid metabolism of individual tissues and cells. The substantial progress made in the field of analytical chemistry is exemplified by the explosion of new information about the potential use of HPLC. Numerous reports emphasize the use of HPLC in amino acid analysis. The application of HPLC reduces the time required for analysis and increases the sensitivity for quantitation of amino acids (see Reference 47). In our laboratory, four automated or semiautomated pre-column derivatization methods are employed for determination of free amino acids in biological fluids, including muscle tissue, by using ortho-phthaldialdehyde (OPA), 9-fluorenylmethyl chloroformate (FMOC-Cl), phenyl isothiocyanate (PITC) and 1-dimethylaminonaphthalene-5-sulphonyl chloride (dansyl-Cl). The methods permit the measurement of 21 to 28 major amino acids and selected dipeptides in 13 to 40 min. The superior sensitivity favours the use of OPA, FMOC-Cl and dansyl-Cl techniques.

Because of instability of the OPA adducts, automated on-line derivatization is required when using this method in general practice. An ultrarapid and sensitive OPA/3-mercaptopropionic acid method has been developed by using 3 μm particle-size reversed phase (RP)-columns, enabling separation of the 26 major tissue free physiological amino acids in the lower picomole range in 12.7 min (still the valid world record).[48] Reliable automated assessments of plasma, muscle, and liver free amino acids are facilitated with the method (Figure 9.2) in biopsy specimens of about 1 mg tissue. The major disadvantage of the OPA method lies in the fact that only primary amines form adducts. This means measurements of proline, hydroxyproline, and cystine are not feasible with this method.

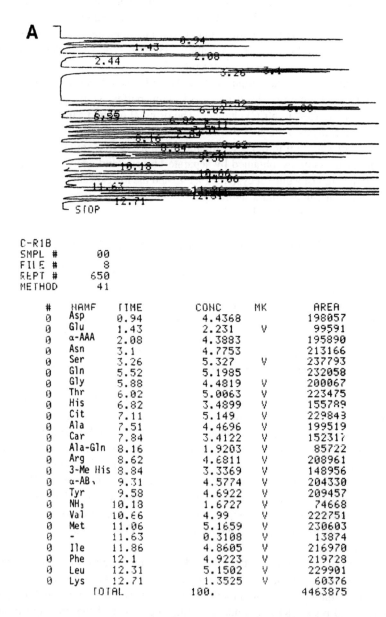

C-R1B
SMPL #   00
FILE #   8
REPT #   650
METHOD   41

#	NAME	TIME	CONC	MK	AREA
0	Asp	0.94	4.4368		198057
0	Glu	1.43	2.231	V	99591
0	α-AAA	2.08	4.3883		195890
0	Asn	3.1	4.7753		213166
0	Ser	3.26	5.327	V	237793
0	Gln	5.52	5.1985		232058
0	Gly	5.88	4.4819	V	200067
0	Thr	6.02	5.0063	V	223475
0	His	6.82	3.4899	V	155789
0	Cit	7.11	5.149	V	229843
0	Ala	7.51	4.4696	V	199519
0	Car	7.84	3.4122	V	152317
0	Ala-Gln	8.16	1.9203	V	85722
0	Arg	8.62	4.6811	V	208961
0	3-Me His	8.84	3.3369	V	148956
0	α-AB	9.31	4.5774	V	204330
0	Tyr	9.58	4.6922	V	209457
0	NH₃	10.18	1.6727	V	74668
0	Val	10.66	4.99	V	222751
0	Met	11.06	5.1659	V	230603
0	-	11.63	0.3108	V	13874
0	Ile	11.86	4.8605	V	216970
0	Phe	12.1	4.9223	V	219728
0	Leu	12.31	5.1502	V	229901
0	Lys	12.71	1.3525	V	60376
	TOTAL		100.		4463875

FIGURE 9.2A   HPLC chromatograms showing the separation of free amino acids in a standard mixture (A), 23 amino acids including the synthetic dipeptide ala-gln . . .

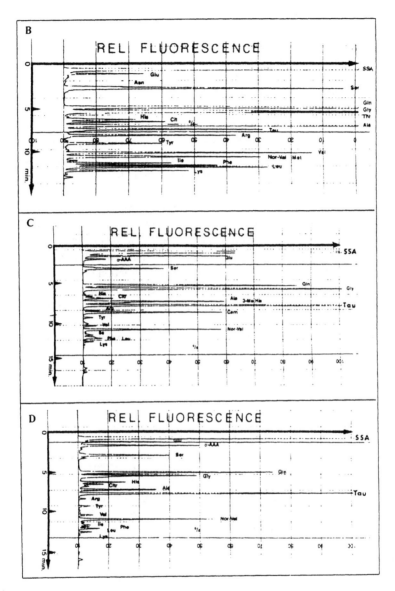

FIGURE 9.2 . . . (**B**) rat plasma, (**C**) muscle, and (**D**) liver tissue [ortho-phthaldialdehyde /3-mercapto-propionic acid (OPA) derivatization].

HPLC conditions:

Column: Spherisorb ODS II, 3 μm, 125 × 4.6 mm, guard column: 10 × 4.6 mm (Waters GmbH, Eschborn, Germany).

Solvents: *A*: 3 % acetonitril in phospha te buffer (pH 7.2, 12.5 mmol/l), *B*: 50% acetonitril in phosphate buffer (pH 7.2, 12.5 μmol/l).

Flow: 1.5 ml/min.

Gradient: 0′, 0% *B*; 6′, 20% *B*; 10′, 42% *B*; 15′, 100% *B*; 18′, 100% *B*; 20′, 0% *B*.

Temperature: Room temperature.

Fluorescence detection: Shimadzu RF 530 (Shimadzu, Tokyo, Japan) Ex. 330 nm, Em. 450 nm.

Injection: 20 μl.

(Reprinted from Reference 48, with kind permission from Academic Press Inc., San Diego, CA)

One ultrasensitive application is the narrow-bore method, employing RP-HPLC columns with internal diameter of 1.8 mm. The sensitivity of the analysis is about 1 pmol of amino acid per injection, and the reproducibility and reliability range between 4 and 8 % (C.V.). The separation of 23 major free amino acids can be accomplished in 22 min. The limit of sensitivity is about 150 fmol at a signal-to-noise ratio of 2.5. A muscle specimen of 1 µg ww is an appropriate sample size. The great advantage of narrow-bore chromatography compared with conventional column technology is the considerably reduced consumption of expensive and polluting organic solvents, the actual use of such reagents with the narrow-bore method being only 15 to 20% of that with conventional RP-HPLC (see Reference 47).

Pre-column derivatization with FMOC-Cl permits the fluorimetric detection of primary and secondary amino acids as stable FMOC adducts, while determination of free tryptophan and cystine is not possible with FMOC-Cl, because the fluorescence of the adducts is quenched. The FMOC-Cl method suffers from the disadvantage that an excess of strong fluorescent reagent has to be extracted manually with pentane, in order to stop the derivatization reaction and to avoid spontaneous hydrolysis of the FMOC adducts. This laborious manual extraction procedure prevents the wide acceptance of this method. This shortcoming, however, might be overcome by using specially designed autosamplers and/or a combination of the FMOC-Cl and OPA methods.[47]

Application of the PITC method, although less sensitive, is useful in clinical chemistry, where sample availability is rarely a problem. Determination of free cystine is not practicable because of poor linearity and reproducibility. In addition, we observed rapid deterioration of the column when analysing tissue material (muscle). This is a serious shortcoming of the PITC method. In our experience, a maximum of 150 physiological analyses per column could be performed in spite of the use of rigorous sample preparation and suitable guard columns containing the same resin.[47]

Dansyl-Cl is a well-known fluorogenic reagent for the determination of primary and secondary amines. The adducts are formed at room temperature in the dark. In contrast to the PITC method, the dansyl-Cl technique shows excellent linearity for cystine and also for cystine-containing short-chain peptides (Figure 9.3). Hence, the dansyl-Cl method appears to offer the only quantitative approach for measuring free cystine in biological material by HPLC techniques.

Overall, we perform ca. 7,500 OPA and 5,000 FMOC-Cl, PITC and dansyl-Cl analyses of biological samples per year. The results obtained with the RP-HPLC methods compare favourably with those derived from conventional ion-exchange amino acid analyses. When the guard column is regularly changed after 120 analyses, the separation remains satisfactory for at least 700 OPA and FMOC-Cl, 150 PITC, and 400 dansyl-Cl analyses. Careful control of factors and limitations inherent to the various methodologies is a prerequisite for proper identification and appropriate quantitations. The sensitivity, errors of the methods, advantages and disadvantages, and problems with certain "difficult" amino acids are summarized in Table 9.2.

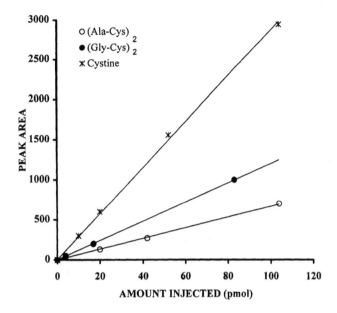

FIGURE 9.3 Linearity obtained with dansyl derivatives of cystine [(Cys)$_2$], bis-glycyl-L-cystine [(Gly-Cys)$_2$] and bis-L-alanyl-L-cystine [(Ala-Cys)$_2$] in the range of 50 to 150 pmol. (Adapted from Reference 47, with kind permission of Elsevier Science-NL, Sara Burgerhartstraat 25, 1055 KV Amsterdam, The Netherlands.)

TABLE 9.2
HPLC Analyses of Free Amino Acids: Comparison of Four Derivatization
Methods. (Reprinted from Reference 47, with kind permission of Elsevier Science-NL, Sara Burgerhartstraat 25, 1055 KV Amsterdam, The Netherlands.)

Parameter	OPA	FMOC-Cl	PITC	Dansyl-Cl
Limit of sensitivity, pmol (Signal-to-noise ratio = 2.5)	0.8	1.0	5.0	1.5
Error of the method (C.V., %) (based on duplicate determinations)	1.0-4.7	1.1-5.9	3.6-7.0	1.7-4.5
Reproducibility (C.V., %)	0.4-2.2	1.9-4.6	2.6-5.5	1.5-4.1
Stable adducts*	N	Y	Y	Y
Detection of secondary amines/cystine*	N/N	Y/N	Y/Y	Y/Y
Laborious	-	+++	++	+
Problematic amino acids	Asp,Trp	His,Trp	Orn,Trp,His, Cystine (Cys)$_2$	His,Asn

* Y = yes, N = no.

9.7.4 DETERMINATION OF PROTEIN-BOUND GLUTAMINE
IN MUSCLE TISSUE

Glutamine is considered to be a conditionally essential amino acid during episodes of catabolic stress and malnutrition. Knowledge of glutamine contents of natural proteins is thus of utmost importance. Quantitative assessment of protein-bound glutamine is, however, hampered by glutamic acid formation during acid hydrolysis, invalidating subsequent distinction between glutamine and glutamic acid residues.

Reliable assessment of the "true" glutamine content might be obtained using laborious and cost-intensive biotechnological methods (cDNA technology), or acquired from sequence analyses (purified protein fragments are requested). Methods focused upon measurement of the amide groups in the polypeptide chain have failed, due to the occurrence of side reactions and the instability of liberated products.

Recently, an easy and rapid procedure for the determination of glutamine in isolated proteins has been developed. It involves a pre-hydrolysis reaction of glutamine residues with bis-(1,1-trifluoroacetoxy)-iodobenzene (BTI) to yield acid stable L-2, 4-diaminobutyric acid (DABA) protein hydrolysis using a microwave technique, and high-performance liquid chromatography (HPLC) after precolumn derivatization of amino acids with dansyl-Cl.[49] Subsequent amino acid analyses are performed with dansyl-Cl derivatisation as described in Section 9.7.3.2. The HPLC analysis of a human muscle specimen is shown in Figure 9.4. DABA and the proteic amino acids could be simultaneously measured with high sensitivity (2.0 pmol/injection; S/N = 3.1) and good reproducibility (C.V = 2.8%). The linearity between DABA formation and glutamine concentration was excellent (r = 0.9996). Unexpectedly, the glutamine content of muscle protein was lower than previously expected (see Table 9.1). About 15 mg of DFFS is required for the complex assessment of glutamine in proteins.

9.8 MUSCLE FREE AMINO ACIDS:
IMPLICATION OF THE METHOD

In 1974, we measured for the first time, reliably, muscle free amino acid concentrations, and calculated the ratio of intra- to extracellular concentrations of 26 amino acids in normal man (Figure 9.5). The majority of the amino acids had a much higher concentration in intracellular water than in plasma. The concentration gradient was especially high for taurine, glutamic acid, and glutamine. The essential amino acids valine, leucine, isoleucine, and phenylalanine, and the non-essential amino acids citrulline and tyrosine, had a gradient below 2. The remainder showed a gradient between 5 and 10.

Direct determinations in man show that 1 kg skeletal muscle contains 230 g dry solids, 120 g extracellular water, and 650 g intracellular water. The total free amino acid concentration in muscle was found to be approximately 35 mmol (5 g/l) intracellular water: taurine is additionally present at a concentration of 15 to 19 mmol/l, and free carnosine at 6 mmol/l. Of the total pool, the eight essential amino acids represent only 8.4%. For a normal man with a body weight of 70 kg and a muscle mass of 400 g/kg body weight, the total volume of intracellular muscle water is 18.2 l; thus, the

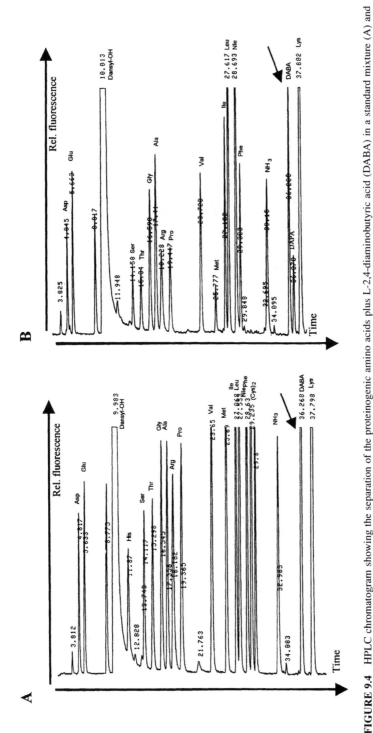

FIGURE 9.4 HPLC chromatogram showing the separation of the proteinogenic amino acids plus L-2,4-diaminobutyric acid (DABA) in a standard mixture (A) and a bis-(1,1-trifluoroacetoxy)-iodobenzene (BTI)-treated muscle protein hydrolysate (B) (dansyl-Cl derivatisation).

HPLC conditions:

Column: Hypersil ODS II, 3 μm, 150 × 4.6 mm (Hypersil, Runcorn, England); Solvents: *A*: 3 % tetrahydrofuran in phosphate buffer (pH 7.2, 12.5 mmol/l), *B*: 60% acetonitril in phosphate buffer (pH 7.2, 12.5 mmol/l); Gradient: 0′, 15% *B*; 15′, 30% *B*; 18′, 30% *B*; 25′, 45% *B*; 30′, 55% *B*; 35′, 60% *B*; 40′, 100% *B*; 43′, 100% *B*; 45′, 15% *B*; Temperature: Room temperature; Flow: 0.9 ml/min; Fluorescence detection: Shimadzu RF 535, Ex. 330 nm, Em. 520 nm; Injection: 20 μl

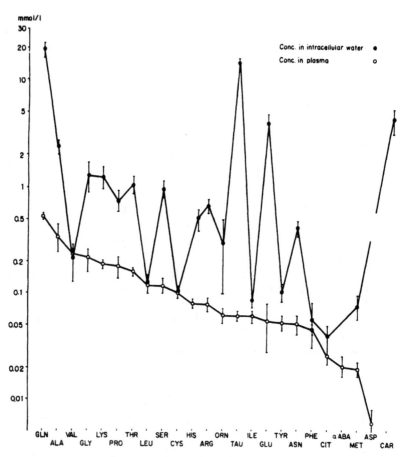

FIGURE 9.5 Comparison between aminograms in plasma water and intracellular muscle water (Means ± SD, n=32). (Reprinted from Reference 11, with kind permission from S. Karger AG, Basel, Switzerland.)

total intracellular amino acid content can be estimated to be 86.5 g. Free amino acid patterns in muscle have been measured in various experimental and pathological conditions (see References 11 and 50).

9.9 MUSCLE BIOPSY AND THE MEASUREMENTS OF TISSUE PROTEIN TURNOVER

The turnover of most functional proteins in the body is a continual process involving the breakdown of proteins by proteolysis and their replacement by protein synthesis. An extensive recent review describes the various techniques which provide quantitative information on the rates of and capacities for protein synthesis and breakdown in tissues.[51] In many of these methods, a single or repeated muscle biopsy is required. Static indices of tissue protein turnover like DNA, ASP, and specific amino acids, were discussed in Section 9.6 (concentrations of individual proteins may be assayed by Western blotting).[52] Yet, the results provide little relevant information about protein turnover.

Total RNA content of a muscle biopsy specimen might be indicative of protein synthesis in the tissue, when expressed per cell (DNA) or per ASP (cell size). Fractional synthesis rate (FSR) expressed per RNA can be interpreted as the efficiency of protein synthesis per synthesis assembly unit.[52] Polyribosome index is a qualitative reflection of protein synthesis. With the polyribosome method, an index of the overall protein synthetic rates in vivo can be estimated using a muscle biopsy specimen of about 50 mg. The technique for the determination of ribosomal concentration and size distribution (density gradient centrifugation) in human skeletal muscle has been described in detail previously.[53] It should be remembered that the proportion of ribosomes and polysomes only provides a relative rate of initiation to elongation, and thus great caution should be exercised when interpreting an increased polyribosome index.[54]

Techniques based on the use of tracers usually necessitate the conduct of one or more muscle biopsy specimens. Protein turnover can be estimated from loss of label from previously labelled proteins, or measured by incorporation of amino acid tracers. These methods are extensively described[51] and a complete comparison of techniques and approaches is outlined in detail in Chapter 3. The use of stable isotopes to label metabolic tracers has dramatically increased the feasibility of carrying out measurements of protein turnover facilitated by muscle biopsy.[51,55]

REFERENCES

1. Duchenne, G.B., Recherches sur la paralysie musculaire pseudohypertrophique ou paralysie myo-sclérosique, I. Symptomatologie. Marche, durée, terminaison, *Arch. gén. Méd*, 11, 179, 1868.
2. Reiffel, L. and Stone, C.A., Neutron activation analysis of tissue: measurements of sodium, potassium and phosphorus in muscle, *J. Lab. Clin. Med.*, 49, 286, 1957.
3. Bergström, J., Muscle electrolytes in man, *Scand. J. Clin. Lab. Invest.*, 14, Suppl. 68, 1962.
4. Bergström, J., Percutaneous needle biopsy of skeletal muscle in physiological and clinical research, *Scand. J. Clin. Lab. Invest.*, 35, 609, 1975.
5. Deeley, T. J., *Needle biopsy*, Butterworth, London, 1974.
6. Dubowitz, V. and Brooke, M. H., *Muscle biopsy: a modern approach*, WB Saunders, Philadelphia, 1973.
7. Edwards, R., Young, A., and Wiles, M., Needle biopsy of skeletal muscle in the diagnosis of myopathy and the clinical study of muscle function and repair, *N. Engl. J. Med.*, 302, 261, 1980.
8. Vondra, K., Rath, R., and Kroupa, Z., Improved needle for muscle biopsy, *Klin. Wochenschr.*, 52, 747, 1973.
9. Young, A., Wiles, C. M., and Edwards, R. H. T., University college hospital muscle-biopsy needle, *Lancet*, 2, 1285, 1978.
10. Edwards, R. H. T., Round, J. M., and Jones, D. A., Needle biopsy of skeletal muscle: a review of 10 years experience, *Muscle Nerve*, 6, 676, 1983.

11. Fürst, P., Direct biochemical analyses of human muscle tissue, *Infusionsther. Transfusionsmed.*, 17, 26, 1990.
12. Bergström, J., Hultman, E., and Saltin, B., Muscle glycogen consumption during cross-country skiing (the Vasa ski race), *Int. Z. angew. Physiol.*, 31, 71, 1973.
13. Edwards, R. H. T., Jones, D. A., Maunder, C., and Batra, G. J., Needle biopsy for muscle chemistry, *Lancet*, March 29, 736, 1975.
14. Bergström, J., Alvestrand, A., Fürst, P., Hultman, E., Sahlin, K., Vinnars, E., and Widström, A., Influence of severe potassium depletion and subsequent repletion with potassium on muscle electrolytes, metabolites and amino acids in man, *Clin. Sci. Mol. Med.*, 51, 589, 1976.
15. Forsberg, A. M., Nilsson, L., Wernerman, J., Bergström, J. and Hultman, E., Muscle composition in relation to age and sex, *Clin. Sci.*, 81, 249, 1991.
16. Fürst, P. and Leweling, H., The interplay between nutrition and body composition, *Asia Pacific J. Clin. Nutr.*, 4, 95, 1995.
17. Bergström, J., Larsson, J., Nordström, H., Vinnars, E., Askanazi, J., Elwyn, D., Kinney, J., and Fürst, P., Influence of injury and nutrition on muscle water and electrolytes; effect of severe injury, burns and sepsis, *Acta Chir. Scand.*, 153, 261, 1987.
18. Lilienthal, J. L., Jr., Zierler, K. L., Folk, B. P., Buka, R., and Riley, M. J., A reference base and system for analysis of muscle constituents, *J. Biol. Chem.*, 182, 501, 1950.
19. Möller, P., Alvestrand, A., Bergström, J., Fürst, P., and Hellström, K., Electrolytes and free amino acids in leg skeletal muscle of young and elderly women, *Gerontology*, 29, 1, 1983.
20. Larsson, L., Grimby, G., and Karlsson, J., Muscle strength and speed of movement in relation to age and muscle morphology, *J. Appl. Physiol.*, 46, 451, 1979.
21. Hedberg, G. and Jansson, E., Skeletal muscle fibre distribution, capacity and interest in different physical activities among students in high school, *Pedagog. Rapporter*, 54, 1975.
22. Nygaard, E. and Hede, K., Physiological profiles of the male and the female, in *Exercise: Benefits, Limits and Adaptations*, Macleod, D., Maughan, R., Nimmo, M., Reilly, T. and Williams, C., Eds., E. and F.N. Spon Ltd., London, 1987, 289.
23. Fitch, C. D. and Shields, R. P., Creatinine metabolism in skeletal muscle. I. Creatine movement across muscle membranes, *J. Biol. Chem.*, 241, 3611, 1966.
24. Bergström, J., Harris, R. C., Hultman, E., and Nordesjö, L-O., Energy rich phosphagens in dynamic and static work, in *Advances in Experimental Medicine and Biology*, Vol. 11., Pernow, B. and Saltin, B., Eds., Plenum Press, New York, 1971, 341.
25. Bergström, J., Fürst, P., Hultman, E., and Vinnars, E., Preliminary studies of energy-rich phosphagens in muscle from severely ill patients, *Crit. Care Med.*, 4, 197, 1976.
26. Edström, L., Hultman, E., Sahlin, K., and Sjöholm, H., The contents of high-energy phosphates in different fibre types in skeletal muscles from rat, guinea pig and man, *J. Physiol.*, 332, 47, 1982.
27. Essén-Gustavsson, B. and Borges, O., Histochemical and metabolic characteristics of human skeletal muscle in relation to age, *Acta Physiol. Scand.*, 126, 107, 1986.
28. Conway, E. J., Nature and significance of potassium and sodium ions in skeletal muscle, *Physiol. Rev.*, 37, 84, 1957.
29. Bolte, H. D., Riecker, G., and Röhl, D., Messungen des Membranpotentials an einzelnen quergestreiften Muskelzellen der Menschen *in situ*, *Klin. Wochenschr.*, 41, 356, 1963.

30. Cunningham, J. N., Jr., Carter, N. W., Rector, F. C., Jr., and Seldin, D. W., Resting transmembrane potential difference of skeletal muscle in normal subjects and severely ill patients, *J. Clin. Invest.*, 50, 40, 1971.
31. Eisenmann, A. J., MacKenzie, L. B., and Peters, J. P., Protein and water of serum and cells of human blood, with a note on the measurement of red blood cell volume, *J. Biol. Chem.*, 116, 33, 1936.
32. Graham, J. A., Lamb, J. F., and Linton, A. L., Measurement of body water and intracellular electrolytes by means of muscle biopsy, *Lancet*, ii, 1172, 1967.
33. Bergström, J., Fürst, P., Noree, L-O., and Vinnars, E., Intracellular free amino acid concentration in human muscle tissue, *J. Appl. Physiol.*, 36, 693, 1974.
34. Gulyassi, P. F., Peters, J. H., and Schoenfeld, P., Hypoalbuminemia and depressed tryptophan binding in chronic uremia, *Abstracts, American Society of Nephrology, Washington D.C.*, 29, 1971.
35. Vinnars, E., Fürst, P., Bergström, J., and Von Francken, I., Intracellular free amino acids in muscle tissue in normal man and in different clinical conditions, in *Metabolism and the Response to Injury*, Wilkinson, A.W. and Cuthbertson, S.D., Eds., Pitman Press, Bath, 1976, 336.
36. Forsberg, A. M., Bergström, J., Lindholm, B., and Hultman, E., Resting membrane potential of skeletal muscle calculated from plasma and muscle electrolyte and water contents, *Clin. Sci.*, 92, 391, 1997.
37. Hodgkin, A. L. and Horowitz, P., The influence of potassium and chloride ions on the membrane potential of single muscle fibres, *J. Physiol.*, 148, 127, 1959.
38. Wilde, W.S., The chloride equilibrium in muscle, *Am. J. Physiol.*, 143, 666, 1945.
39. Sjögaard, G., Adams, R. P., and Saltin, B., Water and ion shifts in skeletal muscle of humans and intense dynamic knee extensions, *Am. J. Physiol.*, 248, R190, 1985.
40. Bergström, J. and Fridén, A. M., The effect of hydrochlorothiazide and amiloride administered together on electrolytes in normal subjects, *Acta Med. Scand.*, 197, 415, 1975.
41. Lowry, O. H., Rosebrough, N. J., Farr, A. L., and Randall, R. J., Protein measurement with folin phenol reagent, *J. Biol. Chem.*, 193, 265, 1951.
42. Giles, K. W. and Myers, A., An improved diphenylamine method for the estimation of DNA, *Nature*, 206, 93, 1965.
43. Munro, H. N. and Fleck, A., Recent developments in measurement of nucleic acids in biological material, *Analyst*, 91, 78, 1966.
44. Schmidt, G. and Tannhauser, S. J., A method for the determination of deoxyribonucleic acid, ribonucleic acid, and phosphoproteins in animal tissues, *J. Biol. Chem.*, 161, 83, 1945.
45. Kedenburg, C-P., A lithium buffer system for accelerated single-column amino acid analysis in physiological fluids, *Anal. Biochem.*, 40, 35, 1971.
46. Spackman, D. H., Stein, W. H., and Moore, S., Automatic recording apparatus for use in the chromatography of amino acids, *Anal. Chem.*, 30, 1190, 1958.
47. Fürst, P., Pollack, L., Graser, Th., Godel, H., and Stehle, P., Appraisal of four precolumn derivatization methods for the high-performance liquid chromatographic determination of free amino acids in biological materials, *J. Chromatogr.*, 499, 557, 1990.
48. Graser, T. A., Godel, H. G., Albers, S., Földi, P., and Fürst, P., An ultra rapid and sensitive high-performance liquid chromatographic method for determination of tissue and plasma free amino acids, *Anal. Biochem.*, 151, 142, 1985.
49. Kuhn, K. S., Stehle, P. and Fürst, P., Quantitative analyses of glutamine in peptides and proteins, *J. Agric. Food Chem.*, 44, 1808, 1996.

50. Fürst, P., Intracellular muscle free amino acids — their measurement and function, *Proc. Nutr. Soc.*, 42, 451, 1983.
51. Smith, K. and Rennie, M. J., Protein Metabolism, in *Baillières Clinical Endocrinology and Metabolism*, Russel-Jones, D. L. and Umpleby, A.M., Eds., Baillière Tindall, London, 1996, 469.
52. Gibson, J. N. A., Smith, K., and Rennie, M. J., Prevention of disuse muscular atrophy by means of electrical stimulation: maintenance of protein synthesis, *Lancet*, ii, 767, 1988.
53. Hammarqvist, F., Strömberg, C., Von der Decken, A., Vinnars, E., and Wernerman, J., Biosynthetic human growth hormone preserves both muscle protein synthesis and the decrease in muscle-free glutamine, and improves whole-body nitrogen economy after operation, *Ann. Surg.*, 216, 184, 1992.
54. Wernerman, J., Von der Decken, A., and Vinnars, E., Size distribution of ribosomes in biopsy specimens of human skeletal muscle during starvation, *Metabolism*, 34, 665, 1985.
55. Rennie, M. J., Metabolic insights from the use of stable isotopes in nutritional studies, *Clin. Nutr.*, 5, 1, 1986.
56. Delaporte, C., Bergström, J., and Broyer, M., Variations in muscle cell protein of severely uremic children, *Kidney Int.*, 10, 239, 1976.
57. Rössle, C., Pichard, C., Roulet, M., Bergström, J., and Fürst, P., Muscle carnitine pools in cancer patients, *Clin. Nutr.*, 8, 341, 1989.
58. Harris, R. C., Hultman, E., and Nordesjö, L-O., Glycogen, glycolytic intermediates and high-energy phosphates determined in biopsy samples of musculus quadriceps femoris of man at rest. Methods and variance of values, *Scand. J. Clin. Lab. Invest.*, 33, 217, 1974.
59. Kuhn, K. S., Schuhmann, K., Stehle, P., and Fürst, P., Determination of protein-bound glutamine in muscle, *JPEN*, 22, S7, 1998.
60. Bergström, J., Fürst, P., Holmström, B., Vinnars, E., Askanazi, J., Elwyn, D. H., Michelsen, C. B., and Kinney, J. M., Influence of injury and nutrition on muscle water and electrolytes. Effect of elective operation, *Ann. Surg.*, 193, 810, 1981.

10 Protein and Amino Acid Metabolism in the Elderly

Naomi K. Fukagawa and Dorothy Y. Fisher

CONTENTS

10.1 INTRODUCTION

Amino acid and protein metabolism is influenced by nutritional status, which in turn is influenced by social, psychological and economic factors. As we grow older, many of these aspects of our lives change, leading to changes in the selection, preparation and consumption of food. Hence, the aging process can have a profound effect on protein, as well as overall nutritional status. Twice as many older adults live in poverty compared to younger adults, as a result of decreases in income and increases in living costs such as medication, specialized aides (hearing, walking), etc. The expense of smaller packaging and high-quality, perishable food can strain an elder's limited budget. In addition, transportation difficulties may influence selection of foodstuffs. Psychological factors may play a significant role in influencing nutritional status. Cognitive deficits may affect an individual's ability to prepare food or even to recognize hunger. Depression and loneliness often lead to decreased appetite and interest in food. Combined with changes in living situations, social roles and support networks, these factors can predispose elders to nutritional deficits.[1,2]

Aging is accompanied by progressive functional declines in many organ systems, which may ultimately result in altered absorption, transport, metabolism and excretion of nutrients.[2] Changes in olfactory and taste acuity may affect food intake. Age-associated changes in the oral cavity and gastrointestinal tract may have a significant

0-8493-9612-3/99/$0.00+$.50
© 1999 by CRC Press LLC

effect on nutritional status. Decreased saliva production, tooth loss or ill-fitting dentures may make it difficult to chew certain foods, such as raw vegetables and meat. In the gastrointestinal tract, age-related decreases in gastric acid and enzyme production may reduce absorption of calcium and proteins, respectively. Altered gastrointestinal motility may contribute to constipation, resulting in poor appetite. The incidence of chronic diseases, which also increases with advancing age, can impair mobility and appetite — thus affecting food intake and, consequently, nutritional status. In addition, the medications frequently used in the treatment of chronic diseases may alter the digestion, absorption and utilization of nutrients. Medications may also affect appetite, taste and smell, as well as cause gastrointestinal upset. Advancing age is accompanied by alterations in body composition, the most striking being the gradual decline in fat-free mass (FFM) and a corresponding increase in fat mass. Studies indicate that this equates to a decline in skeletal muscle with relative preservation of non-muscle lean tissue (Figure 10.1). The mechanisms responsible

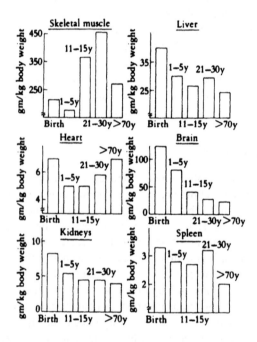

FIGURE 10.1   Relative proportion (gm/kg of body weight) of major organs at various stages of life in humans (Drawn from V. Korenchevsky. *Physiological and Pathological Aging*. New York: Hafner, 1961.) (Reproduced with permission from S. Karger, AG, Basel, Switzerland)

for these changes are numerous, and ways to reverse the trend are the focus of a number of studies.[3] High-intensity strength-training exercises have been shown to counteract some of the effects of age by increasing skeletal muscle mass and decreasing body fat mass, with a concomitant rise in resting metabolic rate.[4]

Protein nutriture is an important factor in an individual's response to injury and stress.[5,6] Concern about the maintenance of body protein status in the elderly must therefore be addressed. Castaneda et al.[7] have reported that low protein intakes in elderly women are associated with a loss in lean body mass, accompanied by impaired immune function and muscle strength. Energy intake is known to decline with advancing age, but the question of protein requirement in the elderly is still debated. Recently, Fereday et al.[8] reported and Millward et al.[9] concluded in a review that the elderly had similar or even lower protein needs as the young. In contrast, Campbell et al.[10] suggested that older persons required more than the present Food and Agriculture Organization of the United Nations/World Health Organization/United Nations University (FAO/WHO/UNU) recommendations for safe protein intakes for adults.

10.2 METHODS FOR ASSESSING PROTEIN TURNOVER AND AMINO ACID KINETICS

Although many of the approaches used to study protein and amino acid metabolism in older individuals are identical to those used in infants, children and young adults (as well as in animals), specific issues related to the elderly will be described in a brief review of these approaches. There are a number of methods available to study protein and amino acid metabolism in humans, as shown in Table 10.1.

TABLE 10.1
Methods to Assess Protein and Amino Acid Metabolism

1. Nitrogen balance technique

2. Precursor methods
      (i) amino acid tracer, administered intravenously or orally
      (ii) measurement of tracer in plasma or urine, or of isotope in CO_2 or urea

3. End-product methods — measurement of tracer excretion in products of N metabolism (e.g., urea or ammonia) or incorporation into specific proteins (e.g., albumin, myosin, fibrinogen)

4. Positron Emission Tomography (PET)

5. Neutron activation analysis

6. Molecular or tissue-specific approaches

10.2.1 NITROGEN BALANCE TECHNIQUE

Nitrogen (N) balance studies are particularly useful in the assessment of overall body protein status. This classic technique is based on a measure of the difference between nitrogen intake and nitrogen output, with positive balance indicating retention of nitrogen; negative balance representing loss of body nitrogen; and zero balance suggesting body nitrogen equilibrium.[11,12] Nitrogen is lost from the body in several ways. Fecal (F) losses are due to unabsorbed protein from the diet, as well as proteins secreted into the lumen of the gastrointestinal tract which are not reabsorbed. End-products of nitrogen metabolism such as urea, ammonia, uric acid and creatinine are excreted in urine (U). Other measurable losses occur from the skin as shed epithelial cells and urea (S). Minor miscellaneous (M) losses include nasal secretions, menstrual fluid, semen and hair clippings. Nitrogen balance (B) may thus be represented by the equation B = I - (U + F + S + M) where I = dietary intake.[11,12]

There are inherent difficulties associated with the nitrogen balance technique, which are often compounded when applied to the older population. Accumulation of errors, both as overestimation of consumption and underestimation of losses, tend to result in a more positive N balance. In addition, losses from cutaneous and other sources are rarely included when the technique is actually applied, because of difficulty measuring these losses accurately. Nutritional status can influence the level of protein at which nitrogen equilibrium is reached. An older person who has been on a low protein diet and has poor protein stores is more likely to reach N equilibrium on a lower protein intake than one whose protein status is optimal. This response reflects the ability of the body to adapt to a lower protein intake, as well as the fact that less N is needed to maintain lower or reduced protein stores. Furthermore, N retention is highly correlated to energy intake, with greater N retention on higher caloric intake. These situations may result in the conclusion that older persons either do not differ or have lower protein requirements than the young. Despite these difficulties, N balance approaches continue to be used, often as an adjunct to other methods.

10.2.2 PRECURSOR METHODS

Assessment of the status of whole-body protein turnover in man reflects an integration of multiple aspects of protein and amino acid metabolism, including the synthesis and breakdown of proteins, and utilization of specific amino acids for non-protein nitrogen containing compounds such as epinephrine, serotonin and polyamines. Measuring whole-body protein turnover *in vivo* often relies on the use of an isotopically labeled amino acid given as a tracer, with measurements of the isotope content in plasma, urine, expired CO_2 or tissue proteins. Different mathematical models are then used to analyze the results and to calculate the components of turnover (synthesis and breakdown). Major assumptions made in the precursor approach include 1) the sampled compartment is representative of the system as a whole; 2) the dilution of the tracer atom must be representative of the infused tracer molecule; and 3) the chosen tracer model should be a representative member of the whole system. The importance of a representative sampling site is also well appreciated (e.g., venous or arterial, plasma or red blood cell), and detailed discussion may be found in several reviews.[12-14]

Isotopic labeling techniques have been utilized over the last two decades to assess human amino acid metabolism, and thus protein status. Stable isotopes, as opposed to radioisotopes, are preferred for use in humans due to safety concerns. Various stable isotopes of hydrogen, oxygen, carbon and nitrogen have been utilized as amino acid tracers. The most widely used probes have been ^{15}N-glycine and L-1-^{13}C-leucine (see Chapter 2). Whole-body protein metabolism is indirectly measured by estimating the flux of a particular amino acid through the metabolic pool. A known quantity of isotopically labeled amino acid is administered either orally or intravenously. The amount of labeled amino acid which is not excreted is assumed to represent that which is incorporated into protein.[12-15] It is assumed that recycling is negligible when studies are conducted over a short time span.[12-14] Studies in the elderly may be complicated by the rigors of the study design. Moreover, deciding on the appropriate denominator for comparing data to younger individuals is a continuing dilemma, since body protein content changes and may not be easily assessed in clinical and/or research situations.

10.2.3 END-PRODUCT METHODS

The classic end-product method was described by Picou and Taylor-Roberts, and based on constant administration of ^{15}N-labeled amino acids (e.g., glycine) and measurement of ^{15}N in urinary urea.[15] By various nitrogen exchange processes, the ^{15}N is assumed to become mixed throughout the body free N pool; after an appropriate time, the pool is sampled to measure dilution of the tracer. Dilution either occurs by dietary N intake or by unlabeled N released as amino acids from protein breakdown. Therefore, by conventional mass balance equations, the latter rate is estimated. Since direct sampling of the body nitrogen pool is difficult, the N pool is indirectly sampled by measuring ^{15}N dilution in urinary urea or ammonia, the major excretory outflows from this pool. A number of assumptions associated with this approach have been described in detail.[15] The importance of recognizing the assumptions and limitations of these methods when applied to studies in older humans is obvious, especially when excretion of urea is measured because of age-related changes in renal function and bladder emptying. Again, the basis for normalizing the data to body weight, fat-free mass (FFM) or body cell mass is critical when comparing different groups.

10.2.3.1 Specific Proteins

The amount of isotopically labeled amino acid incorporated into specific proteins can also be directly measured. This, combined with the precursor pool enrichment and the time course, yields the fractional synthesis rate by using the equation $S_B = k_s {}^* S_1 {}^* t$, where S_B is the isotopically labeled enrichment of the amino acid in the protein; k_s is the fractional rate constant; S_1 is the mean labeled enrichment of the amino acid precursor pool over time, t; and t is the infusion time.[14] This approach is particularly well suited for analysis of muscle where the majority of protein synthesized is not exported. An inherent difficulty with direct measurements of specific protein synthesis rates is that sampling of tissues other than muscle is not normally feasible. However, examination of hepatic or intestinal protein synthesis is technically possible, especially if a patient undergoes these biopsy procedures for clinical purposes. To overcome this limitation, investigators have resorted to sampling representative plasma protein to assess synthesis rates. The choice of the plasma protein is complicated by the secretion rates of the protein, the often low concentration in plasma, and posttranslational modification of the protein of interest. The rapid development in new technology will certainly overcome these issues. A more in-depth discussion of these isotope methods may be found in Chapters 2, 3 and 4 of this book.

In older humans, changes in digestion, absorption and metabolism will influence conclusions obtained in studies utilizing any of these approaches. It is important for the investigator to understand the basis for comparison between groups which vary in the total body protein mass, as well as in metabolic regulation. Assessment of body composition is hence an important aspect of studies as a means to "normalize" the data obtained. The contribution of skeletal muscle to whole-body protein synthesis is small ($< 30\%$); therefore, small changes in muscle protein synthesis rates will not usually be detected in whole-body estimates.[16] Hence, this raises the important issue of assessing synthesis rates of specific organ proteins (e.g., myosin and actin for skeletal muscle; albumin, apolipoprotein B, fibrinogen for the liver, etc.) and the relationship to whole-body protein turnover. Future directions will undoubtedly combine isotope measures with molecular techniques to integrate protein turnover with gene expression and translation.

10.2.4 POSITRON EMISSION TOMOGRAPHY

Positron emission tomography (PET) may be helpful in elucidating some aspects of amino acid metabolism in the brain. Initial work in this area utilized naturally occurring ^{11}C-labeled amino acids. Unfortunately, the accuracy of the determined kinetic rate constants was reduced by the complexity of the metabolic products of the labeled natural amino acids in brain and plasma.[17] Subsequent use of synthetic amino acids circumvented this problem, since the brain does not have the capacity to metabolize them.[17] Studies utilizing synthetic L-(2-^{18}F)-fluorophenylalanine, which utilizes the same carrier system as phenylalanine, have indicated that the rate of neutral amino acid transport into the brain is unaffected by age. Bustany and Comar, utilizing a human model, and others, using a rat model, have reported decreased brain protein synthesis with age.[18,19] Together, these data suggest that any age-related reduction in protein synthesis in the brain is not likely to be due to limited availability of amino acids. The feasibility of PET in assessing protein metabolism is exciting, and the approach could be applied to analysis of functional changes in amino acid transport under various pathological conditions, such as ischemic brain injury and degenerative diseases.

10.2.5 NEUTRON ACTIVATION

The only direct method for assessing the amount of total body protein *in vivo* is neutron activation. This technique involves exposing individuals to a carefully controlled flow of neutron irradiation and detecting the resultant prompt gammas (from the raised activity of nitrogen) with 2 to 4 large-volume NaI detectors. Each subject's body width and thickness are taken into account.[20]

Total body nitrogen (TBN) is calculated from the equation TBN = $k(N_c/H_c)$TBH, where TBH is total body hydrogen, k is a calibration factor derived utilizing an anthropomorphic phantom which contains known amounts of H and N, and N_c and H_c are the net counts for the N and H energy regions in the prompt gamma spectra.[20] The major assumption is that the proportions of carbon, nitrogen and calcium are known and constant with lipid, protein and bone, respectively. It was recently reported that there was no significant gender effect in the hydration and density of fat-free mass, and that there was no significant correlation between the hydration of FFM and age.[21] These findings have important implications for the use of other approaches to assess FFM, a vital component of studies examining protein and amino acid metabolism in the elderly.

10.2.6 MOLECULAR APPROACHES

Slight alterations in protein structure can result in drastic changes in function; thus, a well-tuned synthetic process is crucial for the survival of any organism. Net protein synthesis is known to slow with age; however, this decrease in synthesis may not be equal across all proteins.[22] This emphasizes the importance of assessing specific protein synthesis rates. Molecular approaches have been developed in an effort to understand the regulation of protein metabolism at the level of gene transcription, mRNA translation, peptide synthesis, post-translational protein modification and protein breakdown.

The rate and accuracy of the protein synthetic machinery has been regarded as important in cellular aging. The evidence to date is contradictory, but, in general, studies do not reveal major age-related differences in the number or capacity of ribosomes to accurately translate mRNA. The rate of initiation of protein synthesis also appears to be unaltered by age.[22] Although there may be a slight decrease in total ribosomal number, this is not a rate-limiting factor. Functional changes in ribosomes may occur, but the reasons, as well as the biochemical and biophysical changes influencing translational regulation during aging, are unclear.

Perhaps more important to the aging process is the post-synthetic modifications of proteins, which is beyond the scope of this chapter. However, oxidative modification, glycation, phosphorylation and methylation are some of the processes known to occur and change with advancing age, leading to alterations in protein function.

10.3 RECENT DATA

As individuals age, significant body composition changes occur, the most important being a reduction in active skeletal muscle mass (sarcopenia). This represents a loss in total body nitrogen or protein.[3] Nitrogen balance studies have shed light on this phenomenon. Previous nitrogen balance studies have been recalculated, bearing the above difficulties in mind. These newly calculated data, combined with new data on healthy older men and women has revealed that a safe level of dietary protein intake for older men and women is 1.0 to 1.25 gm high quality protein/kg body weight/day, as compared to the current Recommended Dietary Allowances (RDA) of 0.8 gm/kg/day. Research has shown that many community-dwelling elderly are in negative nitrogen balance. Thus, inadequate dietary protein intake may contribute to sarcopenia.[23] Additional recent reports on protein metabolism in older individuals utilizing stable isotopes have demonstrated that there is 1) an age-related reduction in myosin synthesis;[24] 2) an age-related reduction in mitochondrial protein synthesis;[25] and 3) evidence that changes in body composition, not age or gender per se, influence amino acid and protein turnover.[8,26] Welle et al.[27] also recently demonstrated that slower myofibrillar protein synthesis rates in older muscle are not caused by a reduction in mRNA availability.

In summary, the major difficulty in comparing whole-body protein turnover rates in the young and the old is the basis upon which to report the data. As individuals age, they lose lean body mass (muscle) but gain fat, thus maintaining body weight. This change in body composition often leads to conclusions that turnover is lower in the elderly when expressed per unit of body weight, is not different from the young when expressed per unit of FFM,[8,26] or higher when expressed in terms of body cell mass.[16] Future studies will need to combine classic techniques of assessing whole-body protein metabolism with research on tissue or cell-specific regulation at the molecular level.

Important considerations for studies in the elderly are therefore: 1) appropriate use of body composition data; 2) characterization of the nutritional status prior to study, as subclinical malnutrition contributes to differences in nitrogen utilization, especially energy intake; and 3) recognition that synthesis, modification and turnover of proteins are all interdependent processes, which may be differentially affected by age in different tissues and in different disease states.

REFERENCES

1. Schlenker, E., *Nutrition in Aging,* 2nd Edition, Mosby Year Book, St. Louis, MO, 1993.
2. Chernoff, R., *Geriatric Nutrition: The Health Professional's Handbook*, Aspen Publishers, Inc. Gaithersburg, 1998.
3. Dutta, C., Significance of sarcopenia in the elderly, *J. Nutr.*, 127, 992S, 1997.
4. Fielding, R., Effects of exercise training in the elderly: impact of progressive-resistance training on skeletal muscle and whole-body protein metabolism, *Proc. Nutr. Soc.*, 54, 665, 1995.
5. Kinney, J., Metabolic responses of the critically ill patient, *Critical Care Clinics*, 11, 569, 1995.
6. Kinney, J. M. and Elwyn, D. H., Protein metabolism and injury, *Ann. Rev. Nutr.*, 3, 433, 1983.
7. Castaneda, C., Charnley, J. M., Evans, W. J., and Crim, M. C., Elderly women accommodate to a low-protein diet with losses of body cell mass, muscle function, and immune response, *Am. J. Clin. Nutr.*, 62, 30, 1995.
8. Fereday, A., Gibson, N., Cox, M., Pacy, P., and Millward, D., Protein requirements and ageing: metabolic demand and efficiency of utilization, *Br. J. Nutr.*, 77, 685, 1997.
9. Millward, D., Fereday, A., Gibson, N., and Pacy, P., Aging, protein requirements, and protein turnover, *Am. J. Clin. Nutr.*, 66, 774, 1997.
10. Campbell, W. W., Crim, M., Dallal, G., Young, V., and Evans, W., Increased protein requirements in elderly people: new data and retrospective reassessments, *Am. J. Clin. Nutr.*, 60, 501, 1994.

11. Crim, M. and Munro, H., Proteins and amino acids, *Modern Nutrition in Health and Disease,* 8th Edition, Shils, M., Olson, J. and Shike, M., Eds., Lea and Febiger, Malvern, PA,1994, 3-35.
12. Nissen, S., *Modern Methods in Protein Nutrition and Metabolism,* Academic Press, Inc., San Diego, 1992.
13. Young, V., Fukagawa, N., Bier, D., and Matthews, D., Some aspects of *in vivo* human protein and amino acid metabolism, with particular reference to nutritional modulation, *Proceedings of the 92nd Meeting of the German Society for Internal Medicine,* 92, 640, 1986.
14. Wolfe, R., *Radioactive and Stable Isotope Tracers in Biomedicine: Principles and Practice of Kinetic Analysis,* John Wiley & Sons, 1992.
15. Picou, D. and Taylor-Roberts, T., The measurement of total protein synthesis and catabolism and nitrogen turnover in infants in different nutritional states and receiving different amounts of dietary protein, *Clin. Sci.,* 36, 283, 1969.
16. Nair, K., Muscle protein turnover: methodological issues and the effect of aging, *J. Gerontol. Series A,* 50A, 107, 1995.
17. Ito, H., Hatazawa, J., Murakami, M., Miura, S, Iida, H., Bloomfield, P., Kanno, I., Fukuda, H., and Uemura, K., Aging effect on neutral amino acid transport at the blood-brain barrier measured with L-[2-^{18}F]-fluorophenylalanine and PET, *J. Nuclear. Med.,* 36, 1232, 1995.
18. Bustany, P. and Comar, D., Protein synthesis evaluation in brain and other organs in humans by PET, *Positron emission tomography,* Rivich, M. and Alavi, A., Eds., Alan R. Liss, New York, 1985, 183–201.
19. Hatazawa, J., Itoh, H., Shimosegawa, E., Kanno, I., Murakami, M., Miura, S., Iida, H., Okudera, T., Inugami, A., Ogawa, T., Fujita, H., Satoh, Y., Nagata, K., Hirata, Y., and Uemura, K., Accumulation of L-[2-(F-18)] fluorophenylalanine in peri-infarct area in a patient with acute cerebral infarction, *Ann. Nuclear Med.,* 8, 213, 1994.
20. Vartsky, D., Ellis, K., and Cohns, H., In vivo measurement of body nitrogen by analysis of prompt gammas from neutron capture, *J. Nuclear Med.,* 20, 1158, 1979.
21. Heymsfield, S., Wang, Z., Baumgartner, R., Dilmanian, F., Ma, R., and Yasumura, S., Body composition and aging: a study by in vivo neutron activation analysis, *J. Nutr.,* 123, 432, 1993.
22. Rattan, S., Synthesis, modifications, and turnover of proteins during aging, *Exp. Gerontol.,* 21, 33, 1996.
23. Evans, W., Functional and metabolic consequences of sarcopenia, *J. Nutr.,* 127, 998S, 1997.
24. Welle, S., Thornton, C., Statt, M., and McHenry, B., Postprandial myofibrillar and whole body protein synthesis in young and old human subjects, *Am. J. Physiol.,* 267, E599, 1994.
25. Rooyackers, O., Adey, D., Ades, P., and Nair, K., Effect of age on in vivo rates of mitochondrial protein synthesis in human skeletal muscle, *Proc. Natl. Acad. Sci. U.S.A.,* 93, 15364, 1996.
26. Morais, J., Gougeon, R., Pencharz, P., Jones, P., Ross, R., and Marliss, E., Whole-body protein turnover in the healthy elderly, *Am. J. Clin. Nutr.,* 66, 880, 1997.
27. Welle, S., Bhatt, K., and Thornton, C., Polyadenylated RNA, actin mRNA, and myosin heavy chain mRNA in young and old human skeletal muscle, *Am. J. Physiol.,* 270, E224, 1996.

11 Evaluation of Amino Acid and Protein Metabolism in the Fetus

Patti J. Thureen and William W. Hay, Jr.

CONTENTS

11.1 INTRODUCTION

This chapter describes *in vivo* methods to assess fetal amino acid and protein metabolism. The most basic techniques include chemical composition analysis of the fetus and fetal blood sampling for amino acid and protein concentrations. These methods have been used in animal models and in humans on a selective basis. In large animal models, application of the Fick principle has been used to quantify net placental and fetal uptake and production rates of amino acids. Most recently, tracer methodology has been used to measure placental uptake, metabolism, and transfer to the fetus of individual amino acids and their metabolic products, as well as the metabolism of these amino acids in placenta and fetus to other amino acids, protein synthesis, protein breakdown, oxidation, and glucogenesis. A recent review of nitrogen, amino acid, and protein metabolism in the placenta and fetus provides a summary of data derived from animal models and humans studied by methods described in this chapter.[1]

11.2 NITROGEN AND AMINO ACID BALANCE AT THE WHOLE ANIMAL LEVEL

11.2.1 TOTAL NITROGEN CONTENT

Total body protein content can be estimated from chemical analysis of the whole fetus (post-mortem analysis). This has been done in a variety of species.[1] At the simplest level, both nonfat dry weight and nitrogen content reflect protein mass. In the sheep and guinea pig, approximately 80% of the nitrogen content is found in protein;[2,3] therefore, the following estimate can be made:

Protein content (g) = 0.8 x nitrogen content (g) x 6.25 (g protein/g nitrogen) (1)

11.2.2 WHOLE BODY AMINO ACID ANALYSIS

Total fetal carcass amino acid concentrations have been determined for a variety of species,[2-5] and amino acid concentrations are similar at comparable gestational ages across species. Table 11.1 provides the information required for estimating carbon and nitrogen accretion from amino acid analysis.[6]

11.2.3 GROWTH IN THE FETUS

To estimate fetal protein requirements for growth, both nitrogen accretion and nitrogen losses must be determined. From measurements of nitrogen content in whole fetuses at different gestational ages, the rate of nitrogen accretion in the fetus can be calculated as the change in nitrogen content, divided by the change in gestational age. The nitrogen in the fetus can be divided into that contained in proteins and free amino acids, vs. that present in all other substances in the body including nucleic acids. It is likely that the primary form of nitrogen excretion in the fetus is urea. This has been determined only in the fetal lamb,[7] and does not account for other possible components of fetal nitrogen excretion.

TABLE 11.1
Amino Acid Analysis Data for the Estimation of Carbon and Nitrogen Accretion.*

Amino Acid	Molecular weight	Number of carbon atoms	Number of nitrogen atoms	Percent carbon atoms	Percent nitrogen atoms	Carbon: nitrogen ratio
Essential amino acids						
Lys	146.19	6	2	49.25	19.15	2.57
His	155.16	6	3	46.50	27.07	1.43
Thr	119.12	4	1	40.29	11.75	3.43
Val	117.15	5	1	51.22	11.95	4.29
Met	149.22	5	1	40.21	9.38	4.29
I-Leu	131.18	6	1	54.89	10.67	5.14
Leu	131.18	6	1	54.89	10.67	5.14
Phe	165.19	9	1	65.39	8.48	7.71
Tryp	204.23	11	2	64.63	13.71	4.71
Nonessential amino acids						
Orn	132.16	5	2	45.40	21.19	2.14
Arg	174.21	6	4	41.33	32.14	1.28
Tau	125.15	2	1	19.18	11.19	1.71
Asp	133.10	4	1	36.06	10.52	3.43
Asn	132.14	4	2	31.97	18.65	1.71
Ser	105.09	3	1	34.26	13.32	2.57
Glu	147.13	5	1	40.78	9.52	4.28
Gln	146.15	5	2	41.05	19.16	2.14
Gly	75.07	2	1	31.97	18.65	1.71
Ala	89.09	3	1	40.41	15.71	2.57
Cys	121.15	3	1	29.71	11.56	2.57
Tyr	181.19	9	1	59.61	7.73	7.71
Pro	115.13	5	1	52.11	12.16	4.28
OH-Pro	131.13	5	1	45.76	10.68	4.28
Cit	175.19	6	3	41.13	23.99	1.71

* Reproduced and modified with permission from Frederick Battaglia (University of Colorado) and Academic Press. Inc. Original material in: *An Introduction to Fetal Physiology* Battaglia, 1986, p. 101.

11.3 FETAL BLOOD AMINO ACID CONCENTRATIONS AND MEASUREMENT OF FETAL AMINO ACID UPTAKE FROM THE PLACENTA VIA THE UMBILICAL CIRCULATION

11.3.1 AMINO ACID CONCENTRATIONS

Specific amino acid concentrations provide important information, particularly when the question of interest is a comparison between groups of fetuses that have different nutritional supplies, or between different experimental conditions (i.e., amino acid concentrations at different stages of gestation) within individual fetuses. Interpretation of concentration results requires careful assessment of the physiological stability of the fetus, as amino acid concentrations are affected by numerous experimental factors, including: acute versus steady-state study conditions, maternal anesthesia, and sampling techniques, as well as gestational age and nutritional state. For example, Figure 11.1 shows the arteriovenous amino acid concentration differences in the fetal lamb, at the same gestational age, under acute and chronic study conditions. Certainly, interpretation of amino acid supplies to the fetus under acute, usually stressful, conditions does not provide valid information for normal supply rates of amino acids to the fetus and their relation to fetal requirements for amino acid and protein, and to fetal growth.

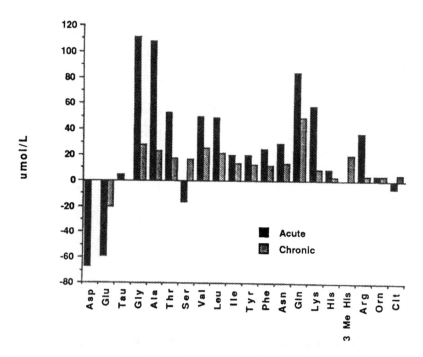

FIGURE 11.1   A comparison of umbilical venous-arterial amino acid differences in fetal lamb studies under acute (solid bars) and chronically catheterized, unstressed (hatched bars) condition. Adapted from Smith, R.M., et al., *Biol. Neonate*, 31, 305-310, 1977, and from Lemons, J.A., et al., *J. Clin. Invest.*, 58, 1428-1434, 1976. Reproduced in modified form with copyright permission of the American Society for Clinical Investigation, and permission from James Lemons (Indiana University Medical Center), and S. Karger AG, Basel.

At present, information on amino acid metabolism in the human fetus is limited to determinations of amino acid concentrations and rare reports of tracer studies (see examples under Section 11.7, "Human Studies," below). *In utero* blood sampling studies have been performed only in the sheep and the human fetus at this point, because of the technical difficulties of blood sampling in small animals. Technical and ethical restraints have further limited experimental assessment of human fetal amino acid and protein metabolism.

11.3.2 UMBILICAL UPTAKES OF AMINO ACIDS

The net rate of uptake of total (as alpha-amino nitrogen) and individual amino acids via the umbilical circulation can be determined by application of the Fick principle as follows:

$$\text{Net umbilical amino acid uptake} = \text{umbilical blood flow } (BF_{umb})$$
$$\text{x whole blood umbilical venous-arterial (v-a)}$$
$$\text{concentration difference of the amino acid} \qquad (2)$$

Measurement of alpha-amino nitrogen uptake by the fetus has been useful for assessment of the effect of maternal nutritional plane on total fetal amino acid supply. It does not, however, provide an assessment of how maternal nutritional plane affects fetal amino acid uptake, nor how placental-fetal amino acid metabolism and exchange interact to provide the unique supply of individual amino acids for fetal amino acid and protein requirements.

Umbilical blood flow has been measured by the transplacental diffusion technique using a variety of indicators, including antipyrine, tritiated water (^3H_2O), and ethanol.[6] The general principle involves use of a relatively inert substance which is rapidly distributed to all body compartments, and which is not rapidly metabolized. ^3H_2O fits these conditions best. Antipyrine has been criticized as a tracer of uterine and umbilical blood flows, because it may increase production of prostaglandins, which might produce independent effects on blood flow. Ethanol also has been criticized as a blood flow indicator, because of potential uteroplacental and/or fetal metabolism. Both antipyrine and ethanol, however, have placental clearances in sheep that are comparable to that of ^3H_2O. Unlike antipyrine or ethanol, because of the permeability of red cells to ^3H_2O, plasma ^3H_2O concentrations require a correction based on the hematocrit level in order to obtain whole blood ^3H_2O concentrations.[8] Microspheres provide accurate flow measurements, but they have the disadvantage of providing few sampling times. In the large animal models, current disposal costs of radioactive microspheres are prohibitive. Colored microspheres may provide an alternative, but there is insufficient experience to define their accuracy vs. blood flows determined by the transplacental diffusion technique or flow probes. Flow probes using electromagnetic or Doppler ultrasonic techniques have been used for uterine blood flow measurements, but so far have not been suitable for umbilical blood flow measurements, particularly in chronic studies.

To measure umbilical blood flow using the transplacental diffusion technique, a tracer such as ^3H_2O is infused into the fetus via a central vein at a fixed rate. In the large animal model, this is accomplished by placement of plastic catheters into the vena cava via forelimb or hindlimb peripheral vessels. Catheters for sampling are also placed into the central aorta near the takeoff of the umbilical artery via a hindlimb artery, and into the common umbilical vein directly or via a branch umbilical vein. Because ^3H_2O is not metabolized, it either accumulates in the fetus or leaves the fetus. The rate of fetal ^3H_2O accumulation can be determined by simultaneous measurement of ^3H_2O concentrations in the umbilical artery and vein over time (e.g., usually 3 to 4 samples at 10- to 20-minute intervals), determining the slope of ^3H_2O concentration vs. time from these values, and multiplying this slope by the fetal volume of distribution of ^3H_2O:

$$\text{rate of fetal } ^3H_2O \text{ accumulation (dpm/min)} = \text{slope of } ^3H_2O \text{ concentration/time} \\ \text{(dpm/ml/min)} \times 0.8 \times \text{fetal wt (g)} \tag{3}$$

where 0.8 is the volume of distribution of ^3H_2O in ml/g of fetal weight. The only significant exit of ^3H_2O from the fetus is presumed to be via transplacental diffusion, which is calculated as:

$$\text{transplacental diffusion rate of } ^3H_2O \text{ (dpm/min)} = {}^3H_2O \text{ infusion rate} \\ \text{(dpm/min)} - \text{fetal } ^3H_2O \text{ accumulation rate (dpm/min)} \tag{4}$$

Thus, umbilical blood flow is calculated as:

$$BF_{umb} \text{ (ml/min)} = \text{transplacental diffusion rate of } ^3H_2O \\ \text{(dpm/min)}/(^3H_2O)_{a\text{-}v} \text{ (dpm/ml)} \tag{5}$$

where a and v are the umbilical artery and vein ^3H_2O concentrations, respectively. Because ^3H_2O is presumed to freely diffuse across the placenta, uterine blood flow (BF_{Ut}) can be calculated as:

$$BF_{Ut} \text{ (ml/min)} = \text{transplacental diffusion rate of } ^3H_2O \\ \text{(dpm/min)}/(^3H_2O)_{V\text{-}A} \text{ (dpm/ml)} \tag{6}$$

where V and A are the uterine vein and artery ^3H_2O concentrations, respectively. To date, umbilical blood flows have been measured in the pregnant sheep, cow, horse, and pig, whereas uterine blood flows have been measured in a larger variety of species where catheterization of the maternal uterine circulation has been possible.[9-12] For most amino acids, uterine and umbilical whole-blood extraction coefficients (i.e., the percentage change in the amino acid concentration across the uterus and the fetus, respectively) are <10%. This has required very careful attention to the accuracy and precision of amino acid analytical techniques. One reason for the relatively small whole blood concentration differences of amino acids across the uterine circulation is that the amino acids carried by adult ovine red cells do not contribute significantly to the rapid amino acid exchange between body organs and circulation.[13] The exchange is virtually limited to the plasma compartment. The same is also true for amino acid exchange between fetal red cells and plasma.[14] The accuracy of uterine and umbilical amino acid uptakes has been improved recently by using plasma amino acid concentration differences, provided that plasma is separated from red cells within a few minutes of sampling.

The only species in which complete amino acid uptakes have been determined is the fetal sheep. Measurements in smaller animals have not been possible, because of the difficulty in putting catheters into the fetal vasculature. In the sheep, this technique has allowed for study of fetal metabolism in both acute and chronic steady-state conditions from mid-gestation to term. The first study of umbilical uptake of individual amino acids was performed by Lemons and coworkers,[15] and demonstrated a nitrogen uptake that was approximately 160% of fetal nitrogen requirement. Improvements in amino acid chromatography and use of plasma concentrations and plasma flow in subsequent studies have shown equivalence of fetal nitrogen uptake and requirements.[14,16]

11.4 MEASUREMENT OF FETAL PROTEIN TURNOVER, SYNTHESIS AND BREAKDOWN

11.4.1 PROTEIN SYNTHESIS AND TURNOVER

In numerous species, it has been demonstrated that fetal protein synthesis and breakdown are dynamic processes operating at high rates. In the growing fetus, protein synthesis exceeds protein breakdown, producing protein accretion; thus,

$$\text{Protein accretion rate} = \text{protein synthetic rate - protein breakdown rate} \quad (7)$$

Using tracer methodology, a single amino acid selected for its reflection of protein metabolism can be labeled and used to study protein metabolism in the fetus. The most commonly used amino acids for this purpose have been two of the essential amino acids, leucine and lysine, labeled with either radioactive or stable isotopes.

The fractional protein synthetic rate (K_s, fraction per day) of the fetus can be estimated by infusing a tracer amino acid at a constant rate into the fetus, until a plasma steady state for both tracer and tracee is reached. At this time, the plasma tracee specific radioactivity (SA_{plasma} for radioactive tracers) or isotopic enrichment (E_{plasma} for stable isotopic tracers) is constant. The fetus is sacrificed at a known time, which determines the total time of tracer infusion (t, as a fraction of the day). The mean specific radioactivity or stable isotopic enrichment of the tracer amino acid at the time of sacrifice is measured in whole body proteins ($SA_{proteins}$ or $E_{proteins}$) that are produced by acid precipitation of a whole body homogenate:[17,18]

$$K_s = t^{-1} (SA_{proteins} / SA_{plasma}) \quad (8)$$

This equation does not account for back flow of the tracer amino acid into the fetal plasma as a result of fetal protein breakdown. This can be calculated using the formula:

$$K_s = -t^{-1} \, ln \, [1-(SA_{proteins} / SA_{plasma})] \quad (9)$$

The above equation assumes that steady state is reached immediately. To further correct for the initial period when steady state has not been achieved, Swick's equation can be used.[19] In studies of the ovine fetus from mid-gestation to term, there has been good agreement between leucine and lysine tracers in the estimate of K_s[17,18,20]. The rate of protein synthesis (PR_s, g/day) can be estimated from the following equation:

$$PR_s = {}^{LEU}R_s \times 1440 \times \text{molecular wt of tracer amino acid} \times$$
$$(\text{grams protein/g tracee amino acid in the fetus}) \qquad (10)$$

where ${}^{LEU}R_s$ is the rate at which fetal plasma tracee leucine enters fetal protein synthesis in µmol/min and is calculated as:

$$^{LEU}R_s = K_s \times (\text{amount of tracee leucine in fetal proteins}$$
$$\text{in µmol /1440 minutes per day}) \qquad (11)$$

Grams protein/g tracee amino acid in the fetus can be assumed as a fixed ratio (i.e., 590 µmol leucine/g protein), or it can be determined as a function of gestational age since the protein composition of the fetus does change with growth. This latter method can be determined by measuring the total protein/tracer ratio in homogenates of the fetal carcass at different gestational ages.[17]

In the living animal, the rate of protein synthesis can be estimated if the fetal protein content and amino acid composition are known from prior studies, and the tracer label is not incorporated into other amino acids. If these assumptions are met, then ${}^{LEU}R_s$ (µmol/min) is calculated during a fetal tracer leucine infusion as:

$$^{LEU}R_s = (I_{f,o} - \text{tracer losses from the fetus})/ {}^{leu}SA_a \qquad (12)$$

where $I_{f,o}$ is the rate of tracer infusion from the outside (o) into the fetus (f), and tracer losses occur as the sum of tracer leucine loss to CO_2 via oxidation plus diffusional loss of tracer leucine to the placenta. Using a carbon tracer that labels CO_2 by oxidation, tracer loss to CO_2 by oxidation (${}^{CO2}r_{p,f}$) is calculated by the Fick principle as:

$$^{CO2}r_{p,f} = BF_{umb} \times [{}^{14}CO_2]_{a-v} \qquad (13)$$

where ${}^{CO2}r_{p,f}$ is the flux of tracer-labeled ${}^{14}CO_2$, which results from oxidation of tracer leucine infused into the fetus; the ${}^{14}CO_2$ produced then diffuses from the fetal circulation into the placenta and the uterine circulation, from which it is expired by the mother. Diffusional loss of tracer leucine from the fetus into the placenta (${}^{leu}r_{p,f}$) is determined as:

$$^{leu}r_{p,f} = BF_{umb} \times [leu]_{a-v} \qquad (14)$$

11.4.2 PROTEIN BREAKDOWN

Many amino acids are delivered to the fetus in amounts that are in excess of their rates of accretion,[15] and estimates of fetal urea production rates are quite high.[6,7] This implies considerable oxidation of amino acids. Estimation of protein and amino acid oxidation by measurement of net excretion of urea from the fetus has not been possible using the Fick principle, because the umbilical venous-arterial concentration differences for urea are too small (at least in the pregnant sheep model) to be determined with accuracy. Using tracer methodology, however, Gresham et al. developed a method for determining fetal urea production from placental urea clearance measurements.[7] Human, rhesus monkey, and sheep measurements of placental urea clearance per fetal weight are all similar. Furthermore, the placenta does not readily produce urea from ammonia. Thus, fetal urea production has been equated with placental urea excretion into the uterine circulation of the mother. During a fetal infusion of [^{14}C]urea:

$$\text{Fetal urea production} = \text{Placental urea excretion into the} \atop \text{maternal (uterine) circulation} \qquad (15)$$

$$\text{Fetal (= Placental) urea excretion} = BF_{umb} \times ([^{12}C]urea)_{a\text{-}v} \qquad (16)$$

$$\text{Fetal (= Placental) } [^{14}C]urea \text{ excretion} = BF_{umb} \times ([^{14}C]urea)_{a\text{-}v} \qquad (17)$$

$$\text{Placental } [^{12}C]urea \text{ clearance} = \text{Placental } [^{14}C]urea \text{ clearance} \qquad (18)$$

$$\text{Placental } [^{12}C]urea \text{ clearance} = \text{Placental } [^{12}C]urea \text{ excretion}/([^{12}C]urea)_{a\text{-}A}$$
$$= BF_{umb} \times ([^{12}C]urea)_{a\text{-}v}/([^{12}C]urea)_{a\text{-}A}$$
$$= \text{Placental } [^{14}C]urea \text{ clearance} = \text{Placental } [^{14}C]urea \text{ excretion}/([^{14}C]urea)_{a\text{-}A}$$
$$= BFumb \times ([^{14}C]urea)_{a\text{-}v}/([^{14}C]urea)_{a\text{-}A} \qquad (19)$$

$$\text{Fetal urea Production} = \{BF_{umb} \times ([^{14}C]urea)_{a\text{-}v} / ([^{14}C]urea)_{a\text{-}A}\}$$
$$\times ([^{12}C]urea)_{a\text{-}A} \qquad (20)$$

Plasma [^{12}C]urea concentrations in the fetal artery (a) and the uterine artery (A) are sufficiently different to allow [^{12}C]urea$_{a\text{-}A}$ to be measured accurately, as are the [^{14}C]urea concentrations in the umbilical artery and vein, allowing accurate measurement of [^{14}C]urea$_{a\text{-}v}$.

11.5 TRACER METHODS FOR STUDYING FETAL-PLACENTAL-MATERNAL METABOLIC INTERACTION

11.5.1 FETAL AMINO ACID METABOLISM

A variety of radioactively or stable isotopically labeled amino acids has been infused into the fetal sheep to model fetal amino acid metabolism. Leucine has been studied principally, as it is an essential amino acid. Thus, its net entry into fetal plasma comes only from fetal protein breakdown, and from the placenta via net uptake by the umbilical circulation; its only net disposal out of fetal plasma is into fetal protein synthesis and oxidation. At steady state:

Leucine net umbilical uptake plus leucine from fetal protein breakdown =
Leucine oxidation plus leucine incorporation into fetal protein synthesis   (21)

During a fetal infusion of tracer leucine, it also is the case that the tracer will exchange with placental leucine, producing a net loss of tracer leucine to the placenta. This occurs because the leucine transporter on both maternal-facing and fetal-facing surfaces of the placental trophoblast is bidirectional, and because the tracer concentration is greater in the fetal plasma (where it is infused) than in the trophoblast or the maternal circulation (where it diffuses to). Thus, net irreversible disposal of tracer leucine from the fetal plasma includes oxidation to labeled CO_2 (assuming a carbon labeled tracer), incorporation into protein synthesis, and net uptake by the placenta via the umbilical circulation. At steady state, fetal plasma disposal rate of leucine ($^{LEU}DR_f$) into fetal protein synthesis ($^{LEU}R_s$) and oxidation ($^{LEU}R_{CO2}$) is proportional to the tracer leucine infusion rate minus the net rate of tracer uptake by the placenta. Thus:

$$^{LEU}DR_f = (^{LEU}R_s) + (^{LEU}R_{CO2}) = \{^{leu}I_f - (BF_{umb} \times leu_{a\text{-}v})\}/\, ^{leu}SA_a \qquad (22)$$

Fetal leucine utilization for protein synthesis is then calculated according to Equations (12), (13), and (14). At steady state, leucine derived from protein breakdown is calculated as net leucine disposal rate into protein synthesis and oxidation, according to Equation (21), minus net umbilical leucine uptake rate according to Equation (2). Leucine incorporation into protein accretion is calculated according to Equation (7) as leucine incorporation into protein synthesis minus leucine derived from protein breakdown. Finally, most investigators also use plasma α-ketoisocaproate (KIC) specific activity to derive fetal leucine disposal rates, as plasma KIC specific activity is considered approximately equal to that of intracellular KIC, the final product of cellular leucine metabolism after deamination and prior to oxidation.

11.5.2 FETAL-PLACENTAL-MATERNAL AMINO ACID METABOLISM

While fetal metabolism of individual amino acids can be traced with a fetal tracer infusion, this is not so for many amino acids when the amino acid tracer is infused into the mother, as many of the amino acids undergo considerable metabolism in the placenta. In such cases, fetal tracer-specific activity or enrichment may not be directly related to the umbilical uptake of the tracer from the placenta. Several recent studies have examined placental-fetal metabolic interactions for selected amino acids, including leucine, serine, glycine, glutamine, glutamate, alanine, and threonine. To demonstrate the complexity of this type of analysis, an example will be used from the work of Ross and co-workers in their study of leucine metabolism in the ovine fetus and placenta.[21]

In this study, the metabolic experiments were conducted 1 to 2 weeks after recovery from surgical placement of maternal, uterine, umbilical, and fetal sampling and infusion catheters. Leucine plasma fluxes were determined during simultaneous infusion of L-[1-^{13}C]leucine into the mother and L-[1-^{14}C]leucine into the fetus. Umbilical and uterine blood flows were determined by the steady-state transplacental diffusion method, using ^3H_2O as the blood flow indicator (see above). Fluxes into and out of the uteroplacenta and fetus were calculated for leucine, α-ketoisocaproic acid (KIC) which is produced from leucine in the placenta by deamination, and labeled leucine and KIC.[21,22] Figure 11.2 shows the fluxes determined by combining tracer and tracee data. The calculations are described below for fluxes numbered I-XIII in Figure 11.2. All flux rates are expressed in units of μmol/min. Note that in this model, in contrast to the model in Section 11.5.1 for fetal leucine metabolism, total fetal plasma leucine disposal rate is the principal measure of fetal leucine metabolism; in addition, both net and unidirectional fluxes between fetal plasma and placenta, and between fetal plasma and fetal tissues, are included.

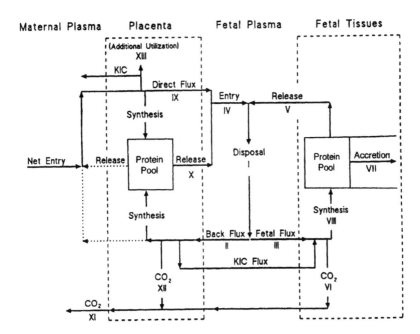

FIGURE 11.2 Model of maternal-fetal-placental fluxes of leucine and ketoisocaproic acid (KIC) estimated by mass balance of tracer and tracee data. Each Roman numeral represents a flux, with equations for each flux described in the text. From Ross, J.C., et al., *Am. J. Physiol.*, 270, E491-E503, 1996. Reproduced with permission from the American Physiological Society.

Flux I. Fetal plasma tracee leucine disposal rate ($^{LEU}DR_f$, μmol/min). Leucine disposal from the fetal plasma is calculated as the ratio between fetal tracer L-[1-^{14}C] leucine infusion rate ($^{leu}I_{f,o}$, dpm/min) and the fetal arterial tracer leucine specific activity $^{leu}SA_a$ (dpm/μmol) at steady state. It is equal to the sum of the two rates of leucine entry into the fetal plasma, leucine unidirectional back flux into the placenta from the fetus (Flux II), and leucine unidirectional flux into fetal tissues from fetal blood (Flux III). Disposal of leucine from the fetal plasma pool is chosen because this is the sampled pool, and the one fetal pool into which leucine, KIC, tracer leucine, and labeled KIC enter from the placenta and the fetal tissues, and from which these same substances leave to enter fetal tissues and the placenta.

$$^{LEU}DR_f = {}^{leu}I_{f,o} / {}^{leu}SA_a = \text{Flux II} + \text{Flux III} \tag{23}$$

Flux II. Tracee leucine unidirectional back flux into the placenta, from the fetus.

$$\text{Flux II} = {}^{LEU}DR_f \times ({}^{leu}frac_{umb}) \tag{24}$$

where $^{leu}frac_{umb}$ is the fraction of tracer leucine infused into the fetus that is taken up by the placenta.

Flux III. Tracee leucine unidirectional flux into fetal tissues, from fetal blood.

$$\text{Flux III} = {}^{LEU}DR_f \times (1-{}^{leu}frac_{umb}) \tag{25}$$

where $1-{}^{leu}frac_{umb}$ is the fraction of tracer leucine infused into the fetus that is taken up by the fetal tissues.

Flux IV. Tracee leucine flux into fetal blood, from placenta. The net flux of leucine into the fetus from the placenta ($^{LEU}R_{f,p}$) is the difference between the unidirectional flux of leucine into the fetal plasma from the placenta (Flux IV) and the unidirectional back flux of leucine into the placenta from the fetus. Therefore,

$$\text{Flux IV} = {}^{LEU}R_{f,p} + \text{Flux II} \tag{26}$$

Flux V. Tracee leucine released into fetal blood, from fetal proteins by protein breakdown.

$$\text{Flux V} = {}^{LEU}DR_f - \text{Flux IV} \tag{27}$$

because leucine entry rate (Flux IV + Flux V) = leucine disposal rate (Flux II + Flux III) under steady-state conditions.

Flux VI. CO_2 produced by the fetus, from fetal plasma carbon-1 of leucine.

$$\text{Flux VI} = {}^{LEU}DR_f \times {}^{CO2}frac_{umb} \tag{28}$$

where $^{CO2}frac_{umb}$ is the fraction of infused tracer leucine carbon excreted as $^{14}CO_2$ via the umbilical circulation.

Flux VII. Tracee leucine and KIC flux into fetal protein accretion, from fetal blood. The combined flux of fetal plasma leucine and KIC into fetal protein accretion is the difference between net leucine and KIC uptakes by fetal tissues and CO_2 production from carbon-1 of fetal plasma leucine (i.e., Flux VI).

$$\text{Flux VII} = (^{LEU}R_{f,p} + {}^{KIC}R_{f,p}) - \text{Flux VI} \tag{29}$$

Flux VIII. Tracee leucine flux into fetal protein synthesis, from fetal blood. Under steady-state conditions, leucine flux into fetal protein synthesis is equal to the leucine incorporated into fetal protein accretion plus the leucine that is released from fetal protein by breakdown.

$$\text{Flux VIII} = \text{Flux VII} + \text{Flux V} \tag{30}$$

Flux IX. Flux of maternal leucine into fetal circulation.

$$\text{Flux IX} = {}^{LEU}DR_f \times ({}^{leu}MPE_a / {}^{leu}MPE_A) \tag{31}$$

where $^{leu}MPE_a$ and $^{leu}MPE_A$ are the molar percent excesses of maternally infused tracer L-[1-^{13}C]leucine in fetal ($_a$) and maternal ($_A$) arterial plasma, respectively.

Flux X. Tracee leucine released into fetal blood, from placental proteins. This is calculated as the difference between the unidirectional flux of leucine into the fetal plasma from the placenta and the direct flux of maternal leucine into the fetal circulation.

$$\text{Flux X} = \text{Flux IV} - \text{Flux IX} \tag{32}$$

Flux X is an approximation. It assumes that direct flux of maternal leucine into the fetal systemic circulation is equal to the flux of maternal leucine into the umbilical circulation. This assumption is not fully true, however, because the fetal liver, which also is perfused by umbilical venous blood, takes up some leucine for fetal hepatic metabolism, producing a slightly lower leucine concentration in the fetal plasma.

Flux XI. CO_2 produced by pregnant uterus, from fetal plasma carbon-1 of leucine.

$$\text{Flux XI} = {}^{LEU}DR_f \times {}^{CO2}frac_{Ut} \tag{33}$$

where $^{CO2}frac_{Ut}$ is the fraction of infused leucine tracer carbon excreted as $^{14}CO_2$ via the uterine circulation.

Flux XII. CO_2 produced by placenta, from fetal plasma carbon-1 of leucine.

$$\text{Flux XII} = \text{Flux XI} - \text{Flux VI} = {}^{LEU}DR_f \times ({}^{CO2}frac_{Ut} - {}^{CO2}frac_{umb}) \tag{34}$$

Flux XIII. Additional leucine utilization by uteroplacenta.

$$\text{Flux XIII} = {}^{LEU}R_{p,m} - ({}^{KIC}R_{p,m} + \text{Flux XI} + \text{Flux VII}) \tag{35}$$

where ${}^{LEU}R_{p,m}$ is the net leucine uptake by the pregnant uterus from the mother. In normal pregnant sheep, Flux XIII is as much as one third of fetal plasma leucine disposal rate, but it is negligible in cases of severe intrauterine growth restriction (IUGR). Thus, it represents a pathway of leucine metabolism in the placenta that is variable and can decrease to preserve the entry of leucine into the fetus.

11.6 TRACER METHODS FOR STUDYING FETAL ORGAN AMINO ACID METABOLISM

The majority of the work in this area has involved study of the fetal hepatic and skeletal muscle metabolism, as a result of successful catheterization of the fetal hepatic and hindlimb circulations,[23] which, in combination with tracer methodology, allows for organ-specific fetal metabolic studies. Liver blood flow has been measured using labeled microspheres and indicator dilution techniques. For downstream sampling, catheters have been inserted into both left and right hepatic veins directly through the thoracic inferior vena cava, following thoracotomy. Upstream sampling is from the fetal abdominal aorta, the umbilical vein, and the portal vein. Hindlimb blood flow, primarily representing blood flow to skeletal muscle in the fetus, has been measured by positioning a flow probe around the distal iliac artery of the studied hindlimb. Upstream sampling is via a catheter placed into the external iliac artery of the non-study limb, and downstream sampling is via a catheter placed into the external iliac vein of the study limb through the pudendoepigastric venous trunk branch. As in whole animal studies, further experimental control has been developed using substrate (e.g., glucose, amino acid mixtures) and hormone (e.g., insulin) clamps to produce steady-state conditions.

11.7 HUMAN STUDIES

With the advent of percutaneous umbilical blood sampling (or cordocentesis) of the human fetus in the mid-1980s,[24] it has been possible to perform limited studies of human fetal amino acid metabolism.

11.7.1 CONCENTRATION DATA

Several studies have demonstrated a reduction in the plasma concentrations of most amino acids, particularly the branched chain amino acids, in growth-restricted fetuses.[25-27] These studies also demonstrated that for most essential amino acids maternal concentrations were greater, and maternal-fetal amino acid concentration differences were significantly less, than normal.[28] Such results indicate a less-than-normal rate of transfer of these amino acids from the maternal to the fetal circulation. To provide normal fetal amino acid concentration data, such studies have relied on approval to perform umbilical cord sampling primarily for genetic indications. Samples are used for normal values when the genetic tests on the fetus prove normal, and the sampled fetus subsequently delivers at term as a normal infant. Samples from intrauterine growth-restricted fetuses are approved for research purposes after clinical indications are considered essential for clinical management (i.e., to determine fetal physiological status as part of fetal surveillance procedures, anticipating early delivery if fetal condition is poor and deteriorating). Umbilical sampling is only acceptable from the umbilical vein, as fetal loss has been unacceptably high after hemorrhage and vasoconstriction from umbilical arterial puncture.

11.7.2 TRACER STUDIES

Several investigators have infused amino acid tracers into the pregnant mother and sampled the umbilical circulation at elective Cesarean delivery,[29] including sampling after exposure of the fetus but prior to cord clamping.[30] However, extrapolation of metabolic studies at the time of delivery to represent normal fetal conditions probably is not accurate. Under more normal *in utero* conditions, Cetin et al.[31] performed the first *in utero*, human study of transplacental amino acid transport in pregnancies scheduled for elective cordocentesis for genetic or infectious disease diagnostic purposes. These investigators employed a nonsteady-state approach, infusing a bolus of stable isotopic tracers of leucine and glycine into the mother over 5 minutes, followed by frequent maternal arterialized venous blood sampling over 15 minutes and 1 to 2 fetal samples by cordocentesis. They found limited glycine transport but rapid leucine transplacental transport (Figure 11.3).[31] Similar observations have been made in the pregnant sheep, with more thorough sampling of maternal arterial and umbilical arterial and venous blood.[32]

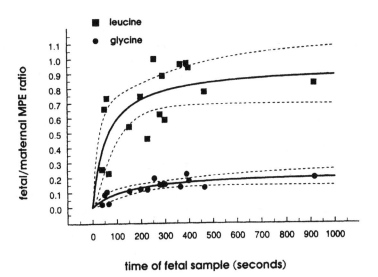

FIGURE 11.3 Venous fetal/maternal enrichment ratios for leucine (squares) and glycine (circles) vs. time of fetal sampling after maternal administration of tracers. From Cetin, I., et al., *Pediatr. Res.*, 37, 571-575, 1995. Reproduced with permission from George Lister, M.D., editor-in-chief, *Pediatric Research*.

REFERENCES

1. Hay, W. W., Jr., Fetal requirements and placental transfer of nitrogenous compounds, in *Fetal and Neonatal Physiology,* 2nd Edition, Polin, R. A. and Fox, W. W., Eds., W. B. Saunders, Philadelphia, 1977, chap. 62.
2. Sparks, J. W., Girard, J. R., Callikan, S., and Battaglia, F. C., Growth of the fetal guinea pig: physical and chemical characteristics, *Am. J. Physiol.,* 248, E132, 1985.
3. Meier, P., Teng, C., Battaglia, F. C., and Meschia, G., The rate of amino acid nitrogen and total nitrogen accumulation in the fetal lamb, *Proc. Soc. Exp. Biol. Med.,* 167, 463, 1981.
4. Southgate, D. A. T., The accumulation of amino acids in the products of conception of the rat and in the young animal after birth, *Biol. Neonate,* 19, 272, 1971.
5. Widdowson, E. M., in *Maternal Nutrition During Pregnancy and Lactation,* Aebi, H., and Whitehead, R., Eds., Berne, H. Huber, 1980, 39.
6. Battaglia, F. C. and Meschia, G., *An Introduction to Fetal Physiology,* Academic Press, Orlando, 1986.
7. Gresham, E. L., Hames, E. J., Raye, J. R., Battaglia, F. C., Makowski, E. L., and Meschia, G., Production and excretion of urea by the fetal lamb, *Pediatrics,* 50, 372, 1972.
8. van Veen, L. C. P., Hay, W. W., Jr., Battaglia, F. C., and Meschia, G., Fetal CO_2 kinetics, *J. Dev. Physiol.,* 6, 359, 1984.
9. Myers, S. A., Sparks, J. W., Makowski, E. L., Meschia, G., and Battaglia, F. C., Relationship between placental blood flow and placental and fetal size in guinea pig, *Am. J. Physiol.,* 243, H404, 1984.
10. Rosenfeld, C. R., Distribution of cardiac output in ovine pregnancy, *Am. J. Physiol.,* 232, H231, 1977.
11. Johnson, R. L., Gilbert, M., Meschia, G., and Battaglia, F. C., Cardiac output distribution and uteroplacental blood flow in the pregnant rabbit: a comparative study, *Am. J. Obstet. Gynecol.,* 151, 682, 1985.
12. Reynolds, L. P. and Ferrell, C. L., Transplacental clearance and blood flows of bovine gravid uterus at several stages of gestation, *Am. J. Physiol.,* 253, R735, 1987.
13. Lobley, G. E., Connell, A., Revell, D. K., Bequette, B. J., Brown, D. S., and Calder, A. G., Splanchnic-bed transfers of amino acids in sheep blood and plasma, as monitored through use of a multiple U-^{13}C-labelled amino acid mixture, *Br. J. Nutr.,* 75, 217, 1996.
14. Chung, M., Teng, C., Timmerman, M., Meschia, G., and Battaglia, F. C., Production and utilization of amino acids by ovine placenta in vivo, *Am. J. Physiol.,* 274, E13, 1998.
15. Lemons, J. A., Adcock, E. W. I., Jones, M. D. J., Naughton, M. A., Meschia, G., and Battaglia, F. C., Umbilical uptake of amino acids in the unstressed fetal lamb, *J. Clin. Invest.,* 58, 1428, 1976.
16. Marconi, A. M., Battaglia, F. C., Meschia, G., and Sparks, J. W., A comparison of amino acid arteriovenous differences across the liver, hindlimb and placenta in the fetal lamb, *Am. J. Physiol.,* 257, E909, 1989.
17. Kennaugh, J. M., Bell, A. W., Teng, C., Meschia, G., and Battaglia, F. C., Ontogenetic changes in the rates of protein synthesis and leucine oxidation during fetal life, *Pediatr. Res.,* 22, 688, 1976.
18. Meier, P. R., Peterson, R. G., Bonds, D. R., Meschia, G., and Battaglia, F. C., Rates of protein synthesis and turnover in fetal life, *Am. J. Physiol.,* 240, E320, 1981.

19. Zak, R., Martin, A. F., and Blough, R., Assessment of protein turnover by use of radioisotopic tracers, *Physiol. Rev.*, 59, 407, 1979.
20. van Veen, L. C. P., Meschia, G., Hay, W. W., Jr., and Battaglia, F. C., Leucine disposal and oxidation rates in the fetal lamb, *Metabolism*, 36, 48, 1987.
21. Ross, J.C., Fennessey, P. V., Wilkening, R. B., Battaglia, F. C., and Meschia, G., Placental transport and fetal utilization of leucine in a model of fetal growth retardation, *Am. J. Physiol.*, 270, E491, 1996.
22. Loy, G. L., Quick, A. N., Jr., Hay, W. W., Jr., Meschia, G., Battaglia, F. C., and Fennessey, P. V., Fetoplacental deamination and decarboxylation of leucine, *Am. J. Physiol.*, 259, E492, 1990.
23. Wilkening, R. B., Boyle, D. W., Teng, C., Meschia, G., and Battaglia, F. C., Amino acid uptake by the fetal ovine hindlimb under normal and euglycemic hyperinsulinemic states, *Am. J. Physiol.*, 266, E72, 1994.
24. Daffos, F., Capella-Pavlowsky, M., and Forestier, F., Fetal blood sampling during pregnancy with use of a needle guided by ultrasound: a study of 606 consecutive cases, *Am. J. Obstet. Gynecol.*, 153, 655, 1985.
25. Economides, D. L., Nicolaides, K. H., Gahl, W. A., Bernardini, I., and Evans, M. I., Plasma amino acids in appropriate and small-for-gestational-age fetuses, *Am. J. Obstet. Gynecol.*, 161, 1219, 1989.
26. Cetin, I., Corbetta, C., Sereni, L. P., Marconi, A. M., Bozzetti, P., Pardi, G., and Battaglia, F. C., Umbilical amino acid concentrations in normal and growth-retarded fetuses sampled in utero by cordocentesis, *Am. J. Obstet. Gynecol.*, 162, 253, 1990.
27. Pardi, G., Cetin, I., Marconi, A. M., Lanfranchi, A., Bozzetti, P., Ferrazzi, E., Buscaglia, M., and Battaglia, F. C., Diagnostic value of blood sampling in fetuses with growth retardation, *N. Engl. J. Med.*, 328, 692, 1993.
28. Cetin, I., Ronzoni, S., Marconi, A.M., Perugino, G., Corbetta, C., Battaglia, F. C., and Pardi, G., Maternal concentrations and fetal-maternal concentration differences of plasma amino acids in normal and intrauterine growth-restricted pregnancies, *Am. J. Obstet. Gynecol.*, 174, 1575, 1996.
29. Gilfillan, C.A., Tserng, K.-Y., and Kalhan, S.C., Alanine production by the human fetus at term gestation, *Biol. Neonate*, 47, 141, 1985.
30. Chien, P. F. W., Smith, K., Watt, P. W., Scrimgeour, C. M., Taylor, D. J., and Rennie, M. J., Protein turnover in the human fetus studied at term using stable isotope tracer amino acids, *Am. J. Physiol.*, 265, E31, 1993.
31. Cetin, I., Marconi, A.M., Baggiani, A.M., Buscaglia, M., Pardi, G., Fennessey, P. V., and Battaglia, F. C., In vivo placental transport of glycine and leucine in human pregnancies, *Pediatr. Res.*, 37, 571, 1995.
32. Geddie, G., Moores, R., Meschia, G., Fennessey, P., Wilkening, R., and Battaglia, F.C. Comparison of leucine, serine and glycine transport across the ovine placenta, *Placenta*, 17, 619, 1996.

12 Analysis of Proteins in Human Milk

Clemens Kunz

CONTENTS

12.1 INTRODUCTION

Human milk has many unique properties that benefit the breast-fed infant. Several of these attributes reside in the protein fraction of human milk, e.g., host defense factors such as immunoglobulins, lysozyme and lactoferrin, or digestive enzymes, specific binding proteins and growth factors.[1,2] These components are present either as soluble proteins in the whey fraction or as casein micelles. In addition, about 5% of total protein is bound within the fat globule membrane.

Significant information is available on the major milk proteins α-lactalbumin, lactoferrin, immunoglobulins and caseins. Their gelelectrophoretic pattern is shown in Figures 12.1A and 12.1B. However, there are still many other components that need to be identified and characterized. For some of these components, the only information available is their approximate molecular weight, e.g., for mucins (> 200 kD) (Figures 12.1A and 12.1B) or for components with a molecular weight between 10 and 30 kD

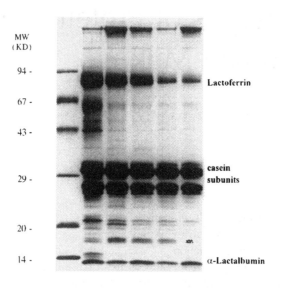

FIGURE 12.1A

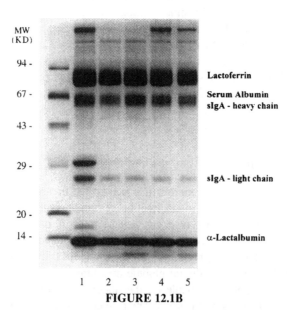

FIGURE 12.1B

FIGURE 12.1 Sodium dodecyl sulfate-gel electrophoresis of proteins in the whey (A) and in the casein fraction (B) of milk from one woman. Before centrifugation (189,000 x g, 4°C, 1 h) fresh milk was treated as follows: lane 2, no pH adjustment; lane 3, pH adjustment to 4.6; lane 4, pH adjustment to 4.3; lane 5, pH adjustment to 4.6 and addition of Ca (60 µmol/L); lane 6, pH adjustment to 4.3 and addition of Ca (60 µmol/L). For more details see Kunz, C. and Lönnerdal, B., *Am. J. Clin. Nutr.*, 49, 464, 1989.[17] (with permission).

in the casein fraction (Figure 12.1B). Many of these proteins stain very faintly with the common dye Coomassie Blue due to their relatively high degree of glycosylation.

The difficulty in analyzing human milk proteins is not the estimation of the total protein content (which can be determined by the Kjeldahl method) but the estimation of a large number of different components. Hence, a general strategy for the separation and characterization of milk proteins is given in this chapter. The final step in the structural analysis of a milk protein, i.e., amino acid sequencing, is the same as for any other protein. Thus, we refer to recent publications in this field, which may also be applied to human milk proteins.[3-5]

After an introduction to some of the physiologic functions of milk proteins and the changes of the milk protein pattern and composition during lactation, the main focus will be analytical procedures such as chromatographic and electrophoretic separation of proteins, as well as the identification of glycoproteins on membranes after Western blotting.

12.2 THE PHYSIOLOGIC ROLE OF MILK PROTEINS

12.2.1 NUTRITIVE AND NON-NUTRITIVE ROLES

Milk proteins are a source of peptides, amino acids and nitrogen for the growing infant. In addition, specific whey proteins are known to be involved in the immune response (immunoglobulins), lactose synthesis (α-lactalbumin), or in the non-immunological defense (lactoferrin).[1,2] Casein phosphopeptides from human milk, as opposed to similar peptides from bovine milk, are thought to enhance the absorption of minerals by keeping them in solution in the intestinal tract.[6] Casein fragments, as digestive degradation products, might be able to regulate intestinal motility (peptides with opioid-like activities). In addition, glycoproteins in human milk, such as kappa-casein, may promote the growth of certain beneficial bacteria, or interact with pathogenic bacteria or viruses to potentially inhibit their adhesion to epithelial cells, and thus prevent infections.[7]

At present, research interest in human milk and lactation is mainly at the cellular level of functional and metabolic aspects. The regulation of changes in milk composition and milk production are important areas for further studies. It is essential to understand the functional aspects of the variety of bioactive substances in milk, and their effects on the recipient infant or on the mammary gland itself. The effects of human milk on brain development, prevention of acute and chronic disease, and long-term programming of body functions are only beginning to be identified.

Studies on animal models have documented the anti-inflammatory effects of milk proteins. Lactoferrin and its potential roles as a growth factor, a bacteriostatic agent, an inflammatory and immunmodulating factor, or its role in iron absorption have recently been discussed.[8] Another major glycoprotein, originating from the mammary gland, is secretory IgA; this does not activate, complement or promote phagocytosis, in contrast to other immunoglobulin isotypes, but protects the host by agglutination of bacteria and inhibition of their attachment.[9]

Milk mucins or their fragments, like other glycoproteins in human milk, may interfere with the attachment of pathogenic bacteria to intestinal tissue, and may therefore be considered as part of the non-immune defense system of the human milk-fed infant.[10,11] Soluble cell adhesion molecules which have recently been detected in human milk[12,13] might belong to these defense factors as well. Selectins are involved in the initial processes of inflammation through the interaction of leukocytes with activated endothelium.[14-16] These interactions cause rolling of leukocytes, allowing their binding to integrins on endothelial cells, followed by extravasation into damaged tissues. Since the uncontrolled invasion of leukocytes may be detrimental, efforts are being made to control this using soluble forms of selectins in patients with some specific diseases. In addition, the selectin ligands, which are carbohydrate-based glycoconjugates, play a crucial role in these interactions.[2,7]

Current research on human milk proteins also includes studies of minor components, such as growth factors or hormones which appear to affect gut maturation and absorption of nutrients.[1,2]

12.2.2 CHANGES DURING LACTATION

It is well known that there are remarkable changes in the total protein content as well as in the protein pattern during lactation (Figure 12.2). An exceptionally high amount of secretory IgA and lactoferrin in the first few days is followed by a decrease over the following few weeks.[17] Casein subunits cannot be detected in milk expressed during the first two days postpartum.[18] The following increase in casein concentration and the concomitant decrease in the concentration of whey proteins during the first days of lactation lead to a changing proportion of casein as a percentage of the total protein. The ratio of whey proteins to casein is high (about 90:10) at the beginning of lactation. However, the ratio changes rapidly during the course of lactation, to a ratio of 60:40 or even 50:50 in mature milk.[19]

The increase in the casein content during lactation is pronounced, and is probably caused by the maturation of the mammary gland. It seems likely that the synthesis of caseins and whey proteins is regulated by different mechanisms, because most whey proteins decrease in concentration during lactation.

Although changes in the protein fraction of milk components during lactation have been well investigated, not much information is available on the differences between the carbohydrate microheterogeneity of individual components in early and mature milk, or between term and preterm human milk.

12.3 SEPARATION OF FAT, WHEY PROTEINS AND CASEINS

The traditional method for classifying milk proteins, developed by Rowland in 1938, was intended primarily for bovine milk proteins.[20] According to this approach, bovine caseins are precipitated at their isoelectric point (pH 4.6). This procedure has also been applied to human milk, but it was found that human casein differs from bovine casein in its physicochemical properties, i.e., the precipitate formed by human casein at pH 4.6 is looser and softer. Proteins such as α-lactalbumin, lactoferrin and serum albumin in human milk coprecipitate with casein at that pH, leading to a large contamination of the whey fraction with casein and vice versa.[6]

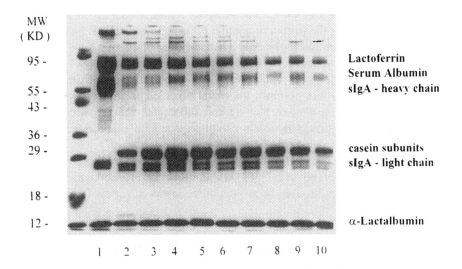

FIGURE 12.2   SDS-gel electrophoresis of delipidated human milk from one mother during lactation. A molecular weight standard is shown on the left. Milk samples were from the following days:

lane	day post partum
1	1
2	3
3	4
4	7
5	9
6	12
7	14
8	27
9	41
10	83

(according to Kunz, C. and Lönnerdal, B., *J. Pediatr. Gastroenterol. Nutr.*, 10, 454, 1990 [42]), (with permission).

Recent studies have shown that lowering the pH to 4.3 and adding calcium apparently achieves an aggregation of the human casein subunits, whereby the whey proteins are excluded.[17,18] Thus, this method is advantageous when compared to previous methods based on pH adjustment to pH 4.6 or no pH adjustment (see Figure 12.1A and 12.1B). It is a rapid and convenient way to isolate casein without significant contamination with whey proteins. After the pH adjustment of whole human milk to pH 4.3 with HCl (1 mol/L), samples are stirred for 10 min and then kept at 4°C for 1 h before centrifugation. If necessary, the pH is readjusted to the original pH-value using NaOH (0.1 mol/L) prior to the addition of $CaCl_2$ (60 mmol/L). Ultracentrifugation (189 000 x g) is carried out for 1 h at 4°C. Whey and casein fractions are separated and kept frozen at -20°C until further analysis.

Milk samples should, whenever possible, be analyzed fresh, or aliquots should be prepared and stored at -20°C. Storage up to 6 months does not affect either the amount of protein or the pattern of specific protein components. Repeated thawing and freezing should be avoided because a redistribution of whey proteins with caseins or with the milk fat would occur.[2,21] Storage conditions and handling of human milk samples have been discussed in detail.[22] The required milk volume depends on the purpose of the study. For example, the characterization of proteins by gel electrophoresis, followed by Western blotting and subsequent staining with antibodies, needs only a few microliters. For a complete structural elucidation, however, a considerably larger volume may be required.

For the isolation of proteins from the milk fat globule membrane, the procedure of Patton and Huston is recommended.[23] Here, fresh milk is underlayered with water before centrifugation, in order to avoid contamination of the fat layer with whey proteins or casein.

12.4 SDS-POLYACRYLAMIDE GEL ELECTROPHORESIS OF MILK PROTEINS

Sodium dodecyl sulfate-polyacrylamide gel electrophoresis (SDS-PAGE) is an easy way to obtain the molecular weight of a specific component, or to compare the protein pattern in milk from different mothers or from one individual during the course of lactation. SDS-PAGE can be performed in 10% polyacrylamide gels, e.g., in a horizontal system such as Multiphor (Pharmacia Biotech, Uppsala, Sweden). Whole milk (10 μL) is diluted with 40 μL sample buffer (Tris-HCl (25 mmol/L), 0. 1% SDS, pH 6.8, 0.25% bromophenol blue, 2.5% β-mercaptoethanol), heated in boiling water for 1.5 min and 5 μL loaded on the gel.[17] To an aliquot (20 μL) of the whey fraction, 75 μL sample buffer is added. Twenty microliters of this solution are loaded on the gel. Lyophilized caseins (1 mg) are dissolved in 1 mL of sample buffer, heated as described above and 15 μL applied to the gel.[18]

Gels are run in tris-glycine buffer (1 mol/L, pH 8.3) with 0.1% SDS at a constant current of 35 mA for about 4 h to 6 h. After fixing the proteins in a mixture of 5'-sulfosalicylic acid, trichloroacetic acid, methanol and water (3/22/22/53; wt/wt/vol/vol) for 30 min under continuous shaking, staining can be carried out overnight in a solution of acetic acid, ethanol and water (8/25/67; vol/vol/vol) containing 0.35 g Coomassie Brilliant Blue. Destaining in ethanol, acetic acid and water (8/25/67; vol/vol/vol) is stopped when a clear background has been reached.

Other electrophoretic separations such as isoelectric focusing or gel electrophoresis without SDS can also be applied.[24, 25]

12.5 FPLC-GEL FILTRATION OF WHEY PROTEINS

The separation of an individual protein component requires the application of several chromatographic procedures. In general, a combination of gel filtration, anion exchange and reversed phase chromatography is necessary. Examples are given below.

Filtered whey (0.45 µm syringe filter, Nalgene Company, Rochester, N.Y., USA) is subjected to fast protein liquid chromatography (FPLC) gel filtration (e.g., Superdex 200, 30 or 10, Pharmacia Biotech, Uppsala, Sweden) using 10 mmol/L imidazole/0.2 mol/L NaCl buffer (pH 7.0) as eluents.[17] Proteins are separated at a flow rate of 1 mL or 0.5 mL/min into various fractions according to their molecular weight. Peak monitoring is carried out continuously at 280 or 254 nm. The sample (e.g., 1 mL) does not need to be diluted with sample buffer prior to the separation.

12.6 FPLC-ANION EXCHANGE OF WHEY PROTEINS

Filtered whey (0.45 µm syringe filter) is subjected to FPLC anion exchange (e.g., Mono Q or Resource Q, Pharmacia Biotech, Uppsala, Sweden) with a linear NaCl gradient.[17] Whey (e.g., 100 µL) is diluted with ethanolamine (20 mmol/L) (e.g., 500 µL) and 500 µL injected. The recommended buffers which should be degased and filtered through 0.45 µm filters are: buffer A, 20 mmol ethanolamine/L (pH 9.5) and buffer B, buffer A containing NaCl (0.3 mmol/L). The following gradient is recommended: from 0 to 3 min, 100% buffer A; from 3 to 60 min, linear gradient to 100% buffer B; from 60 to 65 min, 100% buffer B; from 65 to 70 min, 100% buffer A. The flow rate is 1 mL/min, and peaks are monitored at 280 or 254 nm.

If the resolution of the protein peaks is not satisfactory, the buffer strength (e.g., 0.6 mmol/L NaCl in buffer B) or the gradient (e.g., from 3 to 30 min, linear gradient to 100% buffer B) need to be modified.

12.7 FPLC-ANION EXCHANGE OF CASEIN

Casein pellets are lyophilized and dissolved in ethanolamine (20 mmol/L, pH 9.5; 8 mg casein/mL).[18] Solid urea is added to a final concentration of 6 mol/L. The samples are kept in a waterbath (25°C) with occasional stirring for 0.5 to 1 h. Then the sample is filtered and 500 µL injected onto the column (e.g., Mono-Q HR 5/5 anion-exchange column, Pharmacia Biotech, Uppsala, Sweden) and separated at room temperature using the following conditions: buffer A, ethanolamine (20 mmol/L, pH 9.5) with urea (6 mol/L), and buffer B consisting of buffer A containing NaCl (0.6 mol/L). The following gradient is recommended: from 0 to 3 min, 100% buffer A; from 3 to 57 min, linear gradient to 100% buffer B; from 57 to 62 min, 100% buffer B; from 62 to 67 min, 100% buffer A. The flow rate is 1 mL/min. The column eluant is monitored continuously at 280 or 254 nm.

In contrast to the separation of whey proteins, urea is needed in this case to disassociate the casein subunits which would otherwise spontaneously aggregate to submicelles or micelles. In our studies, we found the use of reducing agents (β-mercaptoethanol or dithiothreitol) unnecessary for the separation of human casein subunits. These reagents are commonly used for bovine casein separation. The FPLC separating conditions might need to be modified with regard to the buffer strength or the gradient.

12.8 FPLC-REVERSED PHASE OF PROTEINS

To further purify proteins, fractions after anion exchange chromatography can be subjected to a C8-column (e.g., ProRPC, Pharmacia Biotech, Uppsala, Sweden) with 0.1% trifluoroacetic acid (TFA) in H_2O as the solvent. The following running conditions are recommended for a sample concentration of 0.1 to 1 mg/20 µL: 0 to 3 min 100% H_2O, followed by a linear gradient of 0 to 100% acetonitrile over the next 22 min, at a flow rate of 1 mL/min. Prior to an amino acid analysis, the purified protein samples should be extensively dialyzed against deionized water at 4°C for 30 to 40 h. For the amino acid determination, please see References 3 to 5.

12.9 INVESTIGATION OF THE GLYCOSYLATION PATTERN

Glycosylation is a major co- and post-translational modification of proteins that generates a potentially large group of glycoforms from a single polypeptide chain. Since glycosylation can play an important role in the biological activity of the protein,[26] there is increasing interest in identifying and characterizing the carbohydrate moieties of glycoproteins. The structural characterization requires the determination of the molecular weight, the type and number of monosaccharides, sequences and pattern of branching, composition of the aglycon fraction, conformation of sugar rings and the anomeric configuration of sugars. Several methods such as high pH anion exchange chromatography with pulsed amperometric detection (HPAEC-PAD), fast atom bombardment-mass spectrometry (FAB-MS) and matrix associated laser desorption mass spectrometry may be used to address these questions.[27-33]

Hardly any detailed information is available about the glycosylation of many milk proteins. For example, it is known that the carbohydrate part of human κ-casein is composed of only a few monosaccharides, i.e., galactose (Gal), N-acetylgalactosamine (GalNAc), N-acetylglucosamine (GlcNAc), N-acetylneuraminic acid (NeuAc) and fucose (Fuc).[6] Further, data on temporal changes in the pattern and branching of oligosaccharides, which might occur during the lactation period, are rare. In human κ-casein, all sugar linkages are of the O-glycan type; no carbohydrate chains linked to asparagine (N-glycan) have been detected. A feature of human κ-casein compared to bovine k-casein is not only the higher amount of carbohydrates (40 to 60% vs. 10%), and therefore the larger variety of possible sugar linkages, but also the presence of up to 10 prosthetic sugar groups in human casein (only one in bovine casein).[34] As noted in the Introduction, there are many glycoproteins in human milk which are currently of great interest, due to the large variety of biological functions they might exert. For studies of the protein part of a glycoprotein, gel electrophoresis and transfer of proteins onto membranes are techniques that are widely used to purify picomole quantities of the components of interest, to minimize preparative losses and to facilitate sample handling for structural analysis. However, until recently, the analysis of the carbohydrate moiety of immobilized glycoproteins, separated by gel electrophoresis, has been mainly limited to the use of lectins.

As detailed below, the procedure for identifying glycoproteins using SDS-PAGE followed by electroblotting onto a polyvinylidene fluoride (PVDF) membrane is given. The transferred protein can either be stained by sugar specific lectins, or the glycoprotein band is excised from the membrane and used for the carbohydrate analysis (Figure 12.3A). This includes acid hydrolysis (which releases monosaccharides for compositional analysis), and a sequential endoglycosidase digestion (Figure 12.3B), which allows the progressive release of oligosaccharides for mapping and tentative structural assignment. Monosaccharides and oligosaccharides can then be analyzed by HPAEC-PAD or FAB-MS.

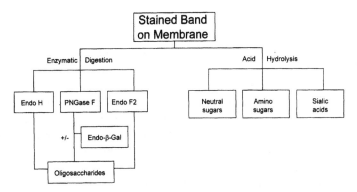

FIGURE 12.3A Scheme for the characterization of membrane-bound glycoproteins. After Western blotting, the bands of interest are excised, and either hydrolyzed in acid for monosaccharide composition or digested with an array of enzymes for oligosaccharide mapping.

Endo H	Endo-glycosidase H (EC 3.2.1.96)
PNGase F	Peptide-N-Glycosidase F (EC 3.5.1.52)
Endo F2	Endo-glycosidase F2 (EC 3.2.1.96)
Endo-ß-Gal	Endo-ß-galactosidase (EC 3.2.1.103)

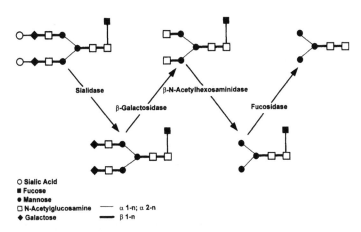

FIGURE 12.3B Diagram showing the sequential enzymatic cleavage of a complex oligosaccharide structure.

12.9.1 IDENTIFICATION OF MEMBRANE-BOUND PROTEINS BY LECTINS

Gel electrophoresis of whole milk, whey proteins, caseins or milk protein fractions after chromatography is performed in a horizontal system as described above. Proteins are then transferred to a nitrocellulose membrane (Western blotting), and incubated with sugar specific lectins (e.g., Maackia amurensis, Sambucus nigra, Galanthus nivalis, Ulex europaeus or Arachis hypogaea) or with antibodies. Bound (digoxigenin-labeled) lectins or antibodies can be detected with alkaline phosphatase or peroxidase-labeled secondary antibodies, with respective substrates for the color reaction.

The use of digoxigenin-labeled lectins (Boehringer, Mannheim, Germany) is described in the following section. However, many unconjugated lectins are available and can also be used. As the recommended dilutions for lectins and antibodies vary between different suppliers, the manufacturer's instructions should be followed carefully.

As an example, Figure 12.4 shows reactions of immobilized glycoproteins with digoxigenin-labeled Sambucus nigra, a lectin that is specific for NeuAc2-6-linked glycoconjugates. Except for lactoferrin, only a small amount of information is available on proteins in the higher molecular weight range. Using various lectins, it is possible to partly characterize a protein with regard to the glycosylation. For example, it can be determined whether N- or O-glycans or both types of linkages are present, or whether lactosamine-type structures predominate over high mannose-type components. Purification of a component by chromatographic means should then allow investigations on the carbohydrate microheterogeneity, or the biological activity of the native or the deglycosylated component.

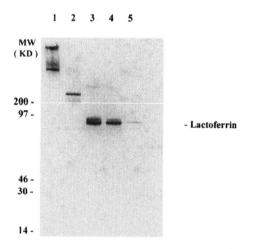

FIGURE 12.4 Western blotting of whey fractions 1 to 5, after FPLC-gel filtration and subsequent incubation of the blotted membrane with the lectin Sambucus nigra (binding specificity: NeuAcα2-6Gal and NeuAcα2-6GalNAc).

The presence of N-acetylneuraminic acid (NeuAc) and/or fucose can easily be demonstrated by performing a mild acid hydrolysis to remove these monosaccharides. The results can then be checked by SDS-PAGE, followed by Western blotting and incubation with different lectins. The hydrolysis conditions are as follows:

Lyophilyzed whey samples are resuspended in water (10 mg/mL) and 10 µL transferred into Wheaton tubes (Fisher Scientific, New Jersey, USA). To each tube, 50 µL H_2SO_4 (0.05 mol/L) is added under nitrogen. The samples are mixed and incubated for 1 h at 80°C. Then, NaOH (0.1 mol/L) is added to the cooled tubes until neutral conditions are achieved. This preparation is verified by protein staining after SDS-PAGE (Coomassie Blue) as well as by Western blotting followed by incubation of the membranes with Sambucus nigra (SNA, specific for NeuAc2-6-R) or Maackia amurensis (MAA, specific for NeuAc2-3-R). For SDS-PAGE and Western blotting, all samples are diluted 1:1 with sample buffer (see above). Furthermore, cleaved NeuAc and fucose can be detected in the hydrolyzed sample by HPAEC-PAD.[27,41]

Quantitation of neutral or acidic monosaccharides by colorimetric assay can be performed as described.[35]

12.9.2 CHARACTERIZATION OF GLYCOPROTEINS ON MEMBRANES

The complete transfer assembly is placed in the electroblotting tank, oriented so that the transfer membrane is between the gel and the positive electrode. The tank is filled with transfer buffer (e.g., Tris, 25 mmol/L; glycine 190 mmol/L, 20% methanol; pH 8.8) and the device cooled by circulating refrigerated water through the equipment. Transfer times at 300 to 400 V vary depending upon thickness and porosity of the acrylamide gel and the size and hydrophobicity of the transferred proteins. Conditions should be optimized empirically. After the transfer is complete, the polyvinylidene fluoride membrane is stained, e.g., in 0.1% Coomassie Brilliant Blue R-250 in water/methanol/acetic acid (5/4/1; v/v/v) for 10 min. The membrane is destained in multiple washes of water/methanol/acetic acid (4/5/1; v/v/v) and finally rinsed in distilled water. It is then dried on a filter paper and stored at 4°C until needed.

Specific membranes for glycoproteins (e.g., PVDF, Immobilon PSQ 15 x 15 cm, 0.1 µm pore size, Millipore Corporation) from different suppliers are available. Some glycoproteins may pass through the membrane during electroblotting if a pore size > 0.1 µm is used. Membranes should be checked for nonspecific reactions. For more information, please see References 36 to 39.

12.9.3 MILD ACID HYDROLYSIS AND ENZYMATIC DIGESTION OF MEMBRANE-BOUND GLYCOPROTEINS

The following conditions for monosaccharide release are suggested as a starting point. A detailed description of hydrolysis conditions for glycoconjugates and oligosaccharides has been published.[41]

1. The stained glycoprotein bands of interest are sliced with a razor blade from the dried, blotted PVDF, wet in 5 to 10 µL methanol, and transferred to capped 1.5 mL polypropylene tubes or to 13 x 100 mm Teflon capped test tubes (acid washed) (Fisher Scientific, New Jersey, USA). For a membrane blank, a band is cut out from an unstained area of the membrane.
2. 200 to 400 µl of either HCl (0.2 mol/L), trifluoroacetic acid (4 mol/L), or HCl (8.0 mol/L) is added for the optimal hydrolysis of sialic acid, neutral sugars or amino sugars, respectively.
3. They are then hydrolyzed for 1 h at 80°C for sialic acids, 2 to 5 hours at 100°C for neutral sugars, or 4 to 6 hours at 100°C for amino sugars.
4. The sample is dried using a Rotovapor or lyophilyzer.
5. The residue is resuspended in a suitable volume of deionized water, and monosaccharide analysis performed as recommended above.

To remove peptides or amino acids, the hydrolysate may be treated with a weak anion exchange resin. However, only basic and neutral monosaccharides can be determined after such resin treatment (acidic sugars will bind to the resin). It has to be noted that sialic acids may be destroyed by a complete evaporation of water during Step 4 (above), as the concentration of HCl may increase up to 12 mol/L.

The determination of monosaccharides in the same solution that is used for amino acid analysis is not recommended. Most of the neutral sugars are destroyed by the highly concentrated solution used for the cleavage of peptide bonds.

In contrast to monosaccharide analysis, oligosaccharide mapping involves the release of carbohydrates from glycoproteins by the use of specific enzymes (see Figure 12.3), followed by an analysis of the liberated oligosaccharides, for example by HPAEC-PAD or FAB-MS. Through digestion with enzymes of differing specificity, various classes of oligosaccharides can be sequentially released from the same immobilized glycoprotein band. As an example, the release of N-linked oligosaccharides is described below: The stained glycoprotein bands of interest are excised from the dried PVDF blot and transferred to capped polypropylene microcentrifuge tubes. The membrane bands are wet with 5 to 10 µL methanol and submerged in 200 µL sodium phosphate buffer (10 mmol/L, pH 7.6) containing 0.1% Triton X-100. Peptide-N-glycosidase F (1 to 5 units) is added and digested at 37°C for 48 h. The released oligosaccharides are now ready for HPAEC-PAD analysis.

For a detailed description of enzymatic digestion of membrane-bound glycoproteins and the analysis of glycoproteins, please see References 33, 35 and 38 to 41.

12.10 CONCLUSIONS

Human milk proteins are not only of nutritive value for the recipient infant but also have many other physiologic functions. Specific proteins are known to be involved in gut maturation, immune responses and non-immunological defense systems. Currently, glycoproteins such as mucins or cell adhesion molecules are of major interest in research on human milk. There is increasing evidence that the protective effect of human milk in preventing gastrointestinal infections is due to specific interactions between pathogenic microorganisms and glycoconjugates, the latter functioning as soluble receptors for many pathogens. The potential roles of glyco-conjugates as ligands for cell adhesion molecules modulating inflammatory pro-cesses have also been noted.

It is certainly relevant to clearly identify the proteins in human milk exerting these biological functions. For most of them, only limited structural information is available. Often, they are not present or there is only a very small amount in bovine milk; hence, they are not detectable in most infant formulas. Before addressing the question of whether these components should be added to a formula, their physio-logic function has to be determined. This will require methods that separate and characterize individual glycoproteins. Due to the very large number of proteins in human milk, the appropriate procedure for the characterization of a specific protein has to be carefully considered.

REFERENCES

1. Atkinson, S. A. and Lönnerdal, B., Eds., *Protein and Non-Protein Nitrogen in Human Milk*, CRC Press, Boca Raton, Florida, 1989, 162–163.
2. Rudloff, S. and Kunz, C., Proteins in human milk, bovine milk and infant formula. Quantitative and qualitative aspects in infant nutrition, *J. Pediatr. Gastroenterol. Nutr*, 24, 328, 1997.
3. Shively, J. E., *Methods of Protein Microcharacterization*, Humana Press, Clifton, New Jersey, 1986.
4. Hugli, T. E., *Techniques in protein chemistry*, Academic Press, San Diego, 1989.
5. Choli, T., and Wittmann-Liebold, B., Protein blotting followed by microsequencing, *Electrophoresis*, 11, 562, 1990.
6. Kunz, C. and Lönnerdal, B., Casein micelles and casein subunits in human milk, in *Protein and Non-Protein Nitrogen in Human Milk*, Atkinson, S. A. and Lönnerdal, B., Eds., CRC Press, Boca Raton, Florida, 1989, 9–27.
7. Kunz, C., Microbial receptor analogs in human milk-structural and functional aspects, in *Probiotics, Other Nutritional Factors and Intestinal Microflora*, Hanson, L.A. and Yolken, R., Eds., Nestlè Nutrition Series, Vol. 42, Raven Press, New York, (in press).
8. Lönnerdal, B. and Iyer, S., Lactoferrrin: molecular structure and biological function, *Annu. Rev. Nutr.*, 15, 93, 1995.
9. Hanson, L.A., Comparative immunological studies of the immune globulins of human milk and of blood serum, *Int. Arch. Allergy Appl. Immunol.*, 18, 241, 1961.
10. Schroten, H., Lethen, A., Hanisch, F. G., Plogmann, R., Hacker, J., Nobis-Bosch, R., and Wahn, V., Inhibition of adhesion of S-fimbriated *Escherichia coli* to epithelial cells by meconium and feces of breast-fed and formula-fed newborns: mucins are the major inhibitory component, *J. Pediatr. Gastroenterol. Nutr.*, 15, 150, 1992.
11. Patton, S., Detection of large fragments of the human milk mucin MUC-1 in feces of breast-fed infants, *J. Pediatr. Gastroenterol. Nutr.*, 18, 225, 1994.
12. Rudloff, S. and Kunz, C., E- and P-selectins in human milk, *FASEB J.*, 8, A578, 1994.
13. Buescher, E. S. and Malinowska, I., Soluble receptors and cytokine antagonists in human milk, *Pediatr. Res.*, 40, 839, 1996.
14. Springer, T. A., Adhesion receptors of the immune system, *Nature*, 346, 425, 1990.
15. McEver, R. P., Role of selectins in leukocyte adhesion to platelets and endothelium, *Ann. New York Acad. Sci.*, 714, 185, 1994.

16. Lasky, A. L., Selectin-carbohydrate interactions and the initiation of the inflammatory response, *Annu. Rev. Biochem.*, 64, 113, 1995.

17. Kunz, C. and Lönnerdal, B., Human milk proteins: Separation of whey proteins and their analysis by polyacrylamide gel electrophoresis, FPLC gel filtration and anion exchange chromatography, *Am. J. Clin. Nutr.*, 49, 464, 1989.

18. Kunz, C. and Lönnerdal, B., Human milk proteins: Analysis of casein and casein subunits by anion exchange chromatography, gel electrophoresis, and specific staining methods, *Am. J. Clin. Nutr.*, 51, 37, 1990.

19. Kunz, C. and Lönnerdal, B., Re-evaluation of the whey protein/casein ratio of human milk, *Acta. Paediatr.*, 81, 107, 1992.

20. Rowland, S. J., The protein distribution in normal and abnormal milk, *J. Dairy Res.*, 9, 47, 1938.

21. Rudloff, S. and Lönnerdal, B., Solubility and digestibility of milk proteins in infant formulas exposed to different heat treatments, *J. Pediatr. Gastroenterol. Nutr.*, 15, 25, 1992.

22. Jensen, R. G., *Handbook of Milk Composition*, Academic Press, San Diego, 1995.

23. Patton, S. and Huston, G. E., A method for the isolation of milk fat globules, *Lipids*, 21, 170, 1986.

24. Dunbar, B. S., *Two-Dimensional Electrophoresis and Immunological Techniques*, Plenum Press, New York, 1987.

25. Westermeier, R., Ed., *Electrophoresis in Practice, A Guide to Methods and Application of DNA and Protein Separation*, 2nd edition, VCH Verlagsgesellschaft mbH, Weinheim, 1997.

26. Varki, A., Biological roles of oligosaccharides: all of the theories are correct, *Glycobiology*, 3, 97, 1993.

27. Kunz, C., Rudloff, S., Hintelmann, A., Pohlentz, G., and Egge, H., High-pH anion exchange chromatography with pulsed amperometric detection and molar response factors of human milk oligosaccharides, *J. Chromatogr. B.*, 685, 211, 1996.

28. Egge, H. and Peter-Katalinic, J., Fast atom bombardment mass spectrometry for the structural elucidation of glycoconjugates, *Mass. Spectrometry Rev.*, 6, 331, 1987.

29. Stahl, B., Thurl, S., Zeng, J., Karas, M., Hillenkamp, F., Steup, M., and Sawatzki, G., Oligosaccharides from human milk as revealed by matrix assisted laser desorption/ionization mass spectrometry, *Anal. Biochem.*, 223, 218, 1994.

30. Stults, J. T., Matrix-assisted laser desorption/ionization mass spectrometry (MALDI-MS), *Curr. Opin. Struct. Biol.*, 5, 691, 1995.

31. Urlaub, H., Thiede, B., Muller, E. C., and Wittmann-Liebold, B., Contact sites of peptide-oligoribonucleotide cross-links identified by a combination of peptide and nucleotide sequencing with MALDI MS, *J. Protein Chem.*, 16, 375, 1997.

32. Eckerskorn, C., Strupat, K., Schleuder, D., Hochstrasser, D., Sanchez, J. C., Lottspeich, F., and Hillenkamp, F., Analysis of proteins by direct-scanning infrared-MALDI mass spectrometry after 2D-PAGE separation and electroblotting, *Anal. Chem.*, 69, 2888, 1997.

33. Hounsell, E. F., *Glycoprotein Analysis in Biomedicine*, Humana Press, Totowa, New Jersey, 1993.

34. Fiat, A-M., Jollès, J., Aubert, J-P., Loucheux-Lefebvre, M-H., and Jollès, P., Localisation and importance of the sugar part of human casein, *Eur. J. Biochem.*, 111, 333, 1980.

35. Beeley, J. G., *Glycoprotein and Proteoglycan Techniques*, Laboratory techniques in biochemistry and molecular biology, Vol. 16, Elsevier, Amsterdam, 1985, 186, 187, 190–191, 204–205.

36. Haselbeck, A. and Hösel, W., Description and application of an immunological detection system for analyzing glycoproteins on blots, *Glycoconjugate J.*, 7, 63, 1990.
37. Ogawa, H., Ueno, M., Uchibori, H., Matsumoto, I., and Seno, N., Direct carbohydrate analysis of glycoproteins electroblotted onto polyvinylidene difluoride membrane from sodium dodecyl sulfate-polyacrylamide gel, *Anal. Biochem.*, 190, 165, 1990.
38. Weitzhandler, M., Kadlecek, D., Avdalovic, N., Forte, J. G., Chow, D., and Townsend, R. R., Monosaccharide and oligosaccharide analysis of proteins transferred to polyvinylidene fluoride membranes after sodium dodecyl sulfate-polyacrylamide gel electrophoresis, *J. Biol. Chem.*, 268, 5121, 1993.
39. Küster, B., Wheeler, S. F., Hunter, A. P., Dwek, R. A., and Harvey, D. J., Sequencing of N-linked oligosaccharides directly from protein gels: In-gel deglycosylation followed by matrix-assisted laser desorption/ionization mass spectrometry and normal-phase high-performance liquid chromatography, *Anal. Biochem.*, 250, 82, 1997.
40. Fukuda, M. and Kobata, A., Eds., *Glycobiology. A Practical Approach.* IRL Press, Oxford University Press, Oxford, 1993.
41. Hardy, M. R., Townsend, R. R., and Lee, Y., Monosaccharide analysis of glycoconjugates by anion exchange chromatography with pulsed amperometric detection, *Anal. Biochem.*, 170, 54, 1988.
42. Kunz, C. and Lönnerdal, B., Casein and casein subunits in preterm milk, colostrum and mature human milk, *J. Pediatr. Gastroenterol. Nutr.*, 10, 454, 1990.

13 Studying Amino Acid and Protein Metabolism in Burn and Other Trauma Patients

Yong-Ming Yu, Colleen M. Ryan, and Wei Cai

CONTENTS

0-8493-9612-3/99/$0.00+$.50
© 1999 by CRC Press LLC

13.1 INTRODUCTION

Since Cuthbertson's [1-2] finding six decades ago that severe trauma patients had greatly increased urinary urea excretion and an accelerated net nitrogen loss from the body, surgeons have tried to further understand the nature of this net nitrogen loss. Many attempts have been made to reverse it, with an expectation for earlier recovery and reduced clinical complications. With the advancement of intensive care and emergency medicine, specifically modern cardiovascular/respiratory support, improved fluid resuscitation, and antibiotics, many acute severely traumatized patients are now able to overcome the initial insult of the injury, and enter a prolonged period of further treatment to battle for survival and recovery.

Nutritional and metabolic support to these patients has become a more prominent issue in critical care.[3] Providing nutrients to these otherwise starving patients can (at least) lessen the extent of malnutrition. Further efforts are now being made in searching for a new approach, via nutritional-pharmacological modulation, to promote host immune system, reduce inflammatory response-induced tissue damage, and support major organ functions. However, we are still far from reaching these goals. In some cases, aggressive nutritional support can promote a whole-body nitrogen balance; however, severe muscle wasting and other nutritional problems still exist in prolonged bedridden burn and septic Intensive Care Unit (ICU) patients, which are closely associated with morbidity and mortality. In addition, the organ-specific nutritional support in relation to organ function in critically ill-patients needs to be further understood. These issues stress the important need for understanding the quantitative dynamic nature and mechanism of metabolic disorders in critically ill patients, with the hope that such knowledge will lead us to newer therapeutic modalities to improve the clinical care of stressed patients.

Research in metabolism and nutrition in severely injured patients serves two general goals: 1) To explore the nature of metabolic alterations in response to severe trauma and injury, in order to develop new treatment modalities based on such understanding, and 2) To test the metabolic response and potential metabolic benefit brought by these modalities during treatment. To serve either of these purposes, it is essential to establish a series of methods which can sensitively quantify metabolic alterations after trauma and with different nutritional support regimes, particularly alterations in amino acid and protein metabolism.

As Wolfe pointed out,[4] the traditional medical research always uses survival rate as its end-point. However, in the case of critically ill patients, burn patients as an example, the severity of the injury and the outcome of the burn patients are determined by multiple factors; varying just one component of nutritional support is unlikely to have a detectable effect on survival in a relatively small number of patients. Furthermore, there is a wide range in the general condition of the burn patients. In some patients, the injury is so severe that they have virtually no chance of survival, while in other patients, the injuries are not life-threatening. Therefore, varying just one aspect of traditional care (e.g., a component of nutritional support) may only affect survival rate in a fraction of the total patient population. Based on these considerations, even though optimal nutritional/metabolic support is an important aspect of clinical care to critically ill patients, the likelihood of demonstrating a dietary effect on survival rate in a single burn unit is extremely small. Therefore, it is necessary to choose outcome variables which are most likely to be directly affected by nutrition and that also can be quantified. The best parameter which can meet these requirements is the quantitative information on the patients' metabolic response to injury and modified nutritional support.

Stable isotope tracer methods are a relatively non-invasive tool to quantify the metabolic response to injury and the potential benefit of modified nutritional support. Furthermore, stable isotope tracer studies can be completed in a relative short period of time; therefore, each patient can serve as his own control, minimizing inter-patient variability. Also, a well-designed and conducted tracer study does not interfere with the routine clinical care. Because of these advantages, tracer techniques have been playing an important role in the metabolic and nutrition research on critically ill patients. Some of the methods, applying tracer techniques to amino acid and protein metabolism in burn patients, are discussed below.

13.2 EVALUATION OF THE DYNAMIC ASPECTS OF WHOLE-BODY PROTEIN AND AMINO ACID METABOLISM IN CRITICALLY ILL PATIENTS

The traditional metabolic research on nitrogen metabolism in patients relied heavily on the measurement of nitrogen balance, i.e., the difference between the dietary nitrogen intake and the total nitrogen output. However, a nitrogen balance only represents the net difference between nitrogen input and nitrogen output, intuitively considered as the net difference of protein synthesis and breakdown; the true metabolic fate of the ingested protein, within the body, remains unknown when using this method alone. An increased nitrogen balance could be the result of increased protein synthesis, with or without changes in protein breakdown; any decreased protein breakdown, with and without changes of protein synthesis; or a combination of the changes at both sides of protein turnover. Therefore, the true metabolic fate of amino acids and proteins inside a human body remains a "black box." There is no information about how the ingested amino acids are utilized for protein synthesis or oxidation, even less on the fate of individual amino acids, nor how the body metabolically responds to injury and various nutritional support regimens. Technically, a classic nitrogen balance study usually requires 6 to 7 days of measurements; hence, it is difficult to compare the effect of nutritional intervention on the same patient, because the patient condition may change during the experimental period. Nitrogen balance studies are even more difficult in patients with renal insufficiency or those suffering from substantial nitrogen loss via routes other than urinary excretion: for example, wound exudation in burn patients. Thus, as Young pointed out, "body N equilibrium does not necessarily reflect an adequate state of organ protein metabolism or of nutritional status because it does not reveal possible alterations in the intensity, quality, and/or distribution of tissue and organ protein metabolism."[5]

The dynamics of protein turnover within the body include two opposite processes: protein synthesis, and breakdown or degradation. Tracer methods provide an opportunity to quantify the kinetics of these opposite processes. The methods used to quantify whole-body protein kinetics can be classified into two major categories: 1) those involving administration of ^{15}N- (or ^{13}C-) labeled tracer and measurement of the label in the end-products of nitrogen metabolism (end-product methods), and 2) those involving administration of specially labeled amino acids and measurements of the tracer in body fluids, e.g., plasma or urine (precursor, plasma or substrate-specific methods). Details of these two approaches have been described in classical literature,[e.g., 6,7,8] books[e.g.,9,10] and reviews.[e.g.,5,11-15] Their applications to studies in critically ill patients are further discussed as follows.

13.2.1 END-PRODUCT METHODS

The end-product method involves the usual administration of ^{15}N-labeled amino acid tracer and quantification of the excretion rate of ^{15}N-labeled end metabolites, usually in the urine (urea and/or ammonia). The protocol can be accomplished by two different procedures: one involves a primed continuous intravenous (IV) infusion or repeated oral ingestion of ^{15}N-labeled glycine [e.g.,16-18] or ^{15}N-alanine,[19] and measurement of plateau level enrichments (over baseline) of ^{15}N-ammonia and/or ^{15}N-urea in the urine; the second procedure involves administering a single dose of isotope tracer followed by continuous urine collection over a period of time, usually 8 to 9 hours, for the measurement of **total** ^{15}N-labeled ammonia and/or urea.[e.g.,20-23] In some instances, ^{13}C-labeled amino acid tracers were used, and the total expired $^{13}CO_2$ was collected as end- product.[24] The advantage of end-product methods is their non-invasive nature, as also detailed in Chapter 2 by El-Khoury. They give reasonable results with respect to the direction of alteration of whole-body nitrogen kinetics in response to various interventions.[12,24] Therefore, they are suitable for studying a large number of patients, especially for repeated measurements of protein kinetics in the recovery or convalescence phase of injured patients when the arterial or venous access for sampling is not available, and more so when the single dose approach is used. However, the kinetic estimate of nitrogen metabolism may not be accurate. Another drawback, which may further hamper this application in clinical studies, is due to the slow turnover of the urea pool: this requires a prolonged period (36 hours or even longer) of tracer administration to reach an isotopic steady state in the end product[16] if the constant infusion approach is used. Thus, the tracer study may either interfere with patient care, or vice-versa; furthermore, it is unlikely that a critically ill patient would remain in a steady state for such a long period. Even more difficult are the cases of acute burn patients, who require multiple surgical procedures of incision and grafting during the initial weeks after hospital admission. These problems have limited the application of end-product methods, particularly those requiring a constant tracer administration, in acutely ill patients.

13.2.2 PRECURSOR, PLASMA, OR SUBSTRATE-SPECIFIC METHODS

In reference to this general category of methods, a tracer-labeled amino acid is administered most often by a continuous intravenous infusion usually preceded by a priming dose to help rapidly achieve an isotopic plateau within the sampled compartment, frequently referring to the plasma free amino acid pool. Alternative procedures include intragastric infusion,[e.g.,25] repeated ingestion of the tracers,[26,27] and both intragastric and intravenous administration of the tracers.[28-31] The enrichment of the tracers is measured in plasma and, when appropriate, the appearance of the label in expired CO_2 is also monitored. The metabolic flux of the amino acid in the sampled compartment (usually plasma pool) is calculated using simple dilution principles.[7-10] Under both metabolic and isotopic steady-state conditions when a nutritionally indispensable amino acid is used as a tracer, the rate of the tracee disappearance via non-oxidative pathways (presumably tracing the rate of protein synthesis) and the rate of amino acid release from whole-body proteolysis can be quantified, provided intake and the oxidation rate of the amino acid are either known or estimated (Figure 13.1) (see also Chapter 2).

$$Q_{in} = Q + i$$

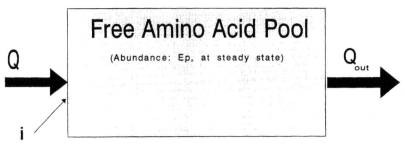

Q

Free Amino Acid Pool

(Abundance: Ep, at steady state)

Q_{out}

i

(Abundance: Ei)

FIGURE 13.1 Model to show the calculation of whole-body amino acid flux (Q) at metabolic and isotopic steady state. The free amino acid is considered in a unified metabolic pool as demonstrated by constant levels of tracee concentration and tracer abundance in plasma pool, when the total input and output of both tracee (Q_{in} and Q_{out}) and tracer are in equilibrium.

Hence,

Mass Balance:	$Q_{in} = Q + i = Q_{out}$
Isotopic Balance:	$i \cdot E_i = E_p \cdot (i + Q)$
Therefore:	$Q = i \cdot [(E_i/E_p) - 1]$

where i is the rate of tracer infusion, E_i is enrichment of tracer infusate, and E_p is the plateau level of tracer enrichment in plasma. Q value is usually expressed in $\mu mol.kg^{-1}.h^{-1}$.

In studying critically ill patients, this method has some advantages:

(i) The study can be completed in a relatively short time. For most of the amino acid tracers (with appropriate priming dose), the isotopic plateau level can be reached within 3 to 4 hours or less. Therefore, it would allow the study to be repeated on the same patient shortly thereafter, and each patient would serve as his/her own control, thus minimizing the inter-subject variability when comparing metabolic data among different therapeutic modalities.

(ii) It allows quantitative determination of the *in vivo* kinetics of individual amino acids and their metabolic fate within the body, including the relationship among these amino acids. This issue will be discussed in more detail later in this chapter.

(iii) It allows the determination of regional amino acid/protein metabolism, also to be discussed later in this chapter.

(iv) It appears that using different labeled amino acid tracers has produced comparable values of protein kinetics. Although there is no "gold standard" for the measurement of protein kinetics *in vivo*, two findings may help substantiate the validity of the method:

(a) In healthy human subjects, Bier[14] has summarized published estimates of whole-body (plasma) flux of specific amino acids in healthy adults (in the postabsorptive fasted state) and compared these with the "relative" concentrations of the amino acids in muscle protein. In the postabsorptive state (as shown in Figure 13.2), the metabolic fluxes of many essential amino acid tracers generally correspond to the average proportion of these essential amino acids in muscle protein. Data in trauma patients have also shown a similar relationship.

(b) Using leucine as a tracer, the rate of net nitrogen loss in healthy subjects[32,33] and burn patients[34] predicted from the measurement of leucine oxidation matched well with the rate of nitrogen excretion.

Therefore, the individual amino acid tracer methods, especially using leucine as a tracer, provide valuable information on the whole-body dynamics of protein metabolism. The tracer methods described above have widened our understanding of the dynamic nature of protein turnover in severely injured patients. This is summarized as follows.

13.2.2.1 Protein Turnover in Response to the Severity of Stress

A summary of the work from O'Keefe et al., Crane et al., Hartigue et al., and Long et al.[35-38] demonstrated that the two opposite processes of protein turnover, protein synthesis and breakdown, vary in relation to the severity of trauma. A lesser trauma seemed to cause a decreased rate of protein synthesis. With more severe trauma, there is an increased rate of protein breakdown, to an extent roughly parallel with the degree of injury. The general response seems to be the same whether the injury is a skeletal muscle trauma,[23] sepsis,[38] burns[18,34,39-42] or systemic infection.[43] Using multiple essential amino acid tracers, Jahoor et al.[40] further demonstrated that after burn injury, the elevated rate of protein breakdown actually lasted for several months during the recovery or even convalescence period of the injury, in spite of aggressive nutritional care. Therefore, with the use of stable isotope techniques, we have gained knowledge on the dynamic nature of protein turnover which accounts for Cuthbertson's findings on the catabolic loss of nitrogen in severe injury and trauma. The approaches to reduce this net nitrogen loss are to increase protein synthesis and/or to reduce the rate of protein breakdown.

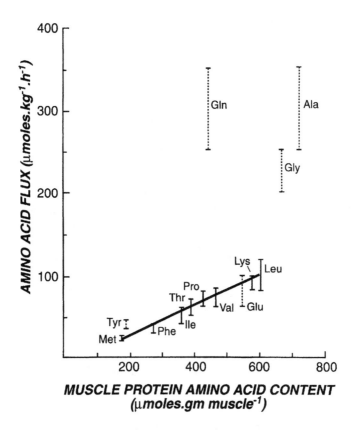

FIGURE 13.2 Relationship between estimated muscle protein amino acid content and representative ranges of plasma amino acid flux. The solid lines are the ranges for the essential indispensable amino acids; the dashed lines reflect the ranges for the nonessential, dispensable amino acids. From Bier, D. M.,[14] Intrinsically difficult problems: the kinetics of body protein and amino acids in man, *Diabetes/Metabolism Reviews*, 5, 111, 1989. Reproduced by permission of John Wiley & Sons, Limited.

13.2.2.2 The Effect of Nutritional Support on Protein Kinetics in Severe Trauma Patients

Accelerated protein breakdown lasts a very long period during the recovery from burn injury, in spite of aggressive nutritional support. Therefore, the observed improved nitrogen balance in burn patients during the recovery stage appears to be due to the increased rate of protein synthesis. The work of Clague et al.[44] also found that adequate nutrient supply to surgical patients caused a rise in protein synthesis, but no significant effect on protein breakdown. In a series of studies on 32 severely burned patients (21 males and 11 females; Mean ± SEM age 44 ± 3; ideal body weight 65 ± 2 kg; total surface of burned area 51 ± 4%; studied on 13 ± 2 post-burn days, with 27 ± 4% of still-open wound surface) using leucine[34,41,42] and methionine[45] as tracers, we also found that total parenteral feeding significantly increased the rate of these tracers' incorporation into proteins, but did not alter the rate of protein breakdown. Therefore, the nitrogen "sparing effect" of nutritional support to these patients is to increase protein synthesis without inhibition of protein breakdown. Based on these findings, it would be even more relevant to use some additional approaches; these include the application of anabolic agents which can selectively decrease the rate of protein breakdown in severely injured patients.

13.2.2.3 The Effect of Anabolic Agents on Protein Turnover

Research on the various hormones and mediators has brought a new dimension to metabolic research with respect to the potential use of various anabolic agents to modulate the stress response of severely injured patients and to promote their early recovery.[46,47] The effect of insulin,[48,49] growth hormone,[50] testosterone,[51] and insulin-like growth factors[52] on whole-body protein turnover have been studied in healthy and diabetic patients. However, relatively few tracer studies thus far have been conducted to explore the effect of these anabolic agents on the nitrogen economy of severely injured patients. It has been reported that long-term use of insulin had the effect of reducing protein breakdown in severely burned patients,[53] and most of the other agents have demonstrated a positive effect on protein synthesis.[e.g.,54] It appears that there is a need for more extensive studies to assess the effect of these anabolic agents in the treatment of severely injured patients. Tracer methods will be a very powerful tool in providing quantitative information on the metabolic effect of these anabolic agents.

13.3 STUDY OF INDIVIDUAL AMINO ACID METABOLISM IN SURGICAL PATIENTS

Burn injury and other trauma alter individual amino acid metabolism; hence, affected patients have specific requirements for some amino acids. Research has been carried out looking for an "ideal" amino acid formula which could "best" support the injured patient. The notion of trauma-induced alteration of individual amino acid metabolism was derived from these findings: 1) trauma patients demonstrated an altered free amino acid concentration profile in plasma and whole blood;[55-58] 2) trauma causes a change in the intracellular amino acid profile;[59,60] and 3) trauma induces changes in the activities of some enzymes which catalyze the metabolism of some amino acids. While these findings are important, quantitative information on the altered fate of amino acid metabolism could not be derived from the above observations. For example, a decline in the plasma concentration of an amino acid could be the consequence of a decrease in its release into the amino acid pool and/or an increased rate of utilization, whether being oxidized, used for protein synthesis, or converted to other substrates (e.g., the conversion of phenylalanine to tyrosine). Furthermore, the altered enzyme activity does not reflect the alteration of total metabolism of its substrate, since the metabolic fate of an amino acid also depends upon its availability. Some examples of using amino acid tracers to evaluate the metabolic fate of these amino acids, hence, the potential requirement for these amino acids, are further discussed below.

13.3.1 BRANCHED CHAIN AMINO ACIDS IN BURN PATIENTS

The treatment of burn and other injured patients with amino acid formulas enriched in branched chain amino acids (BCAA) has been a topic of controversy for years. The rationale for this is based on the following considerations: 1) early *in vitro* studies revealed that BCAA, especially leucine, could promote protein synthesis, and the keto acids of BCAA could inhibit protein breakdown in cultured muscle tissues;[61] 2) some *in vivo* studies also indicated that the peripheral uptake or clearance of BCAA was significantly increased after trauma, presumably as a consequence of increased BCAA oxidation in limb muscle tissue.[62,63] Since burn patients were found to have a compromised utilization of both glucose and fatty acids as energy fuels,[64] it was also hypothesized that BCAA may serve as an alternative fuel after trauma. As a consequence, this may deplete the BCAA pool in the patients, causing a reduced BCAA availability for protein synthesis. Extensive clinical trials have been conducted in various groups of traumatized patients including burn patients, mostly using the nitrogen balance technique.[e.g. 65] Due to large variations in the nature of trauma, the related clinical complications and the timing of the studies conducted, it was not surprising that the results were quite controversial. Furthermore, the technique used above cannot reveal the metabolic fate of BCAA in the body; therefore, the hypothesis with reference to the potential benefit of BCAA-enriched nutritional support has not been tested.

Using a leucine tracer, Wolfe et al.[39] revealed that in burn patients, the rates of leucine oxidation and its utilization for protein synthesis were both significantly increased, though the increase of the latter was much less than the elevation in the rate of leucine release from proteolysis. Therefore, it is unlikely that increased leucine oxidation would competitively reduce its availability for protein synthesis in these patients. We further traced the metabolic fate of leucine during BCAA-enriched enteral feeding and during conventional feeding. It was found that the increased BCAA intake only resulted in an increased rate of leucine oxidation and its utilization for protein synthesis.[66] Similar findings were also reported by Milliken et al.[67] in liver cirrhosis patients receiving BCAA. These studies demonstrated that: 1) injury did increase BCAA oxidation, but there was no evidence that the latter reduces BCAA availability for protein synthesis in burn patients; 2) increased BCAA in enteral feeding did not further promote protein synthesis; 3) most of the increased rate of BCAA uptake was through the pathway of oxidation rather than protein synthesis; and 4) BCAA oxidation accounts for only 2 to 5% of total energy expenditure; increased BCAA supply could not serve as a major energy fuel for the burn patients.[68] These kinetic findings substantiate the more extensive clinical trials of BCAA-enriched formula in critically ill patients, [e.g.,69,70] which failed to provide convincing evidence that these patients would benefit in terms of nitrogen economy or visceral protein synthesis.

13.3.2 Study of Non-Essential Amino Acid Metabolism in Surgical Patients

In addition to disturbing nitrogen economy, the insult of trauma and sepsis altered the relationship between essential and non-essential amino acids. Early studies using the nitrogen balance method have revealed that providing an amino acid solution containing only essential amino acids resulted in a lower nitrogen balance in post-operative surgical patients, as compared to the use of an isonitrogenous essential and non-essential amino acid mixture,[71] indicating that some non-essential amino acids are actually "essential" or "conditionally essential" for these patients. However, the above findings do not provide information with respect to which amino acid is conditionally essential, and how the rate of its *de novo* synthesis and/or its disposal are altered after injury.

Two general approaches have been used to evaluate the rate of *de novo* synthesis of non-essential amino acids.

One approach is based on the model assuming that the total metabolic flux of a non-essential amino acid Q_{NEAA} is contributed by its release from whole-body proteins B_{NEAA}, its *de novo* synthesis S_{denovo}, and the input from enteral or parenteral intake I_{NEAA}.

Thus,

$$Q_{NEAA} = B_{NEAA} + S_{denovo} + I_{NEAA}$$

where Q_{NEAA} is estimated via a primed constant infusion of the particular non-essential amino acid tracer, B_{NEAA} is estimated by measuring the rate of leucine (or another essential amino acid) release from protein breakdown B_{LEU} and the relative concentration of leucine and this non-essential amino acid in whole-body proteins $(R_{NEAA/LEU})$. Thus,

$$B_{NEAA} = B_{LEU} \times R_{NEAA/LEU}$$

The rate of *de novo* synthesis of the non-essential amino acid S_{denovo} can be quantified:

$$S_{denovo} = Q_{NEAA} - B_{NEAA} - I_{NEAA}$$

where I_{NEAA} is the rate of the specific non-essential amino acid (under study) intake from enteral or parenteral nutritional support; when the patient is in the fasting state (or when the feeding solution does not contain this non-essential amino acid), $I_{NEAA} = 0$.

This first approach has been used to quantify the *de novo* synthesis rates of alanine,[72,73] glycine,[73] proline,[74-76] and glutamine [e.g.,77,78] under different patho-physiological conditions, including burn injury.[75]

The second approach is used to evaluate the *de novo* synthesis rate of those amino acids, each of which exclusively *de novo* synthesized from its amino acid precursor. For example, tyrosine is derived from phenylalanine, and arginine is derived from citrulline. Based on the isotope label incorporation from the precursor amino acid to the product amino acid, one can at least quantify the appearance rate of the *de novo* synthesized non-essential amino acid into the plasma pool. This is detailed below.

Assuming 1) amino acid B is exclusively derived from precursor amino acid A, and 2) both free amino acid pools for A and B exist in the plasma (as shown in Figure 13.3), the metabolic flux of amino acid A (Q_A) and B (Q_B) can be estimated by independent primed constant infusions of tracers A^* and B^*. With appropriate isotopic labelling of amino acid A, tracer A^* can be converted to labelled product B^* via the biochemical conversion of amino acid A to B. Assuming that the plateau enrichment in pool A is E_A and that in pool B is E_B (tracer/tracee mole fraction above baseline), when the stoichiometry relationship between A and B is 1:1, and the conversion rate of pool A to pool B is T_{A-B}, then the isotopic appearance rate of tracer B^* in pool B is ($T_{A-B} \cdot E_A$), and the disappearance of tracer B^* from pool B is $[(Q_B + i_B) \cdot E_B]$, where i_B is the infusion rate of an independent tracer of B for the quantitation of Q_B.

Then, the isotopic balance of tracer B^* in amino acid pool B can be shown as:

$$T_{A-B} \cdot E_A = (Q_B + i_B) \cdot E_B$$

Thus, the conversion rate from A to B, $T_{A-B} = \dfrac{(Q_B + i_B) \cdot E_B}{E_A}$

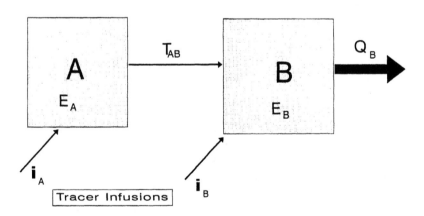

FIGURE 13.3 Model to estimate the rate of metabolic conversion from amino acid A to amino acid B in plasma pool.

Considering both free pools of amino acid A and amino acid B in the body, tracer A is infused into pool A at a rate of i_A, and reaches a plateau enrichment level of E_A. Within the body, the labeled amino acid A yields labeled amino acid B, the latter reaches a plateau enrichment E_B in pool B. The metabolic flux of amino acid B in pool B is estimated by an independent primed constant infusion of a differently labeled tracer B (it usually has a different mass from that of the amino acid A-derived, labeled amino acid B) at an infusion rate of i_B. Detailed derivations of equations are in the text.

This equation may be used for two purposes: 1) quantifying the rate of plasma tyrosine *de novo* synthesis from its precursor phenylalanine, and 2) in some cases, the rate of phenylalanine incorporation into protein S_{PHE} (an indicator of the rate of protein synthesis) can be quantified by:

$$S_{PHE} = Q_{PHE} - T_{P-T}$$

where T_{P-T} is the rate of phenylalanine to tyrosine conversion. This model is particularly useful in evaluating whole-body protein kinetics when collection of expired air (for estimating amino acid oxidation) is not feasible. The latter situation is common in young pediatric patients when they are on high-flow mechanical ventilation.[73] The details of the model and its comparison with the use of other tracers in evaluating whole-body protein kinetics, has been described by Thompson et al.[80]

Based on these approaches, our studies have revealed that in severely burned patients, the *de novo* synthesis rates of proline[75] and tyrosine[81] are compromised; the rate of cysteine formation is also reduced relative to the increased rate of methionine utilization.[45] Others have found a reduced *de novo* synthesis rate of glutamine in patients with extensive small bowel resection.[78] These kinetic findings will aid in improving the amino acid composition of the nitrogen source to be used for the clinical nutritional support of ill patients, especially since most of the currently used parenteral feeding solutions do not contain tyrosine, cysteine, and glutamine.

13.4 STUDY OF PROTEIN METABOLISM IN INDIVIDUAL ORGANS AND TISSUES

In spite of the advances in mechanical and drug-based support to organ functions in the treatment of critically ill patients, the mortality rate for multiple organ failure continues to exceed 90%. Management of organ failure remains the key unresolved issue in critical care medicine. The relationship between various inflammatory-hormonal mediators and other biopharmaceuticals must be considered in perspective with the techniques and specific nutrients in supporting organ metabolic needs and maintaining organ functions. Therefore, quantifying the metabolism of amino acids and proteins in specific organs and tissues *in vivo* is an important aspect of metabolic research in burn and other critically ill patients.

There are several approaches in using tracer techniques to quantify protein and amino acid metabolism in specific organs and tissues, as follows.

13.4.1 COMBINED MEASUREMENTS OF ARTERIO-VENOUS (A-V) TRACER AND TRACEE BALANCE

The general approach is to quantify the metabolic fate of a particular amino acid within an organ and tissue from the disappearance rate of the tracer and the appearance rate of the labeled product across this organ/tissue. For details, see Chapter 3 by Davis et al.. These studies have also been used in evaluating amino acid and protein metabolism in the limbs of healthy and diseased human subjects,[e.g., 82-85] and in some cases, for evaluating protein metabolism in the splanchnic region.[82,83] There are some variations among these models: for the study of the splanchnic bed metabolism in humans, catheterization of the hepatic vein should be perfomed;[82,83] and for limb metabolism, at least a deep vein catheterization is required.[83,85] The invasive nature of these procedures hampers their wide application in critically ill patients.

13.4.2 Stable Isotope Administration Combined with Tissue Biopsy Studies

The general protocol includes a primed constant infusion of a stable isotope labeled tracer amino acid and sequential biopsies of the tissue of interest. The fractional protein synthesis rate is calculated from the increment in the enrichment of amino acid tracer in the protein-bound pool of the sampled tissue and that in the precursor pool. For details, see Chapter 3. In humans, this method is mostly used for quantifying the fractional synthesis rate of limb muscle proteins because of the ease of biopsy procedures.[e.g., 86,89] More recently, this method has been further developed to simultaneously quantify the fractional rate of protein breakdown in the sampled tissues, by timed biopsies of muscle tissue after terminating the tracer infusion.[89] Biolo et al.[90,91] further developed a model applying the approach using A-V concentration of tracer and tracee combined with muscle biopsy to evaluate the kinetics of individual amino acids and proteins in human skeletal muscle. The tracer incorporation approach has provided important quantitative information on muscle protein turnover *in vivo* in burn patients,[53] but the request for use of muscle biopsy in critically ill patients has not been well accepted by many institutions.

13.4.3 A Simultaneous Infusion of Amino Acid Isotopomer Tracers via an Intragastric Route (IG) and an Intravenous (IV) Route

This approach is specifically used for quantifying the metabolic fate of the tracee amino acid in the splanchnic region of human subjects. With this approach, Matthews et al.[31] successfully quantified the rate of leucine entering different metabolic pathways in the whole body and in the splanchnic region. The details of the model have been described.[31] Briefly, the host body can be divided into two major metabolic compartments: the splanchnic pool and the systemic (or non-splanchnic) pool. This method is based on a simultaneous infusion of the isotopomer tracers of the same amino acid via intravenous and intragastric routes. For a detailed example, we refer the reader to our publication by Basile-Filho et al.[27] In this study, this approach was applied to phenylalanine and tyrosine metabolism. For reasons of space, we refer the reader to the Appendix of Reference 27.

This is a much less invasive approach for quantifying amino acid and protein metabolism in the splanchnic and non-splanchnic regions *in vivo*. It is potentially applicable to the study on burn and other critically ill patients, provided an enteral administration route is available. However, the major limitations of this approach include: 1) in evaluating the whole-body metabolic flux and oxidation of the amino acid during the IG infusion, an assumption should be made that the metabolic pools in the splanchnic region and the non-splanchnic region have the same enrichment, i.e., the IG infused tracer is uniformly distributed in both splanchnic and non-splanchnic metabolic pools. This has not been fully verified; 2) conceptually, the metabolism of an amino acid measured by IV tracer infusion is not exclusively the metabolism within the non-splanchnic region. Hence, in stricter terms, the measured difference between data from IG and IV tracer infusion actually represents the first-pass effect and second-pass effect of the splanchnic region in processing the ingested amino acid; and 3) this method cannot separate contributions made by the liver vs. the gut to the metabolism of the amino acid being studied. However, this approach will help to estimate the metabolic fate of the dietary-administered amino acid within these two compartments of the body.[27]

13.5 THE APPLICATION OF THE POSITRON EMISSION TOMOGRAPHY (PET) METHOD IN STUDYING ORGAN AND TISSUE METABOLISM *IN VIVO*

PET is a technique for measuring the concentration of a positron-emitting radio isotope within a three-dimensional body, by external detection of the radiation emitted from the isotopes. The commonly used positron-emitting radio nuclide include ^{11}C, ^{18}F, ^{15}O and ^{13}N. They are made from their particular precursor molecules through bombardment by cyclotron-accelerated, high-energy particles. For example, ^{11}C is made from ^{14}N. The positron-emitting nuclide is unstable and immediately decays to a more stable isotope by either electron capture or positron emission. In the latter process, a proton is converted to a neutron and energy is emitted. The emitted positron immediately undergoes annihilation reaction by combining with an electron in the surrounding tissues (with less than 1 mm of distance). In this process, all the mass of both positron and electron is converted into energy and emitted in the form of two γ-rays, which travel at nearly opposite directions. Detection of these γ-rays outside the body is achieved using a special arrangement of detectors to record the co-incidence events, i.e., only those pairs of γ-rays which are captured between two detectors. Hence, the biochemical activities which take place in a specific location of the body can be detected with the aid of computerized tomography. By imaging the intensity of these reactions, combined with mathematical modeling, the *in vivo* metabolic process of a specific nutrient in a particular tissue or organ of the host can be quantified. Because of the very short-term exposure to radioactivity, PET is thus far the least invasive *in vivo* method for estimating dynamic aspects of metabolism in tissues and organs. In recent years, this method has been applied to the *in vivo* measurement of muscle protein synthesis with [^{11}C]methionine as tracer.[92,93] This method does not require muscle biopsy and it can quantify protein and amino acid metabolism not only in skeletal muscle but also in deep muscles inaccessible to biopsy, such as the peri-spinal muscles. This new technique is potentially useful to explore muscle and other tissue or organ metabolism *in vivo*, in burn and other critically ill patients.

The application of PET to *in vivo* protein and amino acid metabolism is under extensive research and development. The challenging issues for further development include 1) quantitation of the rate of protein breakdown in muscles and other tissues, and 2) extending its measurements of protein synthesis to tissues and organs other than muscle, among which the most challenging development would be the determination of amino acid metabolism in the liver. As discussed earlier, the quantitative *in vivo* information about liver metabolism is very limited due to the difficulty of accessing portal vein blood and the invasive nature of liver biopsy. PET would be the most appropriate approach to investigate metabolism in this organ.

In summary, tracer-based techniques have been and will continue to be a very powerful tool for exploring the quantitative, dynamic nature of altered nitrogen and individual amino acid metabolism in response to trauma and injury. Further development of these techniques will provide more accurate information, which will be used for the development of new therapeutic modalities for the metabolic and nutritional care of critically ill patients.

REFERENCES

1. Cuthbertson, D. P., The influence of prolonged muscle rest on metabolism, *Biochem. J.*, 23, 1328, 1929.
2. Cuthbertson, D. P., The disturbance of metabolism produced by bony and non-bony injury with notes on certain abnormal conditions of bone, *Biochem. J.*, 24, 1244, 1930.
3. Souba, W. W., Nutrition support, *N. Engl. J. Med.*, 336, 41, 1997.
4. Wolfe, R. R., Herman Award lecture, 1996: relation of metabolic studies to clinical nutrition — the example of burn injury, *Am. J. Clin. Nutr.*, 64, 800, 1996.
5. Young, V. R., 1987 McCollum Award lecture: kinetics of human amino acid metabolism: nutritional implications and some lessons, *Am. J. Clin. Nutr.*, 46, 709, 1987.
6. Picou, D. and Taylor-Roberts, T., The measurement of total protein synthesis and catabolism and nitrogen turnover in infants in different nutritional states and receiving different amounts of dietary protein, *Clin. Sci.*, 36, 283, 1969.
7. Matthews, D. E., Motil, K. J., Bohrbaugh, D. K., Burke, J. F., Young, V. R., and Bier, D.M., Measurement of leucine metabolism in man from a primed, continuous infusion of L-[1-^{13}C] leucine, *Am. J. Physiol.*, 238, E473, 1980.
8. Matthews, D. E., Bier, D. M., Rennie, M. J., Edwards, R. H. T., Halliday, D., Millward, D. J., and Clugston, G. A., Regulation of leucine metabolism in man: a stable isotope study, *Science* 214, 1129, 1981.
9. Waterlow, J. C., Garlick, P. J., and Millward, D. J., *Protein turnover in mammalian tissues and in the whole body*, Amsterdam, North-Holland, 1978, 804.
10. Wolfe, R. R., *Radioactive and stable isotope tracers in biomedicine: principles and practice of kinetic analysis*, New York, Wiley-Liss, 1992.
11. Young, V. R. and Bier, D. M., Stable isotopes (^{13}C and ^{15}N) in the study of human protein and amino acid metabolism and requirements, in *Nutritional Factors: Modulating Effects on Metabolic Processes*, Beers, J. F., Jr., and Basset, E. G., Eds., Raven Press, New York, 1981, 267.
12. Waterlow, J. C., Protein turnover with special reference to man, *Q. J. Exp. Physiol.*, 69, 409, 1984.

13. Young, V. R., Yu, Y-M., and Krempf, M., Protein and amino acid turnover using the stable isotopes ^{15}N, ^{13}C, and ^{2}H as probes, in *New Techniques in Nutritional Research*, Whitehead, R. G., and Prentice, A., Eds., Academic Press, New York, 1991, 17.

14. Bier, D. M., Intrinsically difficult problems: the kinetics of body protein and amino acids in man, *Diabetes/Metabolism Reviews*, 5, 111, 1989.

15. Assimon, S. A. and Stein, T. P., [15]N Glycine as a tracer to study protein metabolism in vivo, in *Modern Methods in Protein Nutrition and Metabolism*, Nissen, S., Ed., Academic Press, New York, 1992, chap. 11.

16. Sim, A. J. W., Wolfe, B. M., Suopen, B., Young, V. R., and Moore, F., Nitrogen turnover in man, *JPEN*, 4, 180, 1980.

17. Norton, J. A., Stein, P. T., and Brennan, M. F., Whole-body protein synthesis and turnover in normal man and malnourished patients with and without known cancer, *Ann. Surg.*, 194, 123, 1981.

18. Kien, C. L., Rohrbaugh, D. K., Burke, J. F., and Young, V. R., Whole body protein synthesis in relation to basal energy expenditure in healthy and burned children, *Pediatr. Res.*, 12, 211, 1980.

19. Lapidot, A. and Nissim, I., Regulation of pool sizes and turnover rates of amino acids in humans: ^{15}N-glycine and ^{15}N-alanine single-dose experiments using gas chromatography-mass spectrometry analysis, *Metabolism*, 29, 230, 1980.

20. Glass, R. E., Fern, E. B., and Garlick, P. J., Whole-body protein turnover before and after resection of colorectal tumors, *Clin. Sci.*, 64, 101, 1983.

21. Fern, E. B., Garlick, P. J., Sheppard, H. G., and Fern, M., The precision of measuring the rate of whole-body nitrogen flux and protein synthesis in man with a single dose of [^{15}N]-glycine, *Hum. Nutr. Clin. Nutr.*, 38(1), 63, 1984.

22. Soares, M. J., Piers, L. S., Shetty, P. S., Jackson, A. A. and Waterlow, J. C., Whole body protein turnover in chronically undernourished individuals, *Clin. Sci.*, 86, 441, 1993.

23. Birkhahn, R. H., Long, C. L., Fitkin, D., Jeevanadam, M., and Blakemore, W. S., Whole-body protein metabolism due to trauma in man as estimated by L-[^{15}N]alanine, *Am. J. Physiol.*, 241, E64, 1981.

24. Golden, M. H. N. and Waterlow, J. C., Total protein synthesis in elderly people: a comparison of results with [^{15}N]glycine and [^{14}C]leucine, *Clin. Sci. Mol. Med.*, 53, 277, 1977.

25. De Benoist, B., Abdulrazzak, Y., Brooke, O. G., Halliday, D., and Millward, D. J., The measurement of whole-body protein turnover in the preterm infant with intragastric infusion of L-[1-^{13}C] leucine and sampling of the urinary leucine pool, *Clin. Sci.*, 66, 155, 1984.

26. Basile-Filho, A., El-Khoury, A. E., Beaumier, L., Wang, S. Y., and Young, V. R., Continuous 24-h L-[1-^{13}C]phenylalanine and L-[3,3-[2]H$_2$]tyrosine oral-tracer studies at an intermediate phenylalanine intake to estimate requirements in adults, *Am. J. Clin. Nutr.*, 65, 473, 1997.

27. Basile-Filho, A., Beaumier, L., El-Khoury, A. E., Yu, Y-M., Kenneway, M., Gleason, R. E., and Young, V. R., Twenty-four-hour L-[1-^{13}C]tyrosine and L-[3,3-[2]H$_2$]phenylalanine oral tracer studies at generous, intermediate and low phenylalanine intakes, to estimate aromatic amino acid requirement in adults, *Am. J. Clin. Nutr.*, 67, 640, 1998.

28. Hoerr, R. A., Matthews, D. E., Bier, D. M., and Young, V. R., Leucine kinetics from [[2]H$_3$]- and [^{13}C]leucine infused simultaneously by gut and vein, *Am. J. Physiol.*, 260, E111, 1991.

29. Cortiella, J., Matthews, D. E., Robert, A. H., Bier, D. M., and Young, V. R., Leucine kinetics at graded intakes in young men: quantitative fate of dietary leucine, *Am. J. Clin. Nutr.*, 48, 998, 1988.

30. Pelletier, V., Marks, L., Wagner, D. A., Hoerr, R. A., and Young, V. R., Branched-chain amino acid interactions with reference to amino acid requirements in adult men: leucine metabolism at different valine and isoleucine intakes, *Am. J. Clin. Nutr.*, 54, 402, 1991.

31. Matthews, D. E., Marano, M. A., and Campbell, R. G., Splanchnic bed utilization of leucine and phenylalanine in humans, *Am. J. Physiol.*, 264, E109, 1993.

32. El-Khoury, A. E., Sanchez, M., Fukagawa, N. K., Gleason, R. E., Tsay, R. H., and Young, V. R., The 24-h kinetics of leucine oxidation in healthy adults receiving a generous leucine intake via three discrete meals, *Am. J. Clin. Nutr.*, 62, 579, 1995.

33. El-Khoury, A. E., Ajami, A. M., Fukagawa, N. K., Chapman, T. E., and Young, V. R., Diurnal pattern of the interrelationships among leucine oxidation, urea production, and hydrolysis in humans, *Am. J. Physiol.*, 271, E563, 1996.

34. Yu, Y-M., Young, V. R., Castillo, L., Chapman, T. E., Tompkins, R. G., Ryan, C. M., and Burke, J. F., Plasma leucine kinetics and urea production rates in burn patients, *Metabolism*, 44, 659, 1995.

35. O'Keefe, S. J. D., Sender, P. M., and James, W. P. T., 'Catabolic' loss of body nitrogen in response to surgery, *Lancet*, ii, 1035, 1974.

36. Crane, C. W., Picou, D., Smith, R. and Waterlow, J. C., Protein turnover in patients before and after elective orthopaedic operations, *Bri. J. Surg.*, 64, 129, 1977.

37. Hartig, W., Faust, H., Czarnetzki, H-D., Putziger, J., and Wetzel, K., Studien zum aminosaurenstoffwechsel in Operationsstress, in *Pastaggressionsstoffwechsel*, Heberer, G., Schuutis, K., and Guniher, B., Eds., F. K. Schattauer, Stuttgart, 123.

38. Long, C. L., Jeevanandam, M., Kim, B. M., and Kinney, J. M., Whole body protein synthesis and catabolism in septic man, *Am. J. Clin. Nutr.*, 30, 1340, 1977.

39. Wolfe, R. R., Goodenough, R. D., Burke, J. F., and Wolfe, M. H., Response of protein and urea kinetics in burn patients to different levels of protein intake, *Ann. Surg.*, 197, 163, 1983.

40. Jahoor, F., Desai, M., Herndon, D. N., and Wolfe, R. R., Dynamics of the protein metabolic response to injury, *Metabolism*, 37, 330, 1988.

41. Yu, Y-M., Ryan, C. M., Burke, J. F., Tompkins, R. G., and Young, V. R., Relationships among arginine, citrulline, ornithine and leucine kinetics in adult burn patients. *Am. J. Clin. Nutr.*, 62, 960, 1995.

42. Yu, Y-M., Sheridan, R. L., Burke, J. F., Chapman, T. E., Tompkins, R. G., and Young, V. R., Kinetics of plasma arginine and leucine in pediatric burn patients, *Am. J. Clin. Nutr.*, 64, 60, 1996.

43. Tomkins, A. M., Garlick, P. J., Schofield, W. N., and Waterlow, J. C., The combined effects of infection and malnutrition on protein metabolism in children, *Clin. Sci.*, 65, 313, 1983.

44. Clague, M. B., Keir, M. J., Wright, P. D., and Johnston, I. D. A., The effects of nutrition and trauma on whole body protein metabolism in man, *Clin. Sci.*, 65, 165, 1983.

45. Yu, Y-M., Burke, J. F., and Young, V. R., A kinetic study of L-[1-^{13}C,^{2}H$_3$]methionine metabolism in patients with severe burn injury, *J. Trauma*, 35, 1, 1993.

46. Wilmore, D. W., Catabolic illness: Strategies for enhancing recovery, *N. Engl. J. Med.*, 325, 695, 1991.

47. Ziegler, T. R., Gatzen, C., and Wilmore, D. W., Strategies for attenuating protein-catabolic responses in the critically ill, *Ann. Rev. Med.*, 45, 459, 1994.

48. Frexes-Steed, M., Warner, M. L., Bulus, N., Flakoll, P., and Abumrad, N., Role of insulin and branched-chain amino acids in regulating protein metabolism during fasting, *Am. J. Physiol.*, 258, E907, 1990.

49. Nair, K. S., Ford, C. G., Ekberg, K., Fernqvist-Forbes, E., and Wahren, J., Protein dynamics in whole body and in splanchnic and leg tissues in type I diabetic patients, *J. Clin. Invest.*, 95, 2926, 1995.

50. Horber, F. F. and Haymond M. W., Human growth hormone prevents the protein catabolic side effects of prednisone in humans, *J. Clin. Invest.*, 86, 265, 1990.

51. Urban, R. J., Bodenburg, Y. H., Gilkison, C., Foxworth, J., Coggan, A. R., Wolfe, R. R., and Ferrando, A., Testosterone administration to elderly men increases skeletal muscle strength and protein synthesis, *Am. J. Physiol.*, 269, E820, 1995.

52. Roith, J. S., Insulin-like growth factors, *N. Engl. J. Med.*, 336, 633, 1997.

53. Sakura, Y., Aarsland, A., Herdon, D. N., Chinkes, D. L., Pierre, E., Nguyen, T. T., Patterson, B. W., and Wolfe, R. R., Stimulation of muscle protein synthesis by long-term insulin infusion in severely burned patients. *Ann. Surg.*, 222, 283, 1995.

54. Carli, F., Webster, J. D., and Halliday, D., A nitrogen-free hypocaloric diet and recombinant human growth hormone stimulate postoperative protein synthesis: fasted and fed leucine kinetics in the surgical patient, *Metabolism*, 46, 796, 1997.

55. Cynober, L., Amino acid metabolism in thermal burns, *JPEN*, 13, 196, 1989.

56. Cynober, L., Dinh, F. N., Blonde, F., Saizy, R., and Giboudeau, J., Plasma and urinary amino acid pattern in severe burn patients–evolution throughout the healing period, *Am. J. Clin. Nutr.*, 36, 416, 1982.

57. Siegel, J. H., Relations between circulatory and metabolic changes in sepsis, *Ann. Rev. Med.*, 32, 175, 1981.

58. Jeevanandam, M., Ramias, L., and Schiller, W. R., Altered plasma free amino acid levels in obese traumatized man, *Metabolism*, 40, 385, 1991.

59. Askanazi, J., Carpentier, Y. A., Michelsen, C. B., Elwyn, D. H., Fürst, P., Kantrowitz, L. R., Gump, F. E., and Kinney, J. M., Muscle and plasma amino acids following injury, *Ann. Surg.*, 192, 78, 1980.

60. Stinnett, D. J., Alexander, W. J., Watanabe, C., Macmillan, B. G., Fischer, J. E., Morris, M. J., Trocki, O., Miskell, P., Edwards, L., and James, H., Plasma and skeletal muscle amino acids following severe burn injury in patients and experimental animals, *Ann. Surg.*, 195, 75, 1982.

61. Hedden, M. P. and Buse, M. G., General stimulation of muscle protein synthesis by branched chain amino acids in vitro, *Pro. Soc. Exp. Bio. Med.*, 160, 410, 1979.

62. Elia, M., Farrell, R., Ilic, V., Smith, R., and Williamson, D. H., The removal of infused leucine after injury, starvation and other conditions in man, *Clin. Sci.*, 59, 275, 1980.

63. Desai, S. P., Bistrian, B. R., Moldawer, L. L., Miller, M. M., and Blackburn, G. L., Plasma amino acid concentrations during branched-chain amino acid infusion in stressed patients, *J. Trauma*, 747, 1981.

64. Wolfe, R. R. and Shaw, J. H. F., Glucose and FFA kinetics in sepsis: Role of glucagon and sympathetic nervous system activity, *Am. J. Physiol.*, 248, E236, 1985.

65. Takala, J. and Klossner, J., Branched chain amino acid-enriched parenteral nutrition in surgical intensive care patients, *Clin. Nutr.*, 5, 167, 1985.

66. Yu, Y-M., Wagner, D. A., Walesewski, J. C., Burke, J. F. and Young, V. R., A kinetic study of leucine metabolism in severely burned patients, *Ann. Surg.*, 207, 421, 1988.

67. Milliken, W. J., Jr., Henderson, J., and Galloweay, J. R., *in vivo* measurement of leucine metabolism with stable isotopes in normal subjects and in those with cirrhosis fed conventional and branched-chain amino acid enriched diets, *Surgery*, 98, 405, 1986.

68. Wolfson, A. M. I., Amino acids–their role as an energy source, *Proc. Nutr. Soc.*, 42, 489, 1983.
69. Sanstedt, S., Jorfeldt, L., and Larsson, J., Randomized, controlled study evaluating effects of branched chain amino acids and alpha-ketoisocaproate on protein metabolism after surgery, *Bri. J. Surg.*, 79, 217, 1992.
70. Brennan, M. F., Cerra, F., Daly, J. M., Fischer, J. E., Moldawer, L. L., Smith, R. J., Vinnars, E., Wannemacher, R., and Young, V. R., Report of a research workshop: branched-chain amino acids in stress and injury, *JPEN*, 10, 446, 1986.
71. Tweedle, D. E. F., Spivey, J., and Johnston, I. D. A., Choice of intravenous amino acid solution for use after surgical operation, *Metabolism*, 22, 173, 1973.
72. Robert, J. J., Bier, D. M., Zhao, X. H., Matthews, D. E., and Young, V. R., Glucose and insulin effects on the novo amino acid synthesis in young men: studies with stable isotope labeled alanine, glycine, leucine and lysine, *Metabolism*, 31, 1210, 1982.
73. Yu, Y-M., Yang, R. D., Matthews, D. E., Wen, Z. M., Burke, J. F., Bier, D. M., and Young, V. R., Quantitative aspects of glycine and alanine nitrogen metabolism in postabsorptive young men: effects of level of nitrogen and dispensable amino acid intake, *J. Nutr.*, 115, 399, 1985.
74. Jaksic, T., Wagner, D. A., Burke, J. F., and Young, V. R., Plasma proline kinetics and the regulation of proline synthesis in man, *Metabolism*, 36, 1040, 1987.
75. Jaksic, T., Wagner, D. A., Burke, J. F., and Young, V. R., Proline metabolism in adult male burned patients and healthy control subjects, *Am. J. Clin. Nutr.*, 54, 408, 1991.
76. Miller, R. G., Jahoor, F., and Jaksic, T., Decreased cysteine and proline synthesis in parenterally fed, premature infants, *J. Pediatr. Surg.*, 30, 953, 1995.
77. Darmaun, D., Rongier, M., Koziet, J., and Robert, J-J., Glutamine nitrogen kinetics in insulin-dependent diabetic humans, *Am. J. Physiol.*, 261, E713, 1991.
78. Darmaun, D., Messing, B., Just, B., Rongier, M., and Desjeux, J-F., Glutamine metabolism after small intestinal resection in humans, *Metabolism*, 40, 42, 1991.
79. Castillo, L., Yu, Y-M., Marchini, S., Chapman, T. E., Sanchez, M., Young, V. R., and Burke, J. F., Phenylalanine and tyrosine kinetics in critically ill children with sepsis, *Pediatr. Res.*, 35, 580, 1994.
80. Thompson, G. N., Pacy, P. J., Merritt, H., Ford, G. C., Read, M. A., Cheng, K. N., and Halliday, D., Rapid measurement of whole body and forearm protein turnover using a [^{2}H$_5$]phenylalanine model, *Am. J. Physiol.*, 256, E631, 1989.
81. Yu, Y-M., Chapman, T., Yu, P. R., Cortiella, J., Vogt, J. A., Young, V. R., and Burke, J. F., Increased requirement of tyrosine for burn patients – a kinetic study of aromatic amino acid metabolism, *Proceedings of American Burn Association* 23, 78, 1991.
82. Fong, Y., Matthews, D. E., He, W., Marano, M. A., Moldawer, L. L. and Lowry, S. F., Whole body and splanchnic leucine, phenylalanine, and glucose kinetics during endotoxemia in humans, *Am. J. Physiol.*, 266, R419, 1994.
83. Nair, K. S., Ford, C. G., Ekberg, E., Fernqvist-Forbes, E., and Wahren, J., Protein dynamics in whole body and in splanchnic and leg tissues in type I diabetic patients, *J. Clin. Invest.*, 95, 2926, 1995.
84. Cheng, K. N., Dworzak, F., Ford, G. C., Rennie, M. J., and Halliday, D., Direct determination of leucine metabolism and protein breakdown in humans using L-[1-^{13}C, ^{15}N]-leucine and the forearm model, *Eur J. Clin. Invest.*, 15, 349, 1985.
85. Gelfand, R. A. and Barrett, E., Effect of physiologic hyperinsulinemia on skeletal muscle protein synthesis and breakdown in man, *J. Clin. Invest.*, 80, 1, 1987.

86. Bennet, W. M., Connacher, A. A., Scrimgeour, C. M., Smith, K., and Rennie, M. J., Increase in anterior tibialis muscle protein synthesis in healthy man during mixed amino acid infusion studies of incorporation of [1-^{13}C]leucine, *Clin. Sci.*, 76, 447, 1989.

87. Carraro, F., Stuart, C. A., Hartl, W. H., Rosenblatt, J., and Wolfe, R. R., Effect of exercise and recovery on muscle protein synthesis in human subjects, *Am. J. Physiol.*, 259, E470, 1990.

88. Chinkes, D., Klein, S., Zhang, X-J., and Wolfe, R. R., Infusion of labeled KIC is more accurate than labeled leucine to determine human muscle protein synthesis, *Am. J. Physiol.*, 270, E67, 1996.

89. Zhang, X-J., Chinkes, D. L., Sakurai, Y., and Wolfe, R. R., An isotopic method for measurement of muscle protein fractional breakdown rate in vivo, *Am. J. Physiol.*, 270, E759, 1996.

90. Biolo, G., Chinkes, D., Zhang, X-J., and Wolfe, R. R., A new model to determine in vivo the relationship between amino acid transmembrane transport and protein kinetics in muscle, *JPEN*, 16, 305, 1992.

91. Biolo, G., Fleming, D. R. Y., Maggi, S. P., and Wolfe, R. R., Transmembrane transport and intracellular kinetics of amino acids in human skeletal muscle, *Am. J. Physiol.*, 268, E75, 1995.

92. Hsu, H., Yu, Y-M., Babich, J. W., Burke, J. F., Livni, E., Tompkins, R. G., Young, V. R., Alpert, N. M., and Fischman, A.J., Measurement of muscle protein synthesis by positron emission tomography with L-[methyl-^{11}C]methionine, *Proc. Natl. Acad. Sci. U.S.A.*, 93, 1841, 1996.

93. Young, V.R., Yu, Y-M., Hsu, H., Alpert, N. M., Tompkins, R.G., and Fischman, A.J., Combined stable isotope-positron emission tomography (PET) for *in vivo* assessment of protein metabolism, *Emerging Technology for Nutrition Research*, National Academy Press, Washington, DC, 1997, 1–28.

14 Methods for Investigation of Protein and Amino Acid Metabolism in Diabetes Mellitus

Robert C. Albright, Jr. and K. Sreekumaran Nair

CONTENTS

14.1 INTRODUCTION

Diabetes is a wonderful affection, not very frequent among men, being a melting down of the flesh into urine.

           — Areteus Cappadoceus (A.D. 30–90)[1]

0-8493-9612-3/99/$0.00+$.50
© 1999 by CRC Press LLC

Appreciation of the cachexia associated with untreated insulin-requiring diabetes mellitus has a prolonged history, dating back to ancient Greek writings as the statement above attests. However, it has been only recently that the understanding of some of the mechanisms of protein wasting associated with diabetes have been partially elucidated. There is still much to be learned, and the mechanism of insulin's anticatabolic effect is yet to be completely defined. This chapter will review the methods available to investigate protein and amino acid metabolism in diabetes mellitus.

14.2 METHODS OF ASSESSING PROTEIN METABOLISM

14.2.1 WHOLE-BODY STUDIES

Daily protein turnover occurs at an astonishing rate. In a normal 70 kg adult, about 280 g of protein is synthesized and degraded each day.[2] Multiple techniques are available to investigate body composition and protein kinetics in diabetes mellitus. Interpretation of previous studies (and plans for new investigations) requires close attention to whether the study method(s) evaluated whole-body, regional, or some combination of body compartments or specific proteins. Whether protein accretion or loss occurs depends upon the relative interplay between protein catabolism (breakdown) and protein anabolism (synthesis). The rate of protein breakdown varies widely between different tissue beds and among different proteins. Net increases in splanchnic protein synthesis may offset a smaller net breakdown of protein in skeletal muscle, perhaps leading to an overall increase in protein synthesis in the whole body.[3]

Whole-body studies model the total body protein as one compartment, the mass of which is determined by the balance between synthesis and breakdown (see Chapter 2 by El-Khoury). During the postprandial state, the free amino acid pool is determined by protein synthesis and breakdown, as well as the influences of intake and amino acid oxidation. Most human studies are performed in the postabsorptive state; therefore, exogenous amino acid intake is not considered in the calculations. These models, obviously, greatly simplify a very complex process, and depend upon the uniform mixing and free movement of protein and amino acids between the various pools.

Various labeling techniques have been applied in order to trace and quantify the changes in protein turnover. Both stable and radioactive isotopes have been used. Most human studies are now being performed with stable isotopes, due to the potential hazards involved with radioactive materials, the advances in mass spectrophotometry, the potential of the stable isotope tracers to measure synthesis of proteins with slow rates of turnover, and the potential to label different moities of compounds with different tracers. However, labeled isotope studies are technically demanding and often very expensive. Therefore, in many clinical situations urinary nitrogen and body composition measurements remain useful when properly performed.

14.2.1.1 Nitrogen Balance

Every amino acid has at least one nitrogen atom: hence, the net balance of nitrogen has served as an index of protein balance. Simply, nitrogen balance = nitrogen intake - nitrogen loss. The term nitrogen intake generally reflects the dietary content obtained by dietary records or food analysis. The nitrogen (N) loss reflects stool, urine, skin, hair and other N losses.[4] Urinary nitrogen loss reflects approximately 80% of the total N lost from the body and is measured as a timed collection. The main urinary nitrogen containing compounds are urea and ammonia, comprising 80 to 85% and 5 to 10%, respectively, of total urinary nitrogen. The remaining nitrogen is made up of creatine, creatinine, uric acid, free amino acids and certain polyamines.[5] The relative contribution of ammonia also increases during fasting. Urinary urea is formed as a result of protein catabolism generating amino acids which are transaminated or oxidized to form ammonia, which is then converted to urea in the liver via the ornithine cycle. The urinary urea varies considerably depending on renal function (often a major concern in patients with diabetes), hydration status, certain drug use and, obviously, protein intake and protein breakdown. The urinary ammonia is generated by proximal tubular cells from glutamine and is heavily influenced by the acid-base balance and serum potassium levels, which are often disordered by the Type IV renal tubular acidosis (RTA) associated with diabetes mellitus. The remaining compounds vary little in the setting of normal renal function. While the performance of nitrogen balance evaluations appears to be straightforward, complete measurement of all nitrogen excretion has been difficult, even among studies performed in metabolic wards.[6] Many studies utilize formulae which, after direct measurement of stool and urinary losses, use standard correction factors to account for the remaining N losses.[6]

The urea generation rate in vivo is highly variable, depending upon influences such as physical activity, meals and hydration status. Therefore, prolonged urine collections, often over several days, are required, which have substantial potential for collection and measurement error. Nitrogen balance studies may detect changes in body protein content, but may not truly reflect changes in fat-free mass; therefore, the information may not correlate with the changes in body composition measurement.[7] It must also be recognized that nitrogen balance does not determine the rates of protein synthesis or breakdown. No inferences can be made regarding whether the net gain or loss of N is due to relative increases in synthesis or breakdown in specific tissues.

Nitrogen balance studies, in combination with total body potassium measurements (a reflection of body cell mass) applied both prior to and following initiation of treatment of diabetes mellitus (Type I and II), showed an increase in nitrogen balance and cellular mass with therapy for diabetes (insulin, diet or oral hypoglycemic agents).[8]

Whole-body nitrogen balance studies have also been utilized in studies of protein restriction in diabetic nephropathy,[9,10] artificial beta cell implants,[11] parenteral nutrition regimens[12] and in differing glycemic control models.[13]

14.2.1.2 Urinary 3-Methylhistidine Studies

3-Methylhistidine (3-MH) is a constituent of actin and myosin in human skeletal muscle, and is neither metabolized, reutilized or degraded once released by muscle breakdown.[14] Since muscle accounts for approximately 90% of the body's 3-MH content, measurement of urinary excretion of 3-MH theoretically reflects muscle breakdown.[14] However, in muscle-wasting states, the amount of urinary 3-MH increases, while the creatinine excretion usually decreases in these subjects due to the overall decrease in muscle mass.[15] Recently, the measurements of whole-body 3-MH have been performed without dependence on urinary sampling, using novel isotope labeling techniques; this offers some optimism regarding the use of 3-MH to study muscle protein breakdown.[16] Normalization of 3-MH excretion per unit muscle mass remains problematic, due to the excretion of small amounts of 3-MH from non-muscle tissues such as gut. Arterio-venous balance of 3-MH is an extremely valuable measure of myofibrillar protein breakdown in that specific tissue bed. However, the analytical techniques available to measure 3-MH in plasma are not sufficiently sensitive to detect the small changes often seen.

14.2.1.3 Body Composition Studies

Generally, these techniques are best suited for population-based studies and are less satisfactory for individual quantitative studies. Most of these techniques rely on the ability to determine fat-free mass, and through the application of standard calculations derive measurements of body protein content.

Total body potassium is a measure of cellular mass, while the neutron activation technique can measure the cellular nitrogen content. These two techniques are available only in a few centers.

Imaging techniques, including computed tomography, magnetic and nuclear resonance imaging, dual energy X-ray absorptiometry, anthropomorphometric measurements, total body potassium, dilutometry and bioelectrical impedance have all been utilized in studies of protein metabolism in diabetes mellitus. Lohman's text on body composition is an excellent resource for the specifics of these techniques.[17]

14.2.1.4 Protein Turnover Studies: Precursor Methods

The principles involved in clinical studies of protein kinetics in diabetes mellitus are the same as described in Chapter 2 by El-Khoury for healthy human subjects. However, more specifically, it is important to understand the various precursors and products utilized in the studies which employ stable isotope methodology. Figure 14.1 illustrates the compounds and compartments which are sampled in the studies using L[1-^{13}C] leucine as a tracer.

This approach utilizes the concept of a precursor pool, ideally free of the labeled amino acid at the initiation of the protocol. Infusion of a known amount of labeled

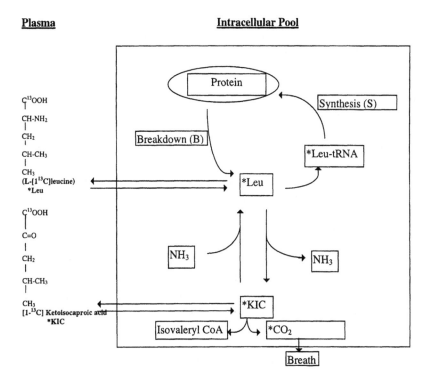

FIGURE 14.1 Leucine kinetic model utilizing L-[1^{13}C] leucine (*Leu). The intracellular and plasma pool are assumed to be completely mixed. Therefore, the leucine pool is a common source for acylation to *leu-tRNA and transamination to 1-[^{13} C] ketoisocaproic acid (*KIC). *KIC has traditionally been used as the intracellular measure of isotopic enrichment of leucine. Note, by additionally labeling the Nitrogen, dual labeled L-[1^{13}C, ^{15}N] leucine can be utilized in order to determine Nitrogen flux concomitantly; see text for details.

amino acid, at a known rate, will eventually reach a steady state of isotope enrichment (i.e., isotopic plateau). A bolus dose of the tracer, administered at initiation of the protocol, will shorten the time required to prime the appropriate pools. Protein turnover can then be calculated from the steady-state isotopic abundance of the labeled amino acid by sampling the various pools of interest over time, including plasma, muscle and interstitial fluid. Waterlow pioneered this precursor pool approach in 1967,[18,19] using [U^{14}C] lysine as the tracer (labeled amino acid). Halliday and McKeran realized the benefits of utilizing non-radioactive tracers in 1975, when they studied protein turnover utilizing L[1-^{13}C] lysine as their tracer.[20] In 1980, Matthews et al. began to utilize intravenous infusions of L[1-^{13}C] leucine with an initial priming bolus to allow achievement of an isotopic plateau much more quickly.[21] Matthews et al.[22] and Schwenk et al.[23] provided the theoretical basis for using plasma [^{13}C] KIC as a surrogate measure of intracellular [^{13}C] leucine for whole-body protein turnover studies. Currently, this technique is the most widely applied method for studying whole-body protein metabolism.

14.2.1.4.1 The Leucine Model

Leucine is an essential amino acid which, by definition, is not synthesized de novo in humans. Leucine is a major component of body proteins representing ~ 6 to 8% of total protein mass. It undergoes reversible transamination, mostly in mammalian skeletal muscle, to an intermediate compound known as ketoisocaproic acid (KIC). KIC then may undergo irreversible decarboxylation via branched chain ketoacid dehydrogenase to isovaleryl CoA and CO_2 (oxidation), or may be reaminated back to leucine. The carboxyl moiety of leucine (the first carbon) is not synthesized in the body; therefore, a label of the carboxyl carbon will allow tracing the ultimate fate of leucine through to the final oxidation to labeled CO_2 which may be measured in the breath. Utilizing [1-^{13}C] leucine as the tracer allows the determination of [^{13}C] KIC, which represents the precursor step prior to oxidation. As previously mentioned (see Chapter 2), $^{13}CO_2$ production in expired air represents oxidation, and must be corrected for bicarbonate recovery data. Computation of whole body leucine (and protein) kinetics are described in Chapter 2.

Nitrogen flux in the labeled leucine model can be additionally determined by applying two labels to the leucine. As doubly labeled leucine (L[1-^{13}C, ^{15}N] leucine) undergoes deamination to [^{13}C] KIC and is subsequently reaminated back to leucine (with naturally occurring ^{14}N), the leucine has lost its ^{15}N label. The differing isotopic enrichments of the dual-labeled leucine ([1-^{13}C,^{15}N] leucine) and single-labeled leucine ([1-^{13}C] leucine) allow us to determine nitrogen flux (representing both transamination and breakdown).

Hence, the use of ([1-^{13}C, ^{15}N] leucine) allows determination of the reversible transamination process that is affected by multiple physiologic and pathophysiologic situations. This allows determination of nitrogen flux (Qn) which may be calculated using [1-^{13}C, ^{15}N] leucine isotopic enrichment in plasma at plateau. Deamination of leucine to KIC (Xo) and subsequent reamination of KIC back to leucine (Xn) may be calculated as follows:

$$Qn - Qc = Xn = Xo - C$$

where Qn is leucine nitrogen flux, Qc is leucine carbon flux, and C is leucine oxidation.

These flux calculations, which are based on a stochastic model, require steady-state conditions and are simplified if performed in the postabsorptive state. The calculations utilized in these models have also been reviewed elsewhere.[15] In an in vivo model, the absolute steady state does not exist. However, when plotting the isotopic enrichment against time the overall slope of this curve should not be significantly different from zero, although it will most likely not be a straight line.

14.3 STUDIES IN DIABETES MELLITUS USING THE LEUCINE MODEL

Multiple studies have documented the increased protein breakdown and protein synthesis using whole-body evaluations in patients with Type I diabetes.[3,24-31]

Increased leucine flux and non-oxidative leucine disposal (NOLD, a putative measure of protein synthesis) were found during insulin deprivation. Increased oxidative disposal of leucine was also found, indicating high amino acid oxidation during insulin deprivation. Insulin replacement reduced protein breakdown and leucine oxidation but also slowed the rate of protein synthesis. The overall net tendency to favor anabolism during insulin replacement likely results from greater reduction of protein breakdown than protein synthesis. Insulin deprivation in patients with Type I diabetes also causes a substantial increase in leucine nitrogen flux, due to increased leucine transamination.

Insulin's secretion increases in the postprandial period, when there is an abundance of dietary amino acids circulating. However, as explained earlier, most previous tracer studies were performed in the postabsorptive (fasting) state in order to simplify the flux calculations. The insulin-induced hypoaminoacidemia which results during these studies[32] may simply indicate a lack of substrate availability as an explanation for the decreased synthesis of protein. Investigators have attempted to clarify this matter by supplementing with amino acids during the insulin replete and deprived states.[28,29,33-36] Overall, the effect of amino acid supplementation on protein synthesis was unclear. Some studies showed an increase in whole-body protein synthesis, as measured by non-oxidative leucine disposal (NOLD) in normal subjects and patients with Type I diabetes mellitus.[29,33,36] However, other investigators failed to confirm any increase in synthesis rate.[28,35] All the above studies showed a decrease in whole-body protein breakdown and increases in leucine oxidation during insulin replacement with amino acid supplementation.

14.4 REGIONAL STUDIES

Information regarding specific muscle and splanchnic protein kinetics is vital in the evaluation of patients with diabetes mellitus. Whereas whole-body measurements may lead the investigator to conclude the catabolism associated with insulin-deprived diabetes is mainly an effect of increased protein breakdown, regional studies have shown the rates of breakdown and synthesis are different among various tissue beds.[3]

14.4.1 ARTERIOVENOUS STUDIES

Arteriovenous studies (see also Chapter 3 by Davis et al., re: animal studies) allow determination of protein turnover in specific tissue beds. These studies may be problematic in human subjects with diabetes, due to the difficulties related to atherosclerosis and vascular access. Careful screening of volunteers and attention to measures which prevent thrombotic complications allow these risks to be minimized.

14.4.1.1 Model for Forearm and Leg Skeletal Muscle Studies

Choices for amino acid tracers include [^{15}N] phenylalanine, or [ring ^{2}H$_5$] phenylalanine, ideally suited for studies across limb skeletal muscle. Because phenylalanine is neither oxidized nor transaminated in peripheral tissues, tracer methodology is greatly simplified. Amino acids such as lysine and tyrosine have similar qualities.

However, lysine has a large intracellular pool which may result in a much longer time to reach isotopic plateau and equilibration among the various pools. Tyrosine's fate is similar to phenylalanine in skeletal muscle, except it is formed from phenylalanine in the liver and has its own catabolic pathway in the liver. Tyrosine, therefore, is not suitable for the simultaneous measurements of protein dynamics in splanchnic and skeletal muscle beds.

As mentioned above, phenylalanine has only one fate in skeletal muscle: incorporation into protein. Conversely, dilution of the venous isotopic enrichment can only occur by entry of naturally occurring phenylalanine derived from protein breakdown. This assumption is valid due to phenylalanine's inability to be synthesized in the body making it an indispensable amino acid. Degradation of phenylalanine occurs only in the liver with the formation of tyrosine. It is mandatory that an isotopic steady state be achieved during the measurement period, and the sampling catheters need to be positioned in a manner such that venous drainage reflects muscle tissue drainage. It is assumed that there is complete mixing of the arterial blood within the muscle cells, and that there is negligible tissue recycling of the phenylalanine label.

Measurements of fractional mixed muscle protein and myosin heavy chain synthetic rates were performed in patients with Type I diabetes mellitus. No difference in muscle protein synthesis was detected between the groups.[37,38] Infusion of substrate (amino acids) also failed to demonstrate any effect of insulin deprivation or supplementation on muscle protein synthesis.[28] The net decreased protein synthesis found in insulin-deprived patients with Type I diabetes, therefore, must be due to the decline in protein synthesis in non-muscle tissues. This was proven by a recent observation, in which it was demonstrated that almost all changes in whole-body protein synthesis occurred in non-skeletal muscle tissue in the insulin-deprived patient with Type I diabetes.[3] Figure 14.2 illustrates the differential effects of insulin on rates of protein breakdown and synthesis found between the splanchnic and skeletal muscle pools. The study illustrated by Figure 14.2 demonstrates an increased protein breakdown occurring in skeletal and splanchnic proteins, in addition to an increased synthesis rate in the splanchnic region during insulin deprivation. The net accretion of protein in the splanchnic bed was confirmed by the balance of essential amino acids (leucine and phenylalanine).[3] The net decline in protein catabolism during insulin repletion was found to be due to a decreased muscle protein breakdown without contribution from the splanchnic region. Further support for the increased splanchnic protein synthesis during insulin deprivation in patients with Type I diabetes was found by DeFeo and colleagues, who demonstrated increased fibrinogen synthesis. This perturbation was reversed with insulin supplementation.[39]

Determination of synthesis rates requires that the amount of tracer delivered be known. Therefore, limb flow rates need to be quantified. Indicator dye techniques with commercially available indocyanine green provide a reliable, accurate method to determine limb blood flow rates; alternatively, plethysmography and thermodilution have been shown to be accurate tools in experienced hands, under controlled conditions.[40,41]

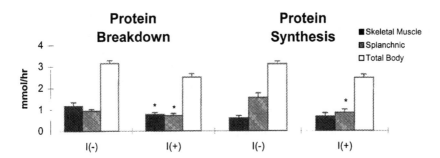

FIGURE 14.2 Changes in skeletal muscle and splanchnic region phenylalanine kinetics. Protein breakdown and protein synthesis were determined by protein to phenylalanine and phenylalanine to protein changes, respectively. Skeletal muscle accounted for 37% of whole-body protein breakdown during insulin deprivation and 30% during insulin supplementation, whereas the splanchnic region accounted for ~ 30% of whole-body breakdown with or without insulin supplementation. However, the splanchnic region accounted for 50% of whole-body synthesis during insulin deprivation, but only 34% during insulin supplementation. Skeletal muscle synthesis accounted for 27% of whole-body synthesis in the insulin replete state, but only 19% during insulin deprivation. Developed using results data in Reference 3.

14.4.1.1.1 Calculations

Phenylalanine balance (PheBal) is calculated as follows:

PheBal = (Phe$_A$ - Phe$_v$) x F

  Phe$_A$, Phe$_V$ = phenylalanine concentration in artery and vein (micromol/l)

  F = limb blood flow (ml/min)

Protein breakdown is indicated by phenylalanine rate of appearance from proteins (Ra Phe$_A$), and is calculated as follows:

Ra Phe$_A$ = Phe$_A$ [(Phe$_{EA}$/Phe$_{EV}$) - 1] x F

  Phe$_{EA}$, Phe$_{EV}$ = phenylalanine isotopic enrichment in arterial and venous blood (molar % excess)

The rate of disappearance of phenylalanine (Rd Phe) represents protein synthesis, and is calculated as follows (two possible methods):

Based on the concept of steady state: Phe Bal = Rd Phe - Ra Phe

Rd Phe = Phe Bal + Ra Phe

Alternatively, calculating directly from the fractional excretion of the tracer:[42]

Rd Phe = [(Phe$_{EV}$ - Phe$_{EA}$/ Phe$_{EA}$) x (Phe$_A$)] x F

The above equation assumes the enrichment of the precursor pool is the arterial enrichment. The argument can be made that, actually, venous enrichment more accurately reflects the precursor pool; by passing through the capillary bed, it has truly been exposed to the muscle cells. Since the venous enrichment is lower than arterial, a higher Rd value will be obtained. However, when comparison was performed with direct measurement of amino acid tRNA (AA- tRNA) levels, both arterial and venous surrogates underestimated protein synthesis.[43] Additionally, the effect of interventions on this model may further compound these mischaracterizations. An ideal study would validate these arteriovenous models with tissue sampling and actual measurement of precursor pool enrichment.

14.4.1.2 Model for Splanchnic Tissues

The same stochastic principles can be utilized when performing studies across the splanchnic tissues. However, these models are complicated by the differing functions, rate of isotope uptake, and pool sizes of the organs in the splanchnic circulation. Additionally, as previously mentioned, direct validation of the arteriovenous methods in humans is complicated by the infeasibility of obtaining tissue from these visceral organs. Most visceral organs drain into the liver, which is in turn drained by the hepatic and portal veins. Unfortunately, portal vein sampling is not possible in human studies, so the entire splanchnic bed is treated as a single pool. The leucine model is applicable across the splanchnic bed utilizing familiar concepts. The phenylalanine model is useful, although it is complicated by the conversion of phenylalanine to tyrosine in the liver, as detailed below.

Selective catheterization of the hepatic vein under fluoroscopic guidance is the standard method for sampling the splanchnic bed.[44] Femoral artery catheterization can be utilized as access to the splanchnic arterial circulation, in order to determine blood flow by standard indocyanine green dilution techniques.[3] The conversion of phenylalanine to tyrosine in the liver means that there are two fates for phenylalanine rate of disappearance (Phe Rd): incorporation into protein and conversion to tyrosine. L[^{15}N] phenylalanine, [ring ^{2}H$_5$] phenylalanine or L[1-^{13}C] phenylalanine can be used as tracers, and their hydroxylation to tyrosine can be monitored by measuring [^{15}N] tyrosine, [^{2}H$_4$] tyrosine and [1-^{13}C] tyrosine, respectively, provided an independent tyrosine tracer (e.g., [ring ^{2}H$_2$] tyrosine) is also used to measure total tyrosine flux.

For example, a primed, continuous infusion of L[^{15}N] phenylalanine is given through a peripheral vein, along with an independent tracer (e.g., [^{2}H$_4$] tyrosine). A priming dose of [^{15}N] tyrosine also must be given to prime the [^{15}N] tyrosine pool, since [^{15}N] tyrosine is generated from the hydroxylation of [^{15}N] phenylalanine and its measurement is crucial to quantify the phenylalanine conversion to tyrosine. Simultaneous samples from the femoral artery and hepatic vein must be analyzed for [^{15}N] phenylalanine, [^{15}N] tyrosine and [^{2}H$_4$] tyrosine.

14.4.1.2.1 Calculations

Ra Phe is calculated using a similar equation as for the limb studies:

$$Ra\ Phe = [(Ph_{EA}\ /\ Phe_{EV})\ -1]\ x\ Phe_A\ x\ F$$

Rd Phe is also computed as previously:

$$Rd\ Phe = Ra\ Phe + Phe\ Bal$$

However, since Rd Phe involves not only protein synthesis but also the disposal of phenylalanine via its conversion to tyrosine, phenylalanine conversion to tyrosine (Ipt) can be calculated as follows:

$$Ipt = ([^2H_4]\ Tyr_{EA}\ /\ [^2H_4]\ Tyr_{EV})\ x\ ([^{15}N]\ Tyr_{EV}\ /\ [^{15}N]\ Phe_{EV}\ )\ -$$
$$([^{15}N]\ Tyr_{EA}\ /\ [^{15}N]\ Phe_{EA})\ x\ Phe\ Rd$$

Phenylalanine incorporation into protein (Phe_S) is then calculated as follows:

$$Phe_S = Phe\ Rd - Ipt$$

Simultaneous measurements of phenylalanine kinetics in skeletal muscle (Leg) could be performed by sampling from the femoral artery, femoral vein and hepatic vein.

14.5 CRITIQUE OF TRACER METHODOLOGY

There are many assumptions involved in the stochastic model. Except for plasma itself, there is no homogenous "pool" of free amino acids into which a tracer is completely and uniformly distributed. However, the plasma pool does not necessarily represent the pool into which unlabeled amino acids are released following protein breakdown. Likewise, the plasma pool does not represent the immediate precursor pool for protein synthesis. In fact, a measurement of tissue fluid, which represents some extracellular (15%) and mainly intracellular fluid (~85%), shows the isotopic enrichment of leucine is higher in the plasma than in the intracellular pool.[45,46] Isotopic enrichment of KIC has been shown to more accurately represent intracellular leucine enrichment than plasma leucine enrichment.[21,22] This is due to the transamination of leucine occurring only intracellularly. However, recent studies demonstrated that plasma KIC enrichment may not exactly be a reliable surrogate measure of leucyl-tRNA and intracellular leucine enrichment in skeletal muscle.[46] This study found that both plasma and tissue fluid KIC and plasma leucine enrichments were significantly greater than those of tissue fluid leucine and leucyl-tRNA. Hence, this suggested that the use of either plasma leucine or plasma KIC as a surrogate measure of leucyl-tRNA would lead to an underestimation of human muscle protein synthesis.[46] In contrast, hepatic venous leucine enrichments under different study conditions are well represented by the KIC enrichment.[47] More studies are needed to further clarify the above question.

Choosing the correct tracee and tracer is also vitally important, as this amino acid must correctly represent the turnover of proteins in the body. Additionally, correct identification and measurement of the pools in which transamination, oxidation and synthesis occur, as well as the site into which breakdown occurs, must be adequately determined. Assumptions regarding adequate mixing of these various pools may not be correct. For example, the acylation of tRNA and transamination of leucine are assumed to occur in a well-mixed intracellular pool. This assumption may not be correct, and some evidence exists supporting the presence of separate pools for both tRNA acylation and leucine transamination.[46,48]

Muscle is the major repository of protein and amino acids in the body; however, it only represents 27% of whole-body protein synthesis. Hence, even a large increase in muscle protein synthesis of ~25% would only reflect an approximately 7% increase in total body protein synthesis rate.[37] This 7% increase is well within the coefficient of variation accepted for these whole-body studies, and may be discounted or go unmeasured. In addition, changes in synthesis rates of protein in non-muscle tissues (such as liver) can occur in a direction opposite that of muscle. Whole-body studies often normalize protein turnover values per unit body weight. Comparisons of obese subjects, lean subjects and subjects with Type I diabetes revealed that when results were normalized for weight alone, leucine turnover was highest in diabetics, followed by lean subjects, with the obese subjects showing the lowest protein turnover. However, when the leucine turnover was normalized for lean body mass, rates of turnover were highest in the diabetic subjects, followed by the obese subjects, with the lean subjects demonstrating the lowest rates of leucine flux.[24] Caution is needed in interpretation of values normalized for lean body mass, as these calculations require the division of the total measured synthesis rate by the lean body mass, which may have decreased by a great deal in certain disease states (e.g., muscle tissue in muscular dystrophy), thus leading to a falsely elevated "corrected" synthesis rate.

The rate of oxidation of protein is calculated based on the production of labeled CO_2.[49] The $^{13}CO_2$ (which carries the [1-^{13}C]label following oxidation) is presumed to exit the cell and be excreted by the lungs. However, the oxidative reaction occurs in the mitochondria, and perhaps quantitation of CO_2 measured from an extracellular source (breath) is not complete. Further information on CO_2 retention is presented in Chapter 2.

14.6 MEASUREMENT OF SYNTHESIS RATE OF TISSUE PROTEIN AND SPECIFIC PROTEINS IN HUMANS

Protein dynamic studies across tissue beds provide valuable information, but limited in that these measurements represent the average of protein synthesis and breakdown of various proteins. There are techniques to measure synthesis rates of specific tissue proteins such as myosin heavy chain,[38,50] and protein fractions such as sarcoplasmic[51] and mitochondrial proteins.[52] Similarly, it is possible to measure synthetic rates of secretory liver proteins such as albumin and fibrinogen[53](see Chapter 4 by Jahoor and Reeds). These techniques are also reviewed elsewhere.[15] They provide valuable tools to study protein metabolism in diabetes.

Circulating proteins of hepatic origin have traditionally been used, including ApoB-100, albumin and fibrinogen.[39,54-56] The VLDL ApoB-100 reaches isotopic plateau more quickly than the other proteins. Hence, ApoB-100 has been proposed as a surrogate for amino acyl-tRNA in liver protein synthesis.[45,57] Immunoaffinity chromatography (IAC) employs highly specific monoclonal antibodies to separate proteins and biologic molecules.[53] IAC was used in the purification and subsequent measurement of tracer amino acid enrichment into ApoB-100, albumin and fibrinogen, from plasma samples, thus providing a measure of hepatic export protein synthesis.[53] Future application of the IAC technique may allow measurement of individual "component" proteins across different tissues.

It is possible with sufficient muscle tissue to measure steady-state mRNA levels of specific proteins, including isoforms of myosin heavy chain (MHC), actin and mitochondrial proteins. Methods which amplify the expression of selected specific mRNA could allow the study of these proteins to be performed on standard-size needle biopsy specimens. Determination of fractional synthetic rates of muscle protein in conjunction with mRNA levels of these proteins will assist in determination of whether a pre-transcriptional or post-transcriptional defect is at fault in disease states which involve muscle wasting.

The observation of muscle wasting associated with diabetes (and with aging) raises questions as to the site of disordered protein metabolism. The possibility that the cumulative damage to muscle mitochondrial DNA which occurs under the influence of aging and perhaps increased oxidative stress (of diverse etiologies) is an interesting hypothesis; this will require the quantitation of mitochondrial DNA in muscle specimens and a reliable means of measuring mitochondrial function. These studies offer exciting opportunities for the further understanding of how human muscle metabolism is regulated in diabetes, aging and in other disease states.[58]

14.7 SUMMARY

Protein breakdown and amino acid oxidation have been convincingly shown to be associated with insulin deficiency in patients with Type I diabetes mellitus. These abnormalities have been shown to be reversed with insulin. However, controversies still exist as to the specific effects insulin deprivation has on specific tissue beds. The investigator needs to be aware of the limitations associated with the methods currently in use, and to be cautious in data interpretation of whole-body studies. Exciting advances in measurement technology and molecular techniques of protein purification offer hope that a much more complete understanding of protein kinetics in diabetes mellitus will soon be possible.

ACKNOWLEDGMENTS

This work was supported by PHS grant RO1 DK41973 and the Murdoch-Dole Professorship.

REFERENCES

1. Reed, J. A. Aretaes, the Cappadocian, *Diabetes*, 419, 1954.
2. Cohn, S. H., Vartsky, D., Yasumura, S., Vaswani, A. N., and Ellis, K. J., Indexes of body cell mass: nitrogen versus potassium, *Am. J. Physiol.*, 244, E305, 1983.
3. Nair, K. S., Ford, G. C., Ekberg, K., Fernqvist-Forbes, E., and Wahren, J., Protein dynamics in whole body and in splanchnic and leg tissues in type I diabetic patients, *J. Clin. Invest.*, 95, 2926, 1995.
4. Heymsfield, S. B. and Williams, P. G., Nutritional Assessment by Clinical and Biochemical Methods, *Modern Nutrition in Health and Disease,* 7th. Edition, Shils, M.E. and Young, V.R., Eds., Lea and Febiger, Philadelphia, 1988, 817.
5. Fuller, N. J. and Elia, M., Inadequacy of urinary urea for estimating nitrogen balance [letter; comment], *Annals of Clin. Biochem.*, 27, 510, 1990.
6. Garrow, J. S., Energy stores: their composition, measurement and control, *Energy Balance and Obesity in Man,* 2nd Edition, Garrow, J. S., Ed., Elsevier/North-Holland Biomedical, Amsterdam, 1978, 13.
7. Waterlow, J. C. and Munro, H. N., The Assessment of Protein Nutrition and Metabolism in the Whole Animal, with Special Reference to Man, *Mammalian Protein Metabolism*, Waterlow, J. C., and Munro, H. N., Eds., Academic, New York, 1969, 325.
8. Walsh, C. H., Soler, N. G., James, H., Harvey, T. C., Thomas, B. J., Fremlin, J. H., Fitzgerald, M. G., and Malins, J. M., Studies of whole body potassium and whole body nitrogen in newly diagnosed diabetics, *Q. J. Med.*, 45, 295, 1976.
9. Brodsky, I. G., Robbins, D. C., Hiser, E., Fuller, S. P., Fillyaw, M., and Devlin, J. T., Effects of low-protein diets on protein metabolism in insulin-dependent diabetes mellitus patients with early nephropathy, *J. Clin. Endo. & Met.*, 75, 351, 1992.
10. Shichiri, M., Nishio, Y., Ogura, M., and Marumo, F., Effect of low-protein, very-low-phosphorus diet on diabetic renal insufficiency with proteinuria, *Am. J. Kidney Dis.*, 18, 26, 1991.
11. Wesson, D. E., Black, P. R., Vlachokosta, F., Aoki, T. T., and Wilmore, D. W., Artificial beta-cell promotes positive nitrogen balance and whole body protein synthesis in insulin-dependent diabetic subjects, *J. Parenteral and Ent. Nut.*, 12, 237, 1988.
12. Overett, T. K., Bistrian, B. R., Lowry, S. F., Hopkins, B. S., Miller, D., and Blackburn, G. L., Total parenteral nutrition in patients with insulin-requiring diabetes mellitus, *J. Am. Coll. Nutr.*, 5, 79, 1986.
13. Lariviere, F., Kupranycz, D. B., Chiasson, J. L., and Hoffer, L. J., Plasma leucine kinetics and urinary nitrogen excretion in intensively treated diabetes mellitus, *Am. J. Physiol.*, 263, E173, 1992.
14. Young, V. R. and Munro, H. N., Ntau-methylhistidine (3-methylhistidine) and muscle protein turnover: an overview, [Review] [70 refs], *Fed. Proceed.*, 37, 2291, 1978.
15. Nair, K. S., Assessment of Protein Metabolism in Diabetes, *Clinical Research in Diabetes and Obesity, Part I: Methods, Assessment and Metabolic Regulation*, Drannin, B. and Rizza, R., Eds., Humana Press, Totowa, NJ, 1998, 137.
16. Rathmacher, J. A., Flakoll, P. J., and Nissen, S. L., A compartmental model of 3-methylhistidine metabolism in humans, *Am. J. Physiol.*, 269, E193, 1995.
17. Lohman, T. G., Ed., Advances in Body Composition Assessment, *Advances in Body Composition Assessment: Current Issues in Exercise Science, Monograph Number 3*, 1.1, Human Kinetics Publishers, Champaign, Illinois, 1992, 1.
18. Waterlow, J. C., Lysine turnover in man measured by intravenous infusion of L-[U-14C]lysine, *Clin. Sci.*, 33, 507, 1967.

19. Waterlow, J. C. and Stephen, J. M., The measurement of total lysine turnover in the rat by intravenous infusion of L-[U-^{14}C]lysine, *Clin. Sci.*, 33, 489, 1967.
20. Halliday, D. and McKeran, R. O., Measurement of muscle protein synthetic rate from serial muscle biopsies and total body protein turnover in man by continuous intravenous infusion of L-(alpha-^{15}N)lysine, *Clin. Sci. Mol. Med.*, 49, 581, 1975.
21. Matthews, D. E., Motil, K. J., Rohrbaugh, D. K., Burke, J. F., Young, V. R., and Bier, D. M., Measurement of leucine metabolism in man from a primed, continuous infusion of L-[1-^{13}C]leucine, *Am. J. Physiol.*, 238, E473, 1980.
22. Nair, K. S., Matthews, D. E., Welle, S. L., and Braiman, T., Effect of leucine on amino acid and glucose metabolism in humans, *Metab.: Clin. & Exp.*, 41, 643, 1992.
23. Schwenk, W. F., Beaufrere, B., and Haymond, M. W., Use of reciprocal pool specific activities to model leucine metabolism in humans, *Am. J. Physiol.*, 249, E646, 1985.
24. Nair, K. S., Garrow, J.S., Ford, C., Mahler, R. F., and Halliday, D., Effect of poor diabetic control and obesity on whole body protein metabolism in man, *Diabetologia*, 25, 400, 1983.
25. Umpleby, A. M., Boroujerdi, M. A., Brown, P. M., Carson, E. R., and Sonksen, P. H., The effect of metabolic control on leucine metabolism in type 1 (insulin-dependent) diabetic patients, *Diabetologia*, 29, 131, 1986.
26. Robert, J. J., Beaufrere, B., Koziet, J., Desjeux, J. F., Bier, D. M., Young, V. R., and Lestradet, H., Whole body de novo amino acid synthesis in type I (insulin-dependent) diabetes studied with stable isotope-labeled leucine, alanine, and glycine, *Diabetes*, 34, 67, 1985.
27. Nair, K. S., Ford, G. C., and Halliday, D., Effect of intravenous insulin treatment on in vivo whole body leucine kinetics and oxygen consumption in insulin-deprived type I diabetic patients, *Metab.: Clin. & Exp.*, 36, 491, 1987.
28. Bennet, W. M., Connacher, A. A., Smith, K., Jung, R. T., and Rennie, M. J., Inability to stimulate skeletal muscle or whole body protein synthesis in type 1 (insulin-dependent) diabetic patients by insulin-plus-glucose during amino acid infusion: studies of incorporation and turnover of tracer L-[1-^{13}C]leucine, *Diabetologia*, 33, 43, 1990.
29. Luzi, L., Castellino, P., Simonson, D. C., Petrides, A. S., and DeFronzo, R. A., Leucine metabolism in IDDM. Role of insulin and substrate availability, *Diabetes*, 39, 38, 1990.
30. Pacy, P. J., Garrow, J. S., Ford, G. C., Merritt, H., and Halliday, D., Influence of amino acid administration on whole-body leucine kinetics and resting metabolic rate in postabsorptive normal subjects, *Clin. Sci.*, 75, 225, 1988.
31. Tessari, P., Amino acid and protein metabolism in diabetes mellitus. [Review] [25 refs], *Ital. J. Gastro.*, 25, 151, 1993.
32. Fukagawa, N. K., Minaker, K. L., Young, V. R., and Rowe, J. W., Insulin dose-dependent reductions in plasma amino acids in man, *Am. J. Physiol.*, 250, E13, 1986.
33. Castellino, P., Luzi, L., Simonson, D. C., Haymond, M., and DeFronzo, R.A., Effect of insulin and plasma amino acid concentrations on leucine metabolism in man. Role of substrate availability on estimates of whole body protein synthesis, *J. Clin. Invest.*, 80, 1784, 1987.
34. Tessari, P., Inchiostro, S., Biolo, G., Trevisan, R., Fantin, G., Marescotti, M. C., Iori, E., Tiengo, A., and Crepaldi, G., Differential effects of hyperinsulinemia and hyperaminoacidemia on leucine-carbon metabolism in vivo. Evidence for distinct mechanisms in regulation of net amino acid deposition, *J. Clin. Invest.*, 79, 1062, 1987.

35. Flakoll, P. J., Kulaylat, M., Frexes-Steed, M., Hourani, H., Brown, L. L., Hill, J. O., and Abumrad, N. N., Amino acids augment insulin's suppression of whole body proteolysis, *Am. J. Physiol.*, 257, E839, 1989.

36. Biolo, G., Tessari, P., Inchiostro, S., Bruttomesso, D., Fongher, C., Sabadin, L, Fratton, M. G., Valerio, A., and Tiengo, A., Leucine and phenylalanine kinetics during mixed meal ingestion: a multiple tracer approach, *Am. J. Physiol.*, 262, E455, 1992.

37. Nair, K. S., Halliday, D., and Griggs, R. C., Leucine incorporation into mixed skeletal muscle protein in humans, *Am. J. Physiol.*, 254, E208, 1988.

38. Charlton, M. R., Balagopal, P., and Nair, K. S., Skeletal muscle myosin heavy chain synthesis in type 1 diabetes, *Diabetes*, 48, 1336, 1997.

39. De Feo, P., Gaisano, M. G., and Haymond, M. W., Differential effects of insulin deficiency on albumin and fibrinogen synthesis in humans, *J. Clin. Invest.*, 88, 833, 1991.

40. Jorfeldt, L. and Wahren, J., Leg blood flow during exercise in man, *Clin. Sci.*, 41, 459, 1971.

41. Proctor, D. N., Halliwill, J. R., Shen, P. H., Vlahakis, N. E., and Joyner, M. J., Peak calf blood flow estimates are higher with Dohn than with Whitney plethysmograph, *J. Appl. Physiol.*, 81, 1418, 1996.

42. Barrett, E. J., Fryberg, D. A., Louard, R. J., and Nair, K. S., Use of Catheterization Methods to Study the Regulation of Muscle Protein Metabolism, *Protein Metabolism in Diabetes Mellitus*, Barrett E.J., Fryburg D.A., Louard R.J., and Nair, K.S., Eds., Smith - Gordon, London, 1992, 91.

43. Biolo, G., Chinkes, D., Zhang, X-J., and Wolfe, R. R., Harry M. Vars Research Award, A new model to determine in vivo the relationship between amino acid transmembrane transport and protein kinetics in muscle, *J. Parenteral & Ent. Nut.*, 16, 305, 1992.

44. Wahren, J., Felig, P., Cerasi, E., and Luft, R., Splanchnic and peripheral glucose and amino acid metabolism in diabetes mellitus, *J. Clin. Invest.*, 51, 1870, 1972.

45. Baumann, P. Q., Stirewalt, W. S., O'Rourke, B. D., Howard, D., and Nair, K. S., Precursor pools of protein synthesis: a stable isotope study in a swine model, *Am. J. Physiol.*, 267, E203, 1994.

46. Ljungqvist, O. H., Persson, M., Ford, G. C., and Nair, K. S., Functional heterogeneity of leucine pools in human skeletal muscle, *Am. J. Physiol.*, 273, E564, 1997.

47. Biolo, G. and Tessari, P., Splanchnic versus whole-body production of alpha-ketoisocaproate from leucine in the fed state, *Metab.: Clin. & Exp.*, 46, 164, 1997.

48. Schneible, P. A., Airhart, J., and Low, R. B., Differential compartmentation of leucine for oxidation and for protein synthesis in cultured skeletal muscle, *J. Biol. Chem.*, 256, 4888, 1981.

49. Irving, C. S., Wong, W. W., Shulman, R. J., Smith, E. O., and Klein, P. D., [^{13}C]bicarbonate kinetics in humans: intra- vs. interindividual variations, *Am. J. Physiol.*, 245, R190, 1983.

50. Balagopal, P., Ljungqvist, O., and Nair, K. S., Skeletal muscle myosin heavy-chain synthesis rate in healthy humans, *Am. J. Physiol.*, 272, E45, 1997.

51. Balagopal, P., Rooyackers, O. E., Adey, D. B., Ades, P. A., and Nair, K. S., Effects of aging on in vivo synthesis of skeletal muscle myosin heavy-chain and sarcoplasmic protein in humans, *Am. J. Physiol.*, 273, E790, 1997.

52. Rooyackers, O. E., Adey, D. B., Ades, P. A., and Nair, K. S., Effect of age on in vivo rates of mitochondrial protein synthesis in human skeletal muscle, *Proc. Natl. Acad. Sci. U.S.A.*, 93, 15364, 1996.

53. Fu, A. Z., Morris, J. C., Ford, G. C., and Nair, K. S., Sequential purification of human apolipoprotein B-100, albumin, and fibrinogen by immunoaffinity chromatography for measurement of protein synthesis, *Anal. Biochem.*, 247, 228, 1997.

54. Ballmer, P. E., McNurlan, M. A., Essen, P., Anderson, S. E., and Garlick, P. J., Albumin synthesis rates measured with [^{2}H$_5$ring]phenylalanine are not responsive to short-term intravenous nutrients in healthy humans, *J. Nutr.*, 125, 512, 1995.

55. Cayol, M., Boirie, Y., Prugnaud, J., Gachon, P., Beaufrere, B., and Obled, C., Precursor pool for hepatic protein synthesis in humans: effects of tracer route infusion and dietary proteins, *Am. J. Physiol.*, 270, E980, 1996.

56. Hunter, K. A., Ballmer, P. E., Anderson, S. E., Broom, J., Garlick, P. J., and McNurlan, M. A., Acute stimulation of albumin synthesis rate with oral meal feeding in healthy subjects measured with [ring-^{2}H$_5$]phenylalanine, *Clin. Sci.*, 88, 235, 1995.

57. Peters, T., Jr., Taniuchi, H., and Anfinsen, C.B., Jr., Affinity chromatography of serum albumin with fatty acids immobilized on agarose, *J. Biol. Chem.*, 248, 2447, 1973.

58. Nair, K. S., Muscle protein turnover: methodological issues and the effect of aging, [Review] [26 refs], *J. Gerontol.*, Series A, Biological, 107, 1995.

Index

Milton Keynes UK
Ingram Content Group UK Ltd.
UKHW040443071024
449327UK00020B/956